LANGUAGE, COMMUNICATION, AND THE BRAIN

Research Publications:
Association for Research in Nervous and Mental Disease
Volume 66

ASSOCIATION FOR RESEARCH IN NERVOUS AND MENTAL DISEASE

Language, Communication, and the Brain

Research Publications:
Association for Research
in Nervous and Mental Disease

Volume 66

Editor

Fred Plum, M.D.

Department of Neurology
The New York Hospital-Cornell Medical Center
New York, New York

Raven Press   New York

Raven Press, 1185 Avenue of the Americas, New York, New York 10036

Made in the United States of America

Library of Congress Cataloging-in-Publication Data

Language, communication, and the brain.

(Research publications / Association for Research in Nervous and Mental Disease ; v. 66)
Based on the 66th Annual Meeting of the Association for Research in Nervous and Mental Disease, held Dec. 5–6, 1986 in New York City.
Includes bibliographies and index.
1. Language disorders—Congresses. 2. Neurolinguistics—Congresses. 3. Brain—Localization of functions—Congresses. I. Plum, Fred. 1924– . II. Association for Research in Nervous and Mental Disease. Meeting (66th : 1986 : New York, N.Y.) III. Series: Research publications (Association for Research in Nervous and Mental Disease) ; v. 66. [DNLM: 1. Brain—physiology—congresses. 2. Communication—congresses. 3. Language Development—congresses. 4. Language Disorders—congresses. W1 RE233P v.66 / WL 340 L2874 1986]
RC423.L333   1988   616.85'5   87-20643
ISBN 0-88167-365-X

9 8 7 6 5 4 3 2 1

RESEARCH PUBLICATIONS: ASSOCIATION FOR RESEARCH IN NERVOUS AND MENTAL DISEASE

Titles marked with an asterisk (*) are out of print in the original edition. Some out-of-print volumes are available in reprint editions from Hafner Publishing Company, 866 Third Avenue, New York, N.Y. 10022.

Preface

Verbal language is the gift that sets our species apart from all others, enabling us to communicate abstract ideas, to learn the accumulated knowledge of our ancestors, and to transmit our discoveries to our descendants. As that wisest of Western books, the Bible, put it, "In the beginning was the Word."

The study of language by neurologists until recently consisted mainly of analyses of aphasia, employing most extensively clinical-pathological and, to a lesser degree, brain stimulation approaches. Those now classic studies originated mainly in Paris during the early nineteenth century as Gall, Spurzheim, and a few other anatomic-functional localizationists began to appreciate that different regions of the cerebrum related to specific, individual motor and sensory functions. By 1825, Bouillaud, Professor of Medicine at l'Hôpital de la Charité, was able to conclude, on the basis of clinical-pathological studies on 114 patients, that the frontal lobes represent "the legislative organs of speech." Broca's famous 1861 lecture set the stage for the modern era, and his influence along with that of Wernicke and others remains with us still. Even now, as illustrated by several chapters in this volume, the neurologic approach of relating carefully observed disturbances of language to meticulously targeted brain stimulation or to anatomic changes deduced from radiographs or postmortem specimens continues to enlarge our understanding.

Recent years have also brought increasing insight into language because of new technical and intellectual approaches to the subject. Chapters in this monograph discuss how recent findings generated by computerized electrophysiology, *in vivo* autoradiography, and the disciplinary approach of developmental neurobiology have illuminated knowledge of the language process.

This volume takes the somewhat innovative step of including considerable material from nonmedical disciplines whose recent scholarship increases our understanding of the language process. Experts in education and psychologists with a variety of particular interests and talents describe and define functional patterns of language that necessarily will constrain any modeling or theorizing that neurology seriously entertains. Much more important, however, they describe some of the functions of the normal brain as it generates speech. Thus, this volume includes chapters on communication in lower species, the nature of linguistic rules, how verbal thought and speech may differ in different human languages, how and when children formulate syntax, and how persons with normal brains apply similar rules to both verbal and nonverbal communication. The results of these approaches take their place along with the findings of anatomy and physiology as elements that require incorporation in any theory that attempts to explain how the cerebral cortex works and, especially, how it creates normal language and thought.

Fred Plum, M.D.

Acknowledgments

The officers and trustees of the Association for Research in Nervous and Mental Disease have seldom turned so widely to fields outside their immediate discipline as they did at their 66th meeting. Isabelle Rapin, Antonio Damasio, and Ivan Bodis-Wollner deserve much of the credit for identifying the speakers who provided this broad scope. The result was a stimulating program, one that rewarded participants and audience alike. We trust that this volume will have a similar effect.

Contents

Contributors

Michael P. Alexander
Aphasia Program
Braintree Rehabilitation Hospital
Braintree, Massachusetts 02184

Doris A. Allen
Saul R. Korey Department of Neurology
Division of Child Psychiatry
Rose F. Kennedy Center for Research in
  Mental Retardation and Human
  Development
Albert Einstein College of Medicine
Bronx, New York 10461

Dorothy M. Aram
Department of Pediatrics
Case Western Reserve University, and
  Rainbow Babies and Children's
  Hospital
Cleveland, Ohio 44106

Elizabeth Bates
Department of Psychology
University of California, San Diego
La Jolla, California 92093

Kathleen Baynes
Burke Rehabilitation Center
Cornell University Medical College
White Plains, New York 10605

Ursula Bellugi
Laboratory for Language and Cognitive
  Studies
The Salk Institute for Biological Studies
La Jolla, California 92037

Sheila E. Blumstein
Department of Cognitive and Linguistic
  Sciences
Brown University
Providence, Rhode Island 02912

Hiram H. Brownell
Aphasia Research Center
Department of Neurology
Boston University School of Medicine,
  and Boston Veterans Administration
  Medical Center
Boston, Massachusetts 02130

Antonio R. Damasio
Department of Neurology
The University of Iowa College of
  Medicine
Iowa City, Iowa 52242

Martha B. Denckla
Neurology Branch
National Institutes of Neurological,
  Communicative Disorders, and Stroke
Bethesda, Maryland 20205

Ranjan Duara
Departments of Radiology and Neurology
University of Miami School of Medicine
Miami, Florida 33101, and
Mount Sinai Medical Center
Miami Beach, Florida 33140

Frank H. Duffy
Department of Neurology
Children's Hospital and
  Harvard Medical School
Boston, Massachusetts 02115

Victoria A. Fromkin
Department of Linguistics
University of California, Los Angeles
Los Angeles, California 90024

Albert M. Galaburda
Department of Neurology
Harvard Medical School, and
Neurological Unit
Charles A. Dana Research Institute and
  Dyslexia Neuroanatomical Laboratory
Beth Israel Hospital
Boston, Massachusetts 02215

Howard Gardner
Aphasia Research Center
Department of Neurology
Boston University School of
 Medicine, and
Boston Veterans Administration Medical
 Center
Boston, Massachusetts 02130

Michael S. Gazzaniga
Division of Cognitive Neuroscience
Cornell University Medical College
New York, New York 10021

Karen Gross-Glenn
Genetics Division
Mailman Center for Child Development
University of Miami School of Medicine
Miami, Florida 33101

Kurt E. Hecox
Project Phoenix of Madison, Inc.
Nicolet Audiodiagnostics
Madison, Wisconsin 53711

Steven A. Hillyard
Department of Neurosciences
University of California, San Diego
La Jolla, California 92093

Audrey L. Holland
Departments of Otolaryngology,
 Psychiatry, and Communications
University of Pittsburgh
Pittsburgh, Pennsylvania 15213

Jane A. Holmes
Department of Psychiatry
Children's Hospital and
 Harvard Medical School
Boston, Massachusetts 02115

William Kimberling
Boys Town National Institute
Omaha, Nebraska 68131

Edward S. Klima
University of California, San Diego
La Jolla, California 92093

Marta Kutas
Department of Neurosciences
University of California, San Diego
La Jolla, California 92093

Herbert A. Lubs
Genetics Division
Mailman Center for Child Development
University of Miami School of Medicine
Miami, Florida 33101

Virginia A. Marchman
Department of Psychology
University of California, San Diego
La Jolla, California 92093, and
University of California, Berkeley
Berkeley, California 94720

John C. Mazziotta
Department of Neurology
Reed Neurologic Institute, and
Division of Nuclear Medicine and
 Biophysics
Department of Radiological Sciences
University of California, Los Angeles
 School of Medicine, and
Laboratory of Nuclear Medicine
Los Angeles, California 90024

Gloria B. McAnulty
Department of Neurology
Children's Hospital and
 Harvard Medical School
Boston, Massachusetts 02115

E. Jeffrey Metter
Department of Neurology
Reed Neurologic Institute, and
University of California, Los Angeles
 School of Medicine
Los Angeles, California 90024, and
Sepulveda Veterans Administration
 Medical Center
Sepulveda, California 91343

Margaret A. Naeser
*CT Laboratory of the Aphasia Research
Center
Psychology Service
Boston Veterans Administration Medical
Center
Boston, Massachusetts 02130, and
Department of Neurology
Boston University School of Medicine
Boston, Massachusetts 02215*

George A. Ojemann
*Department of Neurological Surgery
University of Washington School of
Medicine
Seattle, Washington 98195*

Bruce Pennington
*University of Colorado Medical Center
Denver, Colorado 80262*

Howard Poizner
*Laboratory for Language and Cognitive
Studies
The Salk Institute for Biological Studies
La Jolla, California 92037*

Isabelle Rapin
*Saul R. Korey Department of Neurology
Department of Pediatrics
Division of Child Psychiatry
Rose F. Kennedy Center for Research in
Mental Retardation and Human
Development
Albert Einstein College of Medicine
Bronx, New York 10461*

Shelley Smith
*Boys Town National Institute
Omaha, Nebraska 68131*

Robert T. Wertz
*Veterans Administration Medical Center
Martinez, California 94553*

Sally T. Weylman
*Aphasia Research Center
Department of Neurology
Boston University School of
Medicine, and
Boston Veterans Administration Medical
Center
Boston, Massachusetts 02130*

Association for Research in Nervous and Mental Disease

Members

A

Abrams, Bernard M.
Abrams, Gary M.
Ackerman, Sigurd H.
Adelman, Lester
Adler, Lenard A.
Agranoff, B. W.
Ahuwalia, Brij. M. S.
Aiken, Robert D.
Aita, John F.
Allen, Joseph A.
Allen, Marshall B., Jr.
Allen, Richard
Almaleh, H.
Alter, Milton
Alvord, Ellsworth C., Jr.
Anderson, Milton H.
Anderson, Paul J.
Anderson, William W.
Andriola, Mary
Andy, Orlando J.
Angrist, Burton
Ansari, Khurshed A.
Asbury, Arthur
Auerbach, Sanford
Austin, James
Auth, Thomas L.
Ayala, Giovanni

B

Baker, Robert N.
Baldessarini, Ross J.
Ball, Stanley M.
Ballweg, Gail P.
Bank, Arnold
Barchi, Robert L.
Barclay, Laurie
Barlow, Charles F.
Barlow, John S.
Barnes, Karen L.
Barnett, H. J. M.

Barrett, Robert E.
Barron, Kevin
Bartle, Harvey, Jr.
Baska, Richard E.
Batkin, Stanley
Battista, Arthur A.
Becker, Donald P.
Bell, Robert L.
Bender, Adam N.
Benjamin, Vallo
Berg, Seymour
Bergmann, Kenneth
Berl, Soll
Bick, Katherine L.
Biele, Flora H.
Blankfein, Robert J.
Blass, John Paul
Block, Jerome M.
Bodis-Wollner, Ivan
Bohn, Martha
Boldrey, Edwin B.
Borrus, Joseph C.
Bosley, Thomas McCarthy
Brannon, William, Jr.
Bray, Patrick F.
Breitner, John, C. S.
Brendler, Samuel J.
Bridger, Wagner
Bridgers, Samuel L. II
Brill, A. Bertrand
Brill, Charles B.
Britton, Carolyn Barley
Brodie, Jonathan D.
Broughton, Roger J.
Brown, Dennis
Brown, Lucy L.
Brudny, Joseph
Brust, John C.
Bruun, Bertel
Budabin, Murray
Bullard, Dexter M.

Burger, Andrew
Burke, Robert E.
Buschke, Herman
Busse, Ewald W.
Butler, Ian

C

Cadet, Jean Lud
Cafferty, Maureen S.
Camp, Walter A.
Cancro, Robert
Carmichael, Miriam
Caronna, John J.
Carpenter, William T., Jr.
Carruthers, Richard R.
Carton, Charles A.
Caviness, Verne S., Jr.
Cedarbaum, Jesse M.
Charlton, Maurice H.
Charney, Jonathan Z.
Chase, Richard A.
Chase, Thomas N.
Chawluk, John B.
Chokroverty, Sudhansu
Cicero, Theodore J.
Clark, William K.
Coccaro, Emil F.
Coddon, David R.
Cohan, Stanley L.
Cohen, Bernard
Cohen, Jeffrey
Cohen, Norman
Cohen, Robert A.
Cohen, Sidney M.
Cohen, Wendy Ellen
Cohn, Robert
Cole, Andrew James
Cole, Marvin
Cole, Monroe
Collins, William F., Jr.
Conomy, John Paul

Cook, David G.
Cook, Patricia
Cook, Stuart
Correll, James W.
Cote, Lucien
Couch, James R.
Critides, Samuel D.
Cullis, Paul Anthony
Cummings, Jeffrey L.
Cuthill, John

D

Dale, Robert T.
Damasio, Antonio
Damasto, Hanna
Daroff, Robert B.
Davey, Lycurgus M.
David, Noble
Davis, Kenneth
DeGirolami, Umberto
Delaney, John F.
DeNapoli, Robert A.
Denckla, Martha B.
Derby, Bennett M.
DeVivo, Darryl
Diamond, Mark S.
Diamond, Sidney
DiFiglia, Marian
Dodge, Philip R.
Dodson, William
Donaldson, James O.
Drachman, David
Dreifuss, Fritz E.
Duane, Drake D.
Dubin, Louis L.
Dunstone, David D.
Duvoisin, Roger C.
Dyken, Mark L.
Dyken, Paul R.

E

Earls, Felton James
Easton, J. Donald
Ebers, George C.
Edelson, Alan
Edwards, Diana Dow
Effron, Abraham S.
Eisenberg, Leon
Elizan, Teresita S.
Epstein, Fred
Erba, Giuseppe
Esser, Robert A.

F

Fahn, Stanley
Faillace, Louis A.
Falci, Thomas
Feinberg, Irwin
Feindel, William
Feldman, Daniel S.
Feldman, Martin
Feringa, Earl R.
Ferriss, Gregory S.
Fetell, Michael
Finney, Joseph C.
Fish, Irving
Fishman, Donald
Fishman, Robert A.
Flamm, Eugene S.
Fleming, T. Corwin
Fogelson, M. Harold
Foley, Kathleen M.
Folstein, Marshall
Folstein, Susan
Forrest, David V.
Forster, George
Frazier, Shervert H.
Friedhoff, Arnold J.
Friedman, Richard C.
Frosch, William A.
Funkenstein, H. Harris

G

Gandy, Samuel E.
Garofalo, Michael, Jr.
Garvin, John S.
Gascon, Generoso G.
Geller, Lester M.
Gendelman, Seymour
Gershon, Samuel
Geschwind, Norman
Ghetti, Bernardino
Ghilardi, Maria Felice
Ghobrial, Mona
Gibbs, James
Giblin, Dennis R.
Gillen, H. W.
Gilman, Sid
Gilroy, John
Gold, Arnold P.
Goldberg, Allan
Goldberg, Harold H.
Goldin, Gurston D.
Goldstein, Murray
Grabow, Jack D.

Green, David
Green, Martin A.
Greenberg, Alvin D.
Greenberg, Jack O.
Greenwood, Robert
Greer, Melvin
Gretter, Thomas
Gross, David
Gross, Paul T.
Grossman, Robert
Gumnit, Robert J.
Gutmann, Ludwig
Guynn, Robert William
Guze, Samuel

H

Haase, Gunter R.
Hackett, Earl R.
Haddad, Raef
Hale, Mahlon A.
Hamburg, David
Hamill, Robert W.
Hammill, James F.
Hanna, George R.
Harbison, John W.
Harter, Donald H.
Hass, William Karl
Hauser, W. Allen
Hayward, James Neil
Healton, Edward B.
Hershey, Linda A.
Heyer, Eric
Hinterbuchner, L. P.
Hirano, Asao
Hoehn, Margaret
Hoenig, Eugene M.
Hoff, Julian T.
Hoffman, Julius
Hoffman, Stephen F.
Hogan, Edward L.
Hogan, Patrick A.
Holmes, Gregory L.
Horenstein, Simon
Horowitz, Steven
Housepian, Edgar M.
Hudson, Charles J.

I

Iadecola, Costantino

J

Jacobs, Erwin M.
Jacobs, Lawrence D.

Jacobson, Sherwood A.
Jacquet, Yasuko F.
Jaffe, Joseph
Jammes, Juan L.
Jeub, Robert P.
Joh, Tong H.
Johnson, Anne B.
Johnson, Richard T.
Jonas, Saran
Jones, H. Royden, Jr.
Joynt, Robert J.
Jubelt, Burk

K

Kaelber, William W.
Kandel, Eric R.
Kaplan, Lawrence I.
Kase, Carlos S.
Kattah, Jorge C.
Katzman, Robert
Kaye, Edward M.
Keller, N. J. A.
Kellner, Charles H.
Kennedy, Charles
Kenny, John Thomas
Kessler, Robert M.
Khurana, Ramesh
Kienast, H. W.
Kinkel, William R.
Kirschberg, Gordon
Klass, Donald W.
Klee, Claude Elise
Klein, Donald
Koenig, Harold
Koenigsberger, M. R.
Koeppen, Arnulf H.
Kofman, Oscar
Kolar, Oldrich Jan
Kolodny, Edwin H.
Korein, Julius
Kornfeld, Mario
Krieger, Howard P.
Krinsky, Michael M.
Kupersmith, Mark J.
Kurtzke, John F.

L

Landau, William M.
Lane, Mark H.
Lapovsky, Arthur
Lautin, Andrew
Lavenstein, Bennett

Layzer, Robert
Lederman, Richard J.
Lehrer, Gerard M.
Leiberman, James S.
Leibowitz, Sarah
Lepore, Frederick E.
Lesse, Stanley
Leven, Harvey Steven
Levens, Arthur J.
Leventhal, Carl M.
Levine, Irving M.
Levy, David E.
Levy, Lewis L.
Levy, Susan R.
Levy, Walter J.
Lewis, Linda D.
Liberson, Wladimir
Lightfoote, William
Lipkin, Lewis E.
Lisak, Robert Philip
Liss, Leopold
Livingston, E. Arthur
Livingston, Robert B.
Lombroso, Cesare T.
Lubic, Lowell G.
Lublin, Fred, D.

M

Madow, Michael
Maertens, Paul
Maker, Howard
Malitz, Sidney
Mancell, Elliott L.
Mandel, Martin M.
Maniscalco, Anthony G.
Manyam, Bala
Marcus, Elliott M.
Markham, Charles H.
Marques-Bravo, Jose
Martin, Herbert L.
Martin, Joseph
Martinez, Leonardo
Mashman, Jan
Massey, Edward Wayne
Massey, Janice
Mastri, Angeline R.
Matthysse, Steven
Mattson, Richard
Mayer, Richard F.
Mayeux, Richard
McDowell, Fletcher H.
McGee, Thomas

McGillicuddy, John
McHenry, John T.
McHugh, Paul R.
McIlroy, William J.
McKee, Mary Ann
McKinney, Alexander S.
McKinney, William M.
McMasters, Robert E.
Meisel, Arthur M.
Mendelson, Jack H.
Mendoza, Marina R.
Meyer, John Sterling
Meyerson, Arthur T.
Michels, Robert
Michelson, W. Jost
Mickel, Hubert S.
Miller, Brenda
Miller, Claude
Miller, James R.
Millichap, J. G.
Mohr, J. P.
Mohs, Richard C.
Mondell, Brian
Moore, Donald F.
Moossy, Jon
Mora, Sol M.
Morantz, Robert A.
Morgenstern, Eva
Moros, Daniel A.
Morris, Charles E.
Moshe, Solomon L.
Moskowitz, Michael A.
Mumford, Robert S.
Munsat, Theodore L.
Myers, Gary J.

N

Natelson, Benjamin
Nathanson, Morton
Nilaver, Gajanan
Norsa, Luigia

O

O'Brien, Joseph L.
Okazaki, Haruo
Onofrj, Marco C.
Osborne, Morris

P

Paddison, Richard M.
Pappas, Carol L.
Parr, Justin
Pasik, Pedro

Paul, Norman L.
Pavlakis, Steven
Payne, Richard
Pearl, Richard
Pearlson, Godfrey D.
Pedley, Timothy
Penn, Audrey S.
Penry, J. Kiffin
Perlo, Vincent P.
Petajan, Jack
Peterson, Arthur L.
Peterson, Patti L.
Piepmeier, Joseph
Pietrucha, Dorothy M.
Pincus, Jonathan
Pinney, Edward L., Jr.
Pittman, Hal W.
Pitts, Ferris N., Jr.
Plaitakis, Andreas
Pleasure, David
Plum, Fred
Pollock, George H.
Porrino, Linda J.
Posner, Jerome B.
Posner, Michael
Prensky, Arthur L.
Price, Richard
Prince, David A.
Prioleau, George R.
Prockop, Leon D.
Prohovnik, Isak
Purpura, Dominick P.

R

Raichle, Marcus E.
Raine, Cedric S.
Rainer, John D.
Rakic, Pasko
Ramachandran, Tarakad
Ransohoff, Joseph
Rao, Jayaraman
Rapin, Isabelle
Raskin, Neil H.
Rasmussen, Theodore
Reichlan, Seymour
Reife, Ross A.
Reis, Donald J.
Reivich, Martin
Richards, Nelson G.
Richter, Ralph W.
Rinsley, Donald B.
Roberts, M. P., Jr.
Robinson, Robert G.
Rose, Arthur L.

Rosenbaum, David
Rosenberg, Edwin
Rosenberg, Roger N.
Rosenblum, Jay A.
Rosenthal, Jesse
Rosenthal, Norman E.
Rosomoff, Hubert L.
Ross, Emanuel
Rothballer, Allan
Rovner, Richard
Rowan, A. James
Rowland, Lewis P.
Rubenstein, Alan
Rudolph, Steven
Ruff, Robert L.
Rumberg, Joan

S

Sabshin, James K.
Sackeim, Harold A.
Sackler, Mortimer D.
Sage, Jacob I.
Salmoiraghi, G. C.
Saloman, Michael
Samson, Frederick E., Jr.
Samuels, Stanley
Saper, Joel R.
Sattin, Albert
Sax, Daniel S.
Schaerer, Jacques P.
Schanzer, Bernard
Schapiro, Daniel
Schatz, Norman J.
Schaumburg, Herbert
Schear, Myrna J.
Schildkraut, Joseph J.
Schoenberg, Bruce
Schuelein, Marianne
Schulman, Elliott A.
Seelye, Edward E.
Selby, Roy C.
Selverstone, Bertram
Selzer, Michael E.
Sencer, Walter
Shamoian, Charles A.
Shanzer, Stefan
Shapiro, Mortimer F.
Shapiro, Sidney K.
Shapiro, William R.
Sheremata, William A.
Sherman, David G.
Sherwin, Ira
Shoulson, Ira
Shriver, Joyce

Shuter, Eli R.
Siberstein, Marsha M.
Siberstein, Stephen
Sibley, William A.
Sidell, Alvin
Siekert, Robert G.
Siever, Larry Joseph
Silberberg, Donald H.
Silberfarb, Peter
Siller, Edward J.
Silverstein, Allen
Singer, Robert P.
Singh, Avtar
Singh, Baldev Kaur
Sivak, Mark
Slosberg, Paul S.
Slotwiner, Paul
Small, Iver F.
Smith, G. Bushnell
Smith, Carolyn B.
Smith, Gerard P.
Smith, Michael
Sobin, Allen
Sobol, Norman J.
Sokoloff, Louis
Solomon, Gail
Solomon, Seymour
Spencer, Donald D.
Spencer, Susan
Sroka, Hava
Stadlan, Emanuel M.
Stein, Martin H.
Stein, Marvin
Steiner, Martin R.
Stern, Yakov
Stewart, Bruce
Stewart, James G.
Stiefel, Joseph W.
Stunkard, Albert J.
Sugerman, A. Arthur
Sullivan, Daniel Carl
Summers, David C.
Sumner, Austin J.
Sung, Joo Ho
Suter, Gary G.
Swanson, David W.
Sweeney, Vincent Paul
Sweet, Richard
Syed, Athar

T

Taren, James A.
Tarsy, Daniel
Taylor, Judith M.

Tcheupdjian, Leon
Tejera, Gertrude
Tellez, Isabel
Terry, Robert D.
Thal, Leon J.
Thompson, Hartwell
Thompson, Raymond K.
Thurston, Jean H.
Timberlake, William H.
Tolge, Bruno P.
Tolosa, Edward
Tourian, Ara
Triedman, M. Howard
Tsai, Luke Y.
Tuchman, Alan J.
Tucker, Jolyon S.
Tune, Larry
Twitchell, Thomas E.
Tyler, Richard H.

V

Valsamais, Marius
Van Der Velde, Christian
Van Praag, Herman M.
Vigman, Melvin
Vincent, Frederick M.

W

Walton, Norman
Waltz, Arthur G.
Wanger, Stephen L.
Warner, Carolyn Louise
Waxman, Stephen G.
Webster, Henry De F.
Wechsler, Adam F.
Weinberg, Harold J.
Weinberg, Jessie
Weiner, Herbert
Weinreb, Herman J.
Weiss, Arthur H.
Weissman, William
West, Louis Jolyon
Westbrook, Edward
Wharton, Ralph N.
Whelan, Joseph L.
Whetsell, William O.
Wiener, Jill
Wilk, Ronald
Williams, Robert L.
Williams, Shirley Y.
Wilson, Barbara
Wilson, William P.

Winkler, Howard A.
Winokur, George
Winsberg, Bertrand G.
Wishnow, Donald E.
Wisniewski, Henry
Wolfson, Leslie I.
Wolkin, Adam
Woolsey, Joyce E.
Woolsey, Robert M.
Wright, Jesse H.
Wright, R. Lewis
Wurtman, Richard L.

Y

Yaskin, H. Edward
Yatsu, Frank
Young, Robert C.

Z

Zervas, Nicholas
Ziegler, Dewey
Zier, Adolfo
Zimmerman, Earl A.
Ziskind, Eugene
Zitrin, Arthur

Senior Members

A

Adams, Raymond
Adler, Alexandra
Aird, Robert B.
Airing, Charles D.
Amols, William

B

Badal, Daniel
Bailey, Orville T.
Baker, A. B.
Beach, Frank A.
Bell, H. Craig
Berry, Richard G.
Bertrand, Claude
Binger, Carl
Black, Samuel P. W.
Blau, Abram
Bodian, David
Booth, Carl B.
Borkowski, Winslow J.

Boshes, Louis D.
Botelho, Stella Y.
Brody, Matthew
Brooks, Chandler
Brosin, Henry
Brown, Joe R.
Buckley, Paul

C

Carter, Sidney
Cash, Paul T.
Catell, James P.
Cattanach, George S.
Chambers, William W.
Chusid, Joseph C.
Cobb, Cully A.
Cowen, David
Culleton, James F.

D

Davis, Hallowell
DeFries, Zira

DeJong, Russell N.
Denbo, Elic A.
Denker, Peter G.
Donnelly, John
Dunstone, H. Carter

E

Eberhart, John G.
Echlin, Francis A.
Ecker, Arthur D.
Engisch, Robert R.
Epstein, Samuel H.
Evans, Harrison S.
Everts, William H.

F

Farmer, Thomas W.
Felix, Robert H.
Fields, William S.
Finkelhor, Howard B.
Finley, Knox M.
Flexner, Louis B.

Flicker, David J.
Foley, Joseph M.
Frank, Karl
Friedman, Arnold P.

G

Galbraith, James G.
Gates, Edward
Glaser, Gilbert H.
Glusman, Murray
Goldman, Douglas
Gottschalk, Louis A.
Greene, Justin L.
Greenhill, Maurice H.
Grinker, Roy R., Sr.
Guttman, Samuel A.

H

Hamilton, Francis J.
Hare, Clarence C.
Hasenbush, Lester L.
Heath, Robert G.
Helfer, Louis M.
Herrmann, Christian, Jr.
Hinsey, Joseph C.
Holmes, Thomas
Hovde, Christian A.
Hudson, Robert J.
Hunter, Ralph W.

J

Jarcho, Leonard W.

K

Kabat, Elvin A.
Kalinowsky, Lothar B.
Kaplan, Harold
Kaplan, Harry A.
Karliner, William
Kety, Seymour S.
Kies, Marion W.
King, Arthur
Kolb, Lawrence
Kral, Voitech

L

Larrabee, Martin G.
Lebensohn, Zigmond M.
Levin, Jules
Levy, Daniel
Lipin, Theo
Livingston, Robert E.
Loman, Julius
Lowry, Oliver H.

M

MacPherson, Donald J.

Madonick, Moses
Madow, Leo
Malmo, Robert B.
Masland, Richard L.
McKinney, John M.
McKnight, William K.
McNerey, John C.
Mearin, Robert J.
Menninger, Karl A.
Merlis, Jerome K.
Michael, Stanley
Millikan, Clark
Moore, Matthew T.

N

Nardini, John E.
Nastuck, William L.
Neumann, Meta
Nurnberger, John

O

Oldberg, Eric
Osborne, Raymond L.
Osler, Geoffrey F.

P

Pacella, Bernard
Palmer, Edwin J.
Parker, Joseph
Perret, George
Pasamanick, Benjamin
Pasik, Tauba
Pietri, Raoul
Pisetsky, Joseph
Pope, Alfred

R

Rabiner, A. M.
Randt, Clark T.
Richardson, Edward P.
Richter, Curt P.
Roch, D. McK.
Robb, Preston
Robinson, Franklin
Roizin, Leon
Rose, Augustus S.
Roseman, E.
Ross, Alexander T.
Rottersman, William
Ruesch, Jurgen

S

Sabin, Albert B.
Schlesinger, Edward
Schleziner, Nathan
Schneider, Richard

Schumacher, George
Sciarra, Daniel
Senerchia, Fred F., Jr.
Shenkin, Henry A.
Simon, John
Singer, Marcus
Siris, Joseph H.
Smith, Wilbur K.
Snider, Ray S.
Snyder, Laurence H.
Spotnitz, Hyman
Sprague, James
Sprofkin, Bertram H.
Staley, Robert
Starbuck, Helen L.
Stellar, Stanley
Sweet, William H.

T

Thomas, Madison H.
Thompson, George N.
Thorner, Melvin
Tissenbaum, Morris
Tornay, Anthony
Trufant, Samuel A.
Tucker, Weir M.

V

Vicale, Carmine

W

Waggoner, Raymond
Wagman, Irving H.
Wall, James H.
Wallner, Julius
Wang, S. C.
Ward, Arthur
Warner, Francis
Watson, Robert
Weickhardt, George D.
Williams, Ernest
Wittson, Cecil L.
Woodall, J. Martin
Woodbury, Dixon M.
Woolsey, Clinton H.

Y

Yahr, Melvin D.
Yorshis, Morris

Z

Zubin, Joseph
Zfass, Isadore S.

LANGUAGE, COMMUNICATION, AND THE BRAIN

Research Publications:
Association for Research in Nervous and Mental Disease
Volume 66

Language, Communication, and the Brain, edited by F. Plum.
Raven Press, New York © 1988.

The State of Brain/Language Research

Victoria A. Fromkin

Department of Linguistics, University of California, Los Angeles,
Los Angeles, California 90024

THE HUMAN BRAIN AND THE UNIQUENESS OF LANGUAGE

A volume on "Language, Communication, and the Brain," with contributors from the fields of linguistics, psychology, neuropsychology, neurology, and neuroscience, shows how far we have come since Aristotle suggested that the brain is a cold sponge whose primary action is to cool the blood. It took almost 2,000 years, however, to add substance to the insights of the Greco-Roman physicians, writing in the fifth century B.C., who recognized that the loss of speech and the loss of language could be distinguished and that speechlessness was often associated with paralysis of the right side of the body. We are still looking for evidence to explicate the Hippocratic view that the brain is "the messenger to the understanding" and the organ whereby "in an especial manner we acquire wisdom and knowledge" (1).

It is not surprising that there should have been speculation on the brain/language relationship throughout history. The human brain seems uniquely equipped to acquire and use language. Although in the last few years chimpanzees and gorillas have been shown to have greater cognitive ability than previously thought, they cannot, even with the most intensive human training, learn even 1% of the vocabulary that is acquired by virtually any 3-year-old human child, let alone the complex phonological, morphological, syntactic, and semantic rules that constitute the grammar of all human languages from Akan to Zulu, from Apache to Xhosa (50). To state that the human brain is qualitatively, as well as quantitatively, different is not to deprecate nonhuman primates, just as recognition that certain species of songbirds are innately endowed with the ability to produce songs without any exposure to them is not to demean the human animal who does not have this ability (42).

BIOLOGICAL BASIS OF CHILD LANGUAGE ACQUISITION

The view that the human brain is uniquely suited for the acquisition and use of language is reinforced by the fact that a child, regardless of race, economic status, geographical location, climate, religion, or size, can acquire any language to which he or she is exposed. No language—spoken or signed—used in the community in

1

which the child is born and raised is too difficult for the child to learn. No special talents or skills are needed. Furthermore, children reveal rich and complex knowledge of the language of their community at a very early age despite the deficiency of the stimulus they receive. Highly intelligent children (even geniuses) do not acquire language earlier, more completely, or more easily than do children on the lower scale of intelligence, however measured.

In fact, children diagnosed at birth as mentally retarded acquire language in the same way as those with normal intelligence. Not only can children learn any of the thousands of languages that exist in the world, they do so without being overtly taught. It is difficult, if not impossible, to account for this ability without assuming that the brain is genetically "prewired" for language.

Think of what it means to know a language. It means being able to produce and understand an indefinite number of sentences never spoken or heard before. Thus, the set of sentences in any language—spoken or signed—must be infinite. This is also shown by the fact that, in principle, for every sentence of n length, one can produce a sentence of $n + 1$ in length by virtue of the existence of recursive grammatical rules. The iterative devices or rules that exist in every human language include relativization ("This is the dog that chased the cat that killed the rat that caught the mouse that ate the cheese that . . ."); coordination ("Linguists went to the conference in New York, and neurologists also attended the meeting, and the weather was cold but sunny, and . . ."); and subordination ("I believe that Dr. Plum asked me to tell Dr. Smith that Dr. Jones thought that Dr. Brown had stated that . . ."). Although the child hears only a finite set of utterances, only utterances of finite length, and often only sentence fragments, false starts, and ill-formed strings, he or she acquires the basic rules by a very early age to produce and understand novel sentences and, as experiments have shown, is able to distinguish between well-formed (grammatical) and ill-formed (ungrammatical) sentences.

Knowing a language also means being able to identify any spoken word in less than a third of a second, drawing on the more than 100,000 entries stored in the mental dictionary of a typical monolingual adult. In little more time than it takes to process the sounds themselves, the words are assembled into meaningful sentences that more or less approximate the message intended by the speaker. One cannot perform this feat without knowing a language; although one can know a language but be unable to access that knowledge in speaking or in comprehending, or both, as evidenced by the language deficits of aphasia. The distinction between linguistic knowledge and linguistic processing or behavior, recognized by linguists, is supported by the neurolinguistic data of aphasic patients. More important, one can neither acquire a language nor use it in production and/or comprehension without the brain structures that make this possible.

The attempt to understand the brain mechanisms underlying language acquisition and use relates to what has been called the "innateness hypothesis," which suggests the human animal is born with a genetically determined language faculty, one component of the human mind that to a certain extent specifies the class of humanly accessible grammars (8,10,46). These biologically determined linguistic principles are what Chomsky (7,9) has referred to as the "universal grammar." "The commitment to formulate a restrictive theory of U[niversal] G[rammar] is nothing other than a commitment to discover the biological endowment that makes language acquisition possible and to determine its particular manifestation" (9). This is a view supported by Salvador Luria (36): "Biologists believe that the structure of language is not fully learned by experience but is in part at least embedded in the network of connections of the human brain."

LANGUAGE—AUTONOMOUS OR DERIVATIVE?

The question still remains, however, whether this genetically determined language ability is essentially derivative—a by-product of general cognitive, physiological, and other nonspecific systems underlying human intelligence—or is due to abilities that are specifically and uniquely linguistic (21).

An accumulation of evidence is convincing a growing number of scientists that the human brain is not a "general purpose" computer, but that linguistic capacity to which it gives rise is best viewed as an autonomous, cognitive system governed by its own set of distinct principles. This view is supported by the fact that linguistic abilities can be dissociated developmentally from other cognitive abilities (12,20).

There are numerous case studies of children who have few cognitive skills and virtually no ability to utilize language in sustained, meaningful communication and yet have extensive mastery of linguistic structure. Yamada (53) reports one severely retarded young woman, with a nonverbal IQ of 41 to 44, who lacks almost all number concepts including basic counting principles, draws at a preschool level, and processes an auditory memory span limited to three units, but who could nonetheless produce syntactically complex sentences such as: "She does paintings, this really good friend of the kids who I went to school with last year and really loved" or "Last year at school when I first went there, three tickets were gave out by a police last year." Marta cannot add $2 + 2$. She is not sure of when "last year" is or whether it is before or after "last week" or "an hour ago," nor does she know how many tickets were "gave out" or whether 3 is larger or smaller than 2, but the structure of her sentences reveals sophisticated knowledge of complex syntactic rules. She embeds relative clauses, conjoins verb phrases, produces passives, inflects verbs for number and person to agree with the grammatical subject, and forms past tenses when the time adverbial structurally refers to a previous time. In a sentence imitation task she both detected and corrected surface syntactic and morphological errors. Yet she is unable to tie her shoes.

Marta is one of many examples of children who display well-developed phonological, morphological, and syntactic linguistic abilities, seemingly less developed lexical, semantic, or referential aspects of language, and deficits in nonlinguistic cognitive development (13,14,14a). Furthermore, as shown by Blank et al. (4), grammatical knowledge can be acquired without parallel pragmatic knowledge or "communicative competence." Cases of schizophrenic and autistic children reveal similar disassociation between the ability to acquire the language system and the ability to learn the conventions for the use of the language in social settings (17,24,30).

Such developmental asymmetries argue against the view that linguistic ability derives from more general cognitive "intelligence," since in these cases language develops against a background of deficits in general and nonlinguistic intellectual abilities.

There are also cases of children with little grammar but with other verbal abilities, such as Genie (13,21). This "modern-day wild child" was physically and socially isolated from the world until almost 14 years of age, with no language input during that period. Following her discovery and social emergence, she learned to use a sewing machine and scramble eggs, remembered every face she saw, could go directly to a car parked in a crowded, five-level parking structure after a five- or six-hour interim period, did phenomenally well on the Mooney faces test, and, after her social emergence, acquired very rapidly a large vocabulary. But she never went beyond the rudiments of syntax acquired by a two-year-old child. Her utterances remained ungrammatical, devoid of morphological endings or syntactic operations. This contrast between word lists and grammatical rules is indicative of different and distinct cognitive abilities, and supports the view of language as an autonomous system that, in itself, consists of separate components.

APHASIA: FURTHER EVIDENCE FOR THE MODULARITY OF COGNITIVE SYSTEMS

The clinical studies of aphasia that have been conducted during the last 120 years also support the view that the human brain is "modular" in nature, giving rise to autonomous, independent cognitive systems. If the language system or the grammar (which represents a speaker's linguistic knowledge) and the ability to process this knowledge in speech production and comprehension were not independent of other systems of knowledge and nonlinguistic psychological processing mechanisms, it would be difficult to understand how, following focal brain lesions, language and nonlanguage abilities could be differentially impaired. This asymmetry in both the developing and mature brain suggests a biological basis for human language as a separate system that interacts with other cognitive systems in its acquisition and use.

Role of the Left Hemisphere in Language: Spoken and Signed

Perhaps the most telling and dramatic findings on the brain/language relationship that supports the concept that the brain and mind consist of neurological and cognitive-interactive but autonomous modules are revealed by the research on sign language conducted by Bellugi and colleagues (35,44,45), which is discussed in detail elsewhere in this volume, therefore I will refer briefly to these findings.

The linguistic study of sign language over the last 25 years has already shown that these languages of the deaf have all the crucial properties common to all spoken languages, including highly abstract underlying grammatical and formal principles (35).

Since the same abstract linguistic principles underlie all human languages— spoken or signed—regardless of the motor and perceptual mechanisms that are used in their expression, it is not surprising that deaf patients show aphasia for sign language similar to the language breakdown that hearing aphasics develop following damage to the left hemisphere. Furthermore, although these patients show marked sign language deficits, they can correctly process nonlanguage visual-spatial relationships. The left cerebral hemisphere is thus not dominant for speech, as had been suggested, but for language, the cognitive system underlying both speech and sign (2,34). Hearing and speech are not necessary for the development of left hemispheric specialization for language. This has been a crucial point in determining that the left hemisphere specialization in language acquisition is not due to its capacity for fine auditory analysis, but for language analysis per se. As long as linguists concerned themselves only with spoken languages, there was no way to separate what is essential to the linguistic cognitive system from the constraints imposed, productively and perceptually, by the auditory-vocal modality, that is, to discover the genetically and biologically determined linguistic ability of the human brain (44,45).

Processing of Prosody

Many studies show that linguistic prosody can be destroyed, whereas the ability to comprehend nonlinguistic or affective prosody can be retained and vice versa, depending on which part of the brain has been injured (15,16,33). For example, Emmorey (18) has shown that patients with lesions in the left hemisphere have difficulty in distinguishing contrasts such as the following: *black*board (compound noun with primary stress on first syllable meaning "board to write on that can be black, green, or any other color") and black *board* (noun phrase with primary stress on second syllable meaning "board that is black"). Patients with right hemisphere lesions, however, can process linguistic contrastive stress, but have difficulty with affective intonation reflecting nonlinguistic emotional states. The processing of linguistic prosody, determined by the grammar, is thus a function of the left hemisphere, whereas affective prosody appears to be processed by the right hemisphere.

Studies with normal subjects also support this; the very same stimuli will be processed by either the left or right hemispheres depending on whether the stimuli are considered to be linguistic or nonlinguistic. Two groups of subjects served in an experiment using the dichotic listening technique (51,52). One group consisted of native speakers of Thai, a tone language in which words are contrasted by pitch alone; thus *naa* with a high pitch means something different from *naa* with a low, rising, or falling pitch. The other subjects were speakers of English. The stimuli consisted of the consonant + vowel (CV) syllable *naa* with the four contrasting tones, four CV syllables with contrasting consonants produced with the same pitch on all syllables, and the four pitch contours devoid of segmental context. Thai subjects identified the distinctive tone contrasts on the *naa* syllable and the distinctive consonant CV syllables with significantly greater accuracy when these were presented to the right ear, but not the pitch contours devoid of linguistic context. The English-speaking subjects did better on the CV contrasts but no better with either the *naa* tonal contrasts or the pitch stimuli when these were presented to the right ear. Apparently it is not the physical nature of the stimuli but their functional interpretation that determines which hemisphere will process them.

LOCALIZATION AND MODULARITY

Thus, we find collaborative evidence to support the general tenets of the localization/modularity view of language in the brain, put forth so eloquently by Wernicke in 1874, and now receiving increased interest (19). The French Academy were less insightful than Wernicke when, in 1807, 67 years before his seminal paper, they rejected the nomination for membership of Franz Josef Gall because he suggested that the cortex was involved in thinking (1). Fortunately, that battle appears to be over. As this volume shows, there is now a consensus that the cortex is involved in thinking and, in fact, in different kinds of thinking, i.e., in the different intelligences posed by Gardner (23), one of which is language. But there were detours labeled "equipotentiality" and "antilocalization" on the road that led from the Hippocratic scholars to Gall to Wernicke to Geschwind to this current volume. The observations that there were differences in the aphasias, which were systematically correlated with lesion loci, tended to be ignored, denied, or attributed to the fact that Broca's area lies close to the motor strip, the cortical area that controls articulatory implementation and Wernicke's area that lies close to primary auditory cortex, a view that is insupportable given the recent findings on deaf signer aphasics.

A relationship between areas of the brain and behavior is therefore supported by the data of different focal lesions and differential linguistic breakdown, but we are still far from understanding exactly what that relationship is. The lack of a solution to this problem is not surprising given that the anatomical substrate is a complex interactive network (including the language areas), both sending and receiving information from diverse areas (22). The structure of language, as evidenced by the mental grammar, is also a complex system of interactive components—syntax, phonology, semantics, morphology, the lexicon—with each component itself a complex structure.

CONNECTION BETWEEN THE NOUN PHRASE
AND THE NEURON

Given this complexity, a question posed by Mehler et al. (40)—"What relevance do neurophysiological findings have for psychological models?"—or a slightly altered form of the question—What relevance do neurological and/or aphasia findings have for our understanding of the nature and structure of human language?—is not an easy one to answer, particularly because there does not appear to be "a one-to-one mapping between brain locales and psychological processes."

Marshall (37) stated the problem succinctly:

> Biologists . . . have accumulated a vast body of knowledge concerning the gross anatomy of those parts of the central and peripheral nervous system which seem to be implicated in the acquisition and exercise of linguistic abilities. Some knowledge is even available about the slightly less gross physiology of the relevant brain areas . . . . [In addition] developmental psycholinguists. . . . have amassed alarming amounts of data of the progression from the birth cry to the multiply-embedded relative clause. The problem is . . . found in the simple fact that no-one . . . has the slightest idea how to relate these two domains of inquiry to each other. . . . We have so far failed . . . to construct functional process models (that is, psychological [or linguistic] theories) that could mediate between noun phrases and neurons.

At some level yet to be discovered, there must be a connection between noun phrases and neurons, complex mapping between brain mechanisms, linguistic grammars, and both psychological and linguistic processes. We have neither *a priori* nor empirical evidence of what this mapping will be. The kind of research being reported on in this volume is in line with our search for this knowledge.

In our search we must distinguish between "the use of data from brain-damaged patients (and neurological data from normal subjects) and . . . the activity of mapping psychological functions into the brain" (40). Although the latter activity constitutes a major aim of neuropsychologists and behavioral neurologists, it is the former aspect that is of interest to linguists and psycholinguists. Such data are proving to be of value to linguists testing their hypotheses about the nature of grammars. During the last 30 years, after behaviorism gave way to a more cognitive view of language, a major goal in linguistic theory has been to delimit the class of possible grammars to those that are psychologically and neurologically real, i.e., those that can be acquired, stored, and accessed in speaking and understanding, and that can be impaired following focal brain lesions.

During the 100 or so years since Broca, when neurologists used linguistic data in brain research, few if any linguists considered that neurological data could be of interest in linguistic research. Roman Jakobson (27–29) was the first linguist to conduct research on aphasia using these data to support his ideas on phonological markedness and syntactic theory. For too long a time, only a few insightful linguists, such as Sheila Blumstein (5), followed Jakobson's lead. During the last decade, however, it has become apparent to linguists that such data can aid in linguistic theory construction. Even Chomsky (7) has shown his approval of the possible viability of neurological data, as shown in his statement: "Suppose there is some data from electrical activity of the brain that bears on, say, word boundaries. Why should that be irrelevant? It . . . seems absurd to restrict linguistics to the study of (say) introspective judgments."

On the other side, neurologists are also recognizing that linguistic research can aid in the understanding of the brain and brain functions. It was not long ago that nonlinguists viewed language as a list of words, or syntax as simply a distinction between lexical and grammatical morphemes and the linear ordering of these open and closed classes of words in utterances.

Today, using the linguistic analyses of complex syntactic phenomena (3,5, 6,25,26,31,32,47,48,54), subtle distinctions are being revealed that correlate with different lesion sites. Detailed grammatical as well as linguistic processing analyses of the deficits associated with focal lesions are needed if we are to discover the mapping between brain and language.

No neurological data can provide information on verb subcategorizations, on whether particle movement is the result of an alpha movement rule or generated in the phrase structure rules, tag questions, sentential complements, cleft subject versus cleft object sentences, the validity of the projection principle, or empty categories. To put it somewhat simplistically, aphasia studies cannot tell us that "She went up the stairs in a hurry" is grammatical, whereas "She went the stairs up in a hurry," even though "She called up her sister" and "She called her sister up" are both grammatical. Linguistics, however, provides such data, which are now being used in the analysis of aphasia deficits.

The data collected in these aphasia studies do provide evidence for the construction and testing of linguistic hypotheses and information on the organization of the mental grammar. A question of interest to linguistics, for example, is whether the parts of the language system that are impaired parallel the separate components of grammars posited by linguistic theories. If this is shown to be the case, such findings are important as further support for theories of language and as a first step toward bridging the gap between brain and linguistic mechanisms.

One example may suffice to show how this gap is being bridged by cooperative efforts between linguists and neuroscientists.

For the purposes of linguistic theory that aims at modeling the internalized mental grammar, a lexical entry, e.g., a word, must include everything a speaker knows about that word—its phonological form, morphological structure, syntactic category, semantic representation, subcategorization constraints, selectional features, and, for literate speakers, orthographic shape.

Studies of acquired dyslexia and of various aphasias have provided invaluable information on the form and organization of the mental lexicon. The relevance of such studies to psycholinguistic and linguistic models of normals was shown in the seminal paper by Marshall and Newcombe in 1966 (39) as well as in their later papers (38,41) and has been reinforced by many additional studies (11,43,47–49).

A patient of Newcombe's with whom I have worked during the last five years illustrates the kinds of data that are particularly relevant to lexical representation and access.[1] The subject, Kram, was the victim of a severe traffic accident in 1978 when he was 18 years of age. A long, posttraumatic amnesia of more than a month was recorded, but there were no persistent neurological signs other than that of right, macula-sparing, homonymous hemianopia. Visual acuity was good (J1 and N5 for each eye), and color vision (measured on the Farnsworth Munsell 100-hue test) was unimpaired. A CT scan was performed in January 1981.

The medical record reported (Dr. Philip Sheldon):

> slight but generalized dilation of the left lateral ventricle affecting in particular the left trigonal region and the left temporal horn. In addition, the right temporal horn is slightly dilated. The sulci are slightly more prominent on the left than in the right in particular in the posterior part of the Sylvian fissure. Appearances indicate slight generalised atrophy of the whole of the left hemisphere, in particular the left temporo-parietal region, and of the right temporal region.

The neuropsychological assessments, carried out in 1981, 1982, 1983, and 1985, showed a marked impairment of both verbal (delayed story recall) and nonverbal (maze learning and delayed recall of the Rey Osterrieth pattern) long-term memory. The WAIS verbal and performance IQs were 79 and 90, respectively. Understanding of language was good (Token test 64/66). Picture description and spontaneous speech were fluent and intelligible but with traces of nominal difficulties, which were even more overt on formal object-naming tasks, e.g., 22 of 36 pictures were correctly named on the Oldfield Wingfield test (61). Reading, writing, and oral spelling are disproportionately severely affected (Schonell's reading age 5.5 years, Schonell's spelling age 6.5 years) and his performance is closely analogous in reading and writing.

Table 1 presents examples of Kram's reading and writing to dictation. Kram does not use the orthography to access the phonology and pronunciation. There are some similarities to the spelling and reading errors of children first learning to read and write, particularly in the use of letter names. An examination of school notebooks containing his pre-accident writing show that some but not all of the rules that he now uses to read from written text or write to dictation are those he used when he could not remember the learned spelling/orthography of a word when he was in school.

According to the rules that he has remembered or constructed and that he now uses, all vowels are [+ syllabic], some digraphs are pronounced as clusters, but he does not read letter by letter as is shown by his pronunciation of initial obstruant-liquid clusters /fl/ in "float" and /tr/ in "treat." "Silent" letters, however, are pronounced, e.g., the "h" in "wheel." He has no orthographic representation for the affricates /č/ and /ǰ/ but is aware of the phonemic segment since in writing to dictation he indicates the missing sound by dots. For the most part he writes phonemically, e.g., writing "z" for /z/ rather that using the more common spelling "s" (as in the writing of "busy" /bɪzi/ as "bize," or "goes" /goz/ as "goz."

---

[1] The medical and neuropsychological data were provided by Dr. Freda Newcombe, Neuropsychology Unit, The Radcliffe Infirmary, Oxford.

TABLE 1. *Kram reading aloud and writing to dictation*

Stimulus	Reading pronunciation	Writing to dictation
fame	[fæmi]	FAM
cafe	[sæfi]	KAFA
cape	[sepi]	KAP
tone	[toni]	TON
fight	[fɪg-hɔt]	FiT
goes	[ɡo-ɛs]	GOZ
float	[flo-æt]	FLOT
thing	[tɔhiŋ]	FiNG
charm	[s-ha:m]	...ARM
match	[mæt-kə-hə]	MA...
treat	[tri-æt]	TReT
boost	[bɔ-ɔst] or [dɔ-ɔst]	BUST
wheel	[w-hil]	WeL

Kram's correct spelling of a few items that are exceptions to his own rules implies that some orthographic representations have been spared, or that he can access these but not the majority of words. It is interesting that the spared orthographic representations include grammatical morphemes such as *the* and *that* or the plural *-s*. This provides support for the proposals that grammatical formatives (often referred to as closed-class items) are stored in a separate subcomponent of the lexicon.

Another interesting aspect of his rules is that they reflect his more abstract phonological system rather than the phonetics, as shown by the fact that in writing to dictation when he hears a theta [θ], he writes an "f" and when he hears [ð] (the initial sound in the standard pronunciation of the word *then*, he writes a "v." [θ] and [ð] do not occur in his dialect of English. Note that without a linguistic analysis, the substitution of "f" for "theta" and "v" for "edth" would appear to be random and idiosyncratic errors, as would the spelling of grammatical morphemes.

Figure 1 represents an example of Kram's pre-accident writing. Note that at that time he wrote the "th" of "think" correctly, not the letter "f," showing that at that time he was using a stored orthographic representation rather than constructing the written word on the basis of his own phonological system.

After first meeting with Kram, I made the following prediction, based on the phonemic-orthographic rules I constructed, of how he would write that same letter to dictation. My prediction is given in Fig. 2.

Figure 3 shows how he actually wrote the letter when he next visited the hospital. After further analysis, the revised orthographic-to-phonemic rules that I constructed to account for Kram's errors predict his reading and writing with even fewer errors.

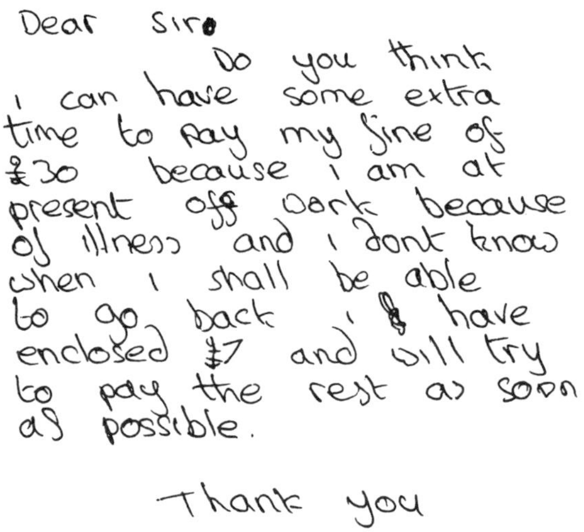

Dear Sir,

Do you think i can have some extra time to pay my fine of £30 because i am at present off oork because of illness and i dont know when i shall be able to go back i have enclosed £7 and will try to pay the rest as soon as possible.

Thank you

FIG. 1. Pre-accident letter written by Kram.

```
D E R       S U R

     D U     Y U     F I N K     i     K A N     A V     S U M     E K S T R A
                                 I

T I˙M     T U     P A     M i     F I N     U V     £30     B E K O Z     i

                                 U
A M     A T     P R E Z E N T     O F     W U R K     B E K O Z     U V

i                                                          i
I L N E S     A N     i     D O N T     N O     W E N     I     S H A L     B E
              A N D

A B U L     T U     G O     B A K     i     A V     E N K L O Z D £7     A N

W I L     T R I     T U     P A     . . U     R E S T     A Z     S U N     A Z

P A S U B U L

                                   F A N K       Y U
```

FIG. 2. V.F. prediction of Kram's postinjury writing.

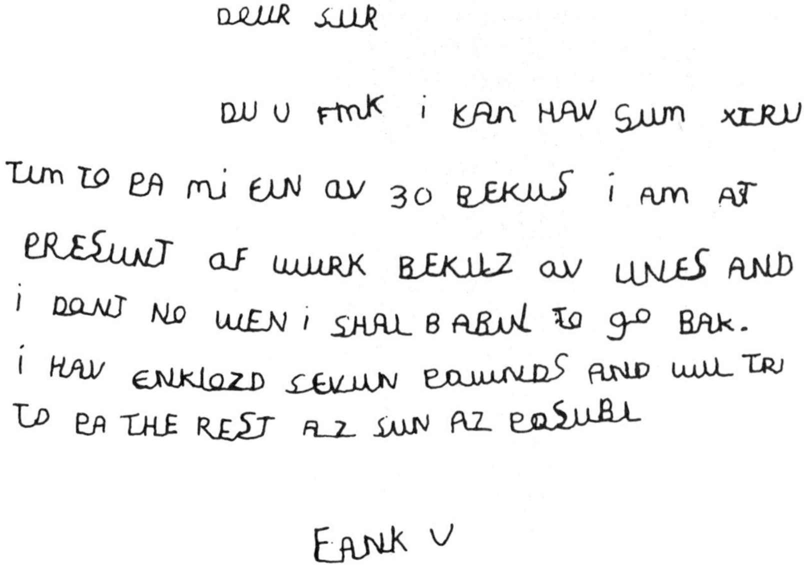

DEUR SUR

DU U FINK i KAN HAV SUM XERU
TUM TO PA mi EUN AV 30 REKUS i AM AT
PRESUNT AV UUURK BEKUZ AV UNES AND
i DANT NO WEN i SHAL B ABUL TO go BAK.
i HAV ENKLOZD SEVUN PAUUNDS AND UUL TRI
TO PA THE REST AZ SUN AZ POSUBL

EANK V

FIG. 3. Postaccident letter written by Kram.

Kram cannot tell from the written representation whether the letters on the stimulus represent a real word. He makes all lexical decisions solely according to his own pronunciation. Thus, if he pronounces a word correctly, he knows it is a word. If he does not, he is at a loss.

Table 2 shows that Kram is only able to comprehend the meaning of a word through the phonology. If his rules used in reading produce a pronunciation that is one of an actual English word in his dictionary, even if it is not the printed word presented to him, Kram provides the meaning of the word he has pronounced. For example, he has a visual difficulty in differentiating between ''d'' and ''b,'' which caused him to read ''rob'' with the pronunciation of ''rod.'' He then gave the meaning as being related to fishing.

The errors that Kram makes in both reading and writing tell us a great deal about the normal process of pronouncing a written word or providing a meaning to a written or spoken word. This is illustrated by the oversimplified model in Fig. 4.

In this model, the lexicon is composed of sublexicons as well as rule components. (In a more complete model, there would also be morphological rules, syntactic category information, subcategorization features, and the like.) Each entry in each of the lexical components is connected to its parallel representation through an addressing system. This is only one way of representing the networking of the phonological, semantic, and orthographic representations. The numerically close addresses are ''on the same street'' or at least ''in the same city.'' This is to account for normal or aphasic speech errors in which semantically related or phonologically similar words are incorrectly selected.

TABLE 2. *Kram: meaning through phonology*

Stimulus	Reading pronunciation	Meaning/use in sentence
sum	[sʌm]	I've got *some* money.
can	[sæn]	I don't know. If it was /m/, it would be "Sam"
hymn	[haj-hi-haj-m-ən]	Hymen?
for	[fɔ]	Four—I have four fingers and a thumb.
rob	[rad]	Fishing?
rib	[rajd]	I know—a motor bike.
son	[son]	If that were a "u" it would be up in the sky.
pig	[pɪg]	Oink oink.
was	[wæs]	Don't know.
so	[so]	*So* you can tell.

Suppose, for example, a speaker intends to say "coat" and says "cape" instead. One might suggest that instead of the semantic address S115, through some noise in the system, he gets to a close but inexact address—S124. This then addresses the phonological address P2007 and the speaker says "cape" (or, phonetically, /kep/).

Note that this model not only accounts for the normal data but also for Kram's errors. One need simply block the arrows or pathways to and from the orthographic lexicon (Fig. 5). There is no orthographic lexicon in the model since there is no evidence that Kram has access to it. The model accounts for the following facts.

1. In reading, Kram does not match the orthographic stimulus to a phonological representation. His pronunciation depends solely on his own grapheme/phoneme rules. Thus he pronounces "cape" as /sæpi/.
2. The normal orthography-to-pronunciation rules are also erased or inaccessible. He uses his own rules.
3. There is no direct route from the orthographic listing to the meaning since he can only provide a meaning for an acoustic signal that sounds like a real word. Since /sæpi/ is not an entry in the phonological lexicon, he cannot provide a meaning.
4. In listening or reading his own writing of "cape," "kap," Kram matches the acoustic signal to the phonological entry and then to the semantic representation permitting him to state its meaning.

Cases such as this, then, provide evidence for the modular organization of the separate components of a grammar. These components appear to form a system whose very origin is independent of other human abilities; that is, the basic structure

Lexical Subcomponents for a Linguistic Processing Model

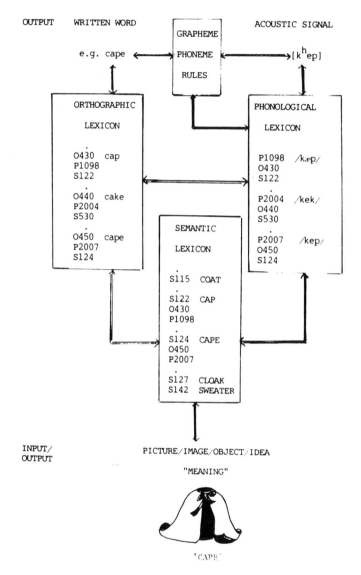

OUTPUT   WRITTEN WORD   ACOUSTIC SIGNAL

                                   GRAPHEME

        e.g. cape ←→   PHONEME ←   →[kʰep]

                                   RULES

            ORTHOGRAPHIC   PHONOLOGICAL

            LEXICON   LEXICON

            .
            O430   cap   P1098   /kæp/
            P1098   O430
            S122   S122
            .   .
            O440   cake   P2004   /kek/
            P2004   O440
            S530   S530
            .   SEMANTIC   .
            O450   cape   P2007   /kep/
            P2007   LEXICON   O450
            S124   S124

                                       .
                                       S115   COAT

                                       .
                                       S122   CAP
                                       O430
                                       P1098

                                       .
                                       S124   CAPE
                                       O450
                                       P2007

                                       .
                                       S127   CLOAK
                                       S142   SWEATER

INPUT/   PICTURE/IMAGE/OBJECT/IDEA
OUTPUT
                                "MEANING"

                                  'CAPE'

FIG. 4. Model of the lexicon and lexical access.

MODEL FOR KRAM READING/WRITING TO DICTION

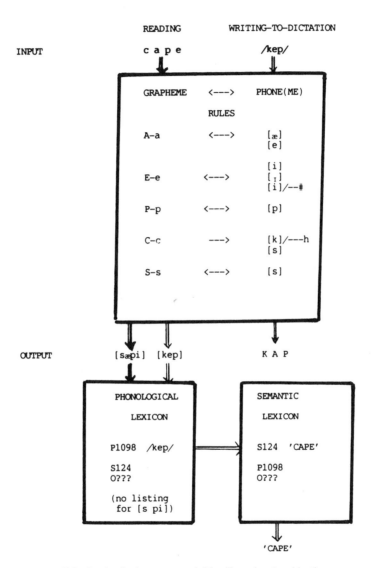

FIG. 5. Lexical access model for Kram (postaccident).

and units of the linguistic system or grammar do not seem to be derived from more general human cognition.

This model could not be constructed without the data provided by aphasia research, nor could it be constructed without the concepts provided by linguistic analysis and theory. Linguistics raises questions for the neurologist and the brain researcher. Aphasia data provide evidence for linguistic constructs. We appear to have established a good working team. Together we may someday actually discover the relationship between the brain and human language.

REFERENCES

1. Arbib, M.A., Caplan, D., and Marshall, J.C. (1982): Neurolinguistics in historical perspective. In: *Neural Models of Language Processes*, edited by M.A. Arbib, D. Caplan, and J.C. Marshall, pp. 5–24. Academic Press, New York.
2. Bellugi, U., Poizner, H., and Klima, E.S. Brain organization for language: Clues from sign aphasia. *Hum. Neurobiol. (in press)*.
3. Berndt, R., and Caramazza, A. (1980): A redefinition of the syndrome of Broca's aphasia: Implications for a neuropsychological model of language. *Applied Psycholinguistics*, 1:225–278.
4. Blank, M., Gessner, M., and Esposito, A. (1979): Language without communication: A case study. *Journal of Child Language*, 6:329–352.
5. Blumstein, S. (1973): *A Phonological Investigation of Aphasic Speech*. Mouton, The Hague.
6. Caplan, D. (1981): Prospects for neurolinguistic theory. *Cognition*, 10:59–64.
7. Chomsky, N. (1982): *On the Generative Enterprise: A Discussion with Riny Hybregts and Henk van Riemsdijk*. Foris, Dordrecht, The Netherlands.
8. Chomsky, N. (1978): On the biological basis of language capacities. In: *Psychology and the Biology of Language and Thought: Essays in Honor of Eric Lenneberg*, edited by A. George and E. Lenneberg, pp. 208–209. Academic Press, New York.
9. Chomsky, N. (1977): *Essays on Form and Interpretation*. Elsevier-North Holland, New York.
10. Chomsky, N. (1972): *Language and Mind*, enlarged ed. Harcourt Brace Jovanovich, New York.
11. Coltheart, M., Patterson, K., and Marshall, J.C. (eds.) (1980): *Deep Dyslexia*. Routledge and Kegan Paul, London.
12. Curtiss, S. Language as a cognitive system: Its independence and selective vulnerability. In: *Developmental Plasticity: Social Context and Human Development*, edited by E.S. Gollin. Academic Press, New York *(in press)*.
13. Curtiss, S. (1977): *Genie: A Psycholinguistic Study of a Modern-Day Wild Child*. Academic Press, New York.
14. Curtiss, S., Kempler, D., and Yamada, J. (1981): The relationship between language and cognition in development: Theoretical framework and research design. *UCLA Working Papers in Cognitive Linguistics*, 3:161–175.
14a. Curtiss, S., Yamada, J., and Fromkin, V. (1979): How independent is language? On the question of formal parallels between grammar and action. *UCLA Working Papers in Cognitive Linguistics*, 1:131–157.
15. Danly, M., and Cooper, W. (1983): Fundamental frequency, language processing, and linguistic structure in Wernicke's aphasia. *Brain Lang.*, 19:1–24.
16. Danly, M., and Shapiro, B. (1982): Speech prosody in Broca's aphasia. *Brain Lang.*, 16:171–190.
17. Elliott, D., and Needleman, R. (1981): Language, cognition and pragmatics: The view from developmental disorders of language. *UCLA Working Papers in Cognitive Linguistics*, 3:199–207.
18. Emmorey, K. The neurological substrates for prosodic aspects of speech. *Brain Lang. (in press)*.
19. Fodor, J.A. (1983): *The Modularity of Mind*. MIT Press, Cambridge, MA.
20. Fromkin, V.A., and Klima, E. (1980): General and special properties of language. In: *Signed and Spoken Language: Biological Constraints on Linguistic Form*, edited by U. Bellugi and M. Studdert-Kennedy, pp. 13–28. Verlag Chemie, Basel.
21. Fromkin, V.A., Curtiss, S., Krashen, S., Rigler, D., and Rigler, M. (1974): The development of language in Genie: A case of language acquisition beyond the "critical period." *Brain Lang.*, 1:81–107.

22. Galaburda, A.M. (1984): The anatomy of language: Lessons from comparative anatomy. In: *Biological Perspectives on Language*, edited by D. Caplan, A.R. Lecours, and A. Smith, pp. 290–302. MIT Press, Cambridge, MA.
23. Gardner, H. (1983): *Frames of Mind: The Theory of Multiple Intelligences*. Basic Books, New York.
24. Goodman, J. (1972): A case study of an autistic savant: Mental function in the psychotic child with markedly discrepant abilities. *J. Child Psychol. Psychiatry*, 13:267–278.
25. Grodzinsky, Y. (1985): On the interaction between linguistics and neuropsychology. *Brain Lang.*, 26:186–199.
26. Grodzinsky, Y. (1984): The syntactic characterization of agrammatism. *Cognition*, 16:99–120.
27. Jakobson, R. (1964): Towards a linguistic typology of aphasic impairments. In: *Disorders of Language*, edited by A.V.S. deReuck and M. O'Connor, pp. 21–41. Little, Brown, Boston.
28. Jakobson, R. (1955): Aphasia as a linguistic problem. In: *On Expressive Language*, edited by H. Werner, pp. 69–81. Clark University Press, Worcester, MA.
29. Jakobson, R. (1940): *Kindersprache, Aohasie and allgemeine Lautgesetze*. Almqvist u. Wilsells, Uppsala. Reprinted as *Child Language, Aphasia, and Phonological Universals*, 1968. Mouton, The Hague.
30. Kanner, L. (1943): Autistic disturbances of affective contact. *Nerv. Child.* 2:217–250.
31. Kean, M.-L. (ed.) (1985): *Agrammatism*. Academic Press, New York.
32. Kean, M.-L. (1980): Grammatical representations and the description of language processing. In: *Biological Studies of Mental Processes*, edited by D. Caplan, pp. 239–268. MIT Press, Cambridge, MA.
33. Kent, R.D., and Rosenbek, J.C. (1982): Prosodic disturbance and neurologic lesion. *Brain Lang.*, 15:259–291.
34. Klima, E.S., Poizner, H., and Bellugi, U. (1983): What the hands reveal about the brain: Evidence from American Sign Language. In: *Brain Organization: Clues from Sign Aphasia*, pp. 3.1–26. The Salk Institute, La Jolla, CA.
35. Klima, E.S., and Bellugi, U. (1979): *The Signs of Language*. Harvard University Press, Cambridge, MA.
36. Luria, S. (1973): *Life: The Unfinished Experiment*. Scribners, New York.
37. Marshall, J.C. (1980): On the biology of language acquisition. In: *Biological Studies of Mental Processes*, edited by D. Caplan, pp. 106–148. MIT Press, Cambridge, MA.
38. Marshall, J.C., and Newcombe, F. (1973): Patterns of paralexia: A psycholinguistic approach. *J. Psycholinguist. Res.*, 2:175–199.
39. Marshall, J.C., and Newcombe, F. (1966): Syntactic and semantic errors in paralexia. *Neuropsychologia*, 4:169–176.
40. Mehler, J., Morton, J., and Jusczyk, P. (1984): On reducing language to biology. *Cognitive Neuropsychology*, 1:83–116.
41. Newcombe, F., and Marshall, J.C. (1985): Reading and writing by letter sounds. In: *Surface Dyslexia*, edited by K. Patterson, J.C. Marshall, and M. Coltheart, pp.35–51. Routledge and Kegan Paul, London.
42. Nottebohn, F. (1984): Vocal learning and its possible relation to replaceable synapses and neurons. In: *Biological Perspectives on Language*, edited by D. Caplan, A.R. Lecours, and A. Smith, pp. 65–95. MIT Press, Cambridge, MA.
43. Patterson, K.E. (1982): The relation between reading and phonological coding: Further neuropsychological observations. In: *Normality and Pathology in Cognitive Functions*, edited by A.W. Ellis, pp. 77–112. Academic Press, New York.
44. Poizner, H., Bellugi, U., and Iragui, V. Apraxia and aphasia in a visual-gestural language. *Am. J. Physiol.* (in press).
45. Poizner, H., Kaplan, E., Bellugi, U., and Padden, C. Hemispheric specialization for nonlinguistic visual-spatial processing in brain damaged signers. *Brain and Cognition* (in press).
46. Rieber, R.W. (ed.) (1983): *Dialogues on the Psychology of Language and Thought: Conversations with Noam Chomsky, Charles Osgood, Jean Piaget, Ulric Neisser and Marcel Kinsbourne*. Plenum Press, New York.
47. Saffran, E.M. (1985): Lexicalization and reading performance in surface dyslexia. In: *Surface Dyslexia*, edited by K.E. Patterson, J.C. Marshall, and M. Coltheart, pp. 53–70. Lawrence Erlbaum, Hillside, NJ.
48. Saffran, E.M., and Marin, O.S.M. (1977): Reading without phonology: Evidence from aphasia. *Q. J. Exp. Psychol.*, 29:307–318.

49. Schwartz, M.R., Saffran, E.M., and Marin, O.S.M. (1980): Fractionating the reading process in dementia: Evidence for word-specific print-to-sound associations. In: *Deep Dyslexia*, edited by M. Coltheart, K. Patterson, and J.C. Marshall, pp. 259–269. Routledge and Kegan Paul, London.
50. Seidenberg, M.S., and Petitto, L.A. (1979): Signing behavior in apes: A critical review. *Cognition*, 7:177–215.
51. Van Lancker, D., and Fromkin, V.A. (1978): Cerebral dominance for pitch contrasts in tone language speakers and in musically untrained and trained English speakers. *Journal of Phonetics*, 6:19–23.
52. Van Lancker, C., and Fromkin, V.A. (1973): Hemispheric specialization for pitch and "tone": Evidence from Thai. *Journal of Phonetics*, 1:101–109.
53. Yamada, J. (1983): The independence of language: A case study. Unpublished Ph.D. dissertation. University of California, Los Angeles.
54. Zurif, E., and Blumstein, S. (1978): Language and the brain. In: *Linguistic Theory and Psychological Reality*, edited by M. Halle, J. Bresnan, and G. Miller, pp. 229–246. MIT Press, Cambridge, MA.

Language, Communication, and the Brain, edited by F. Plum.
Raven Press, New York © 1988.

What Is and Is Not Universal in Language Acquisition

*Elizabeth Bates and * †Virginia A. Marchman

*Department of Psychology, University of California, San Diego,
La Jolla, California 92093, and †Department of Psychology, University of California,
Berkeley, California 94720*

The noted linguist Noam Chomsky has referred to language as a "mental organ" (24). As with other organs, language should therefore develop and mature in predictable ways, with few deviations from a universal embryogenetic course. We argue instead that there is no such thing as normal language development—if by "normal" we mean a single, universal sequence of events that takes place whenever a healthy child acquires his/her native language. Language acquisition is marked, instead, by great diversity, including variations that derive from the language being acquired, and variations that derive from the learning strategies preferred by an individual child. Although the organ metaphor is hard to defend in the face of this diversity, we need not abandon our efforts to characterize language as a biological system. Rather, our attention must shift from a focus on universals to the much more interesting question of *plasticity*, i.e., how many different forms can a biological system take under a range of normal and abnormal conditions?

One widely accepted description of the course of early language development is as follows [(30, p. 79); cf. (8)]:

1. At about 9 to 10 months of age, infants begin to show systematic evidence of language comprehension (for at least a few well-practiced words and phrases).

2. By 12 months of age, most infants begin to use single words—particularly words that name objects.

3. Between 12 and 20 months, there is a sudden burst in expressive vocabulary (usually beginning after the first 50 words are produced). At the same time, there is a shift in the use of single words—from nouns to verbs, adjectives, and other relational terms, and within noun use, from naming and requesting objects to talking about relational meanings (e.g., pointing to Daddy's jogging shoes and saying "Daddy").

4. At 20 months of age, most children begin to produce their first word combinations; these combinations consist primarily of "telegraphic speech," strings of

19

content words stripped of any grammatical morphology (i.e., inflections and function words).

5. Between two and three years of age, there is a burst in grammatical development. Bound morphemes and function words take their places among the major constituents of sentence structure like "ivy growing in between the bricks" (22); complex syntactic structures begin to come in during this period, and grammatical development is for all intents and purposes complete by the age of four.

This is a fair description of group means, averaged over many children and many languages. But social psychologists have become rightfully suspicious of group means: No single Vassar graduate has 2.5 children, and few suburban families have three-quarters of a dog (A.R. Damasio, *this volume*). Recent evidence suggests that the textbook view of language milestones is just as misleading. If we take a careful look at cross-linguistic data and at individual differences within English, it is difficult to make a case for universal sequences of development.

Some researchers (69) clearly understood this all along. For many others, the diversity that is possible in language acquisition has come as something of a surprise. In the 1960s, most psycholinguists were convinced that the important aspects of language development occur at the same time and in the same sequence in every natural language (55). Of course, the strongest version of this argument has always been untenable. Some children are slow learners and some are fast; some learn Italian and some learn Arabic. Differences in rate of development have always been expected and differences in *particular* content and structure are necessarily determined by the language that a particular child must learn. But there were nevertheless good reasons to believe that universal patterns lay beneath all this "local" diversity.

Faith in a universal and innate Language Acquisition Device derived primarily from the finding that children are active and creative participants in the acquisition process. They make errors (e.g., "goed," "comed") and innovations (e.g., "I broomed it, Mommy!") that cannot be found in their linguistic environment. These overgeneralizations have been used as evidence for the existence of rules that children have abstracted in an apparent effort to construct a coherent, albeit temporary and erroneous, theory of their language (11,41,42). Investigators may continue to debate about the *exact* nature of children's intermediate theories (47,53,54,66), but few would argue with the premise that they somehow go beyond the data provided by their caretakers.

Children can operate on their language as a "formal problem space" (41,42), creating intermediate theories, because they are equipped with prior clues about the possible forms that a natural language can take. In other words, language is something that all humans are *predisposed* to learn. In fact, this conclusion is just as valid as ever; we do not intend to challenge it here. The current debate focuses not on the existence or nonexistence of predispositions for language, but on their nature. Does the child come into the world with constraints on learning that are specific to the domain of language (13)? Or does s/he apply more general cognitive principles to the specific problems posed by language acquisition (5)? For present purposes, we will simply stipulate that predispositions for language do exist. These prior constraints can, in turn, be used to argue in favor of a biological substrate for language (25,31,45,71).

The point that we want to make is that the child's predispositions for language are *not* realized in universal sequences of development. Psycholinguists at one time hoped to factor out the relevant "local details" of acquisition within and across natural languages, laying bare a linguistic embryogenesis with all the predictability that we have come to expect of mental and physical organs. More than anything else, this naive belief in universals may show just how little psychologists and linguists know about biology. The relationship between genotype and phenotype is rarely direct. Furthermore, genes may be responsible for variations as well as constants in development. In this chapter, we review current evidence against universal patterns of acquisition. We begin with a brief overview of cross-linguistic evidence; then we provide an even more rapid review of evidence for individual differences in the acquisition of English. Our hope is not to discourage those who seek the biological foundations of language, but to encourage a more realistic view of language development as a complex and highly plastic biological system.

CROSS-LINGUISTIC EVIDENCE

Most developmental psycholinguists hope that the patterns uncovered by their research will generalize across linguistic and cultural environments. Nevertheless, the bulk of what we know about acquisition has come from studies of children acquiring English. Such unfortunate limitations in the data base often resulted in the premature elevation of idiosyncratic facts about English to the status of universals. Cross-language comparisons, pioneered by Slobin and his colleagues (70,72,73), offer a powerful tool for separating universal from particular, like wheat from chaff.

Does the textbook story of acquisition hold up under the scrutiny of cross-language comparisons? If we focus on early meanings, then it appears that all children talk about the same things in the early stages of language acquisition. They begin by talking about objects in their immediate environment. In fact, the onset of reference, i.e., the understanding that things have names, is crucial for the young child to make contact with his/her social world, regardless of which language learning community s/he is about to join (8,76). After naming is firmly established, children then go on to talk about a common stock of relational meanings—again, regardless of the language being learned (19,70). Some of these meanings have to do with the presence, absence, ownership, desire, and/or refusal of objects: "Allgone!", "More!", "Mine!", "No!", and the like. Other meanings concern the structure of simple events (e.g., agents, actions, things acted on, as in "Mommy go" and "Cut finger") and simple scenes (e.g., states and/or locations of objects, as in "Hot coffee!" or "Teddy up dere").

However, universal *meanings* are not necessarily reflected in universal *means* for expressing those meanings. Marked and interesting differences have been noted from one language to another in the exact nature of those first words and word combinations even in the earliest stages of grammar (1,19,50). As a result, terms that have been used to describe "what all children do" have been seriously called into question.

Much of this work is summarized in a massive two-volume work by Slobin (73), and in a forthcoming book by MacWhinney and Bates (51). We try to make the point more succinctly here, examining how four proposed universals have held up to cross-linguistic evidence. Two of them are drawn from evidence on language production; the other two come from studies of language comprehension. These four examples will show not only what current cross-linguistic research has revealed about the nature of the language learning process, but also how the "old" universalism can be revised to account for acquisition data.

Universal #1:   Children proceed from single words, to ordered but uninflected word combinations, to word combinations with grammatical inflections and function words.

This is an abbreviated version of the textbook description that we presented earlier. Above all, it involves the claim that children universally go through a stage of *telegraphic speech*, i.e., strings of words without grammatical inflections. This may be a valid description for children acquiring word-order languages such as English (at least some subset of English children—an issue that we address later). However, the telegraphic speech hypothesis does not qualify as a universal. Turkish children seem to make productive use of case inflections from the very beginning of multiword speech—and according to some reports, they may be able to inflect a few words correctly early in the single-word stage (at about 14 months of age) (73). In fact, Turkish children seem to master all of the basic case morphology contrasts in their language by 24 months of age (72). The same pattern of acquisition seems to hold, to a lesser extent, for children acquiring Hindi (79) and Polish (82,83).

Turkish children complete acquisition of grammatical morphology in their language at approximately the same point at which normal English children launch their first attack on noun and verb endings (i.e., between 2 and 2½ years). This is a striking contrast—but the contrast with Russian and Serbo-Croatian children is even more striking. These children are also acquiring a case-marked language, but do not reach the level of performance demonstrated by Turkish two-year-olds before six or seven years of age. They seem to avoid acquiring grammatical morphology until they have exhausted a series of other possibilities. For example, some Russian or Serbo-Croatian children act as though they were acquiring a rigid word-order language like English, using only one or two of the many word order possibilities in their language (68,71). This can be contrasted with the performance of Finnish children, who produce a wide variety of word orders in the early stages even though they have not yet mastered the adult system of case inflections (17). Hence at least three distinct routes into grammatical morphology are possible: (a) productive inflection from the beginning, even in the one-word stage; (b) rigidly ordered telegrams without grammatical morphology; and (c) uninflected word combinations that nevertheless occur in a range of different orders (19).

How can these cross-language differences be reconciled with the notion that there are "universal" patterns of acquisition? One explanation can be found by looking more closely at the nature of the languages that children in these various language communities must acquire. English has an extremely regular set of word-order principles, but relatively little grammatical morphology. Given this situation, English children zero in on word order at an early age, and postpone the acquisition of noun and verb endings for several months. Turkish, according to many linguists and historians, has the most regular, clear, and semantically transparent inflectional system of any language studied to date. Turkish children apparently agree with this assessment, given the speed with which they complete morphological development. By contrast, Russian and Serbo-Croatian have very irregular and arbitrary inflectional systems. As a result, children who are learning these languages often begin to talk by using nouns and verbs in their uninflected form, only later attempting to apply grammatical markings.

In short, the array of strategies elected by small children makes perfect sense from the point of view of the languages being acquired. We have to reject Universal #1. But there *is* a universal tendency underlying all of this variation: Children are biased to pick up clear and regular structures before they learn arbitrary and/or irregular forms. This bias toward clear and regular forms may reflect the application of language-specific predispositions—but may also reflect the application of general perceptual/cognitive strategies to the domain of language learning.

Universal #2: Children tend to omit verbs from their first multiword combinations.

It has been noted that children are particularly likely to omit verbs during the stage when they first put words together (14). At least two different explanations have been offered for this pattern:

1. Verbs are morphologically more complex than nouns, and hence avoided until the problems of morphology are worked out.
2. Verbs express complex semantic relationships that are acquired relatively late in development. Because these relations are so cognitively complex, the child first expresses verb meanings in a syncretic, unanalyzed form by simply naming one or more of the associated nouns (e.g., "mommy sock").

These statements offer plausible explanations for the original verb-omission finding, each focusing on complexity in relation to the development of general information processing capabilities—in one case, the morphological system, and in the other, the semantic domain. Much research has since been devoted to elucidating the relative contribution of the semantic (or meaning) component of language compared with the structural (or formal) aspects of the system to the acquisition process. Unfortunately, new evidence suggests that this debate may have been misguided, because the supposedly universal pattern of verb omission does not hold across all languages.

In a cross-linguistic study designed to address this issue, MacWhinney and Bates (50) showed that there are differences in the frequency with which children learning various languages omit the verb from their productions. In an experimental situation in which children were describing the same set of pictures, Italian two- to three-year-olds were significantly less likely to omit the verb than their English-speaking counterparts. Instead, Italian children were more likely to omit the subject of the sentence. Hungarian children showed yet another pattern—a tendency to omit the object of the verb. As discussed by Bates and MacWhinney (4), similar differences in lexicalization and ellipsis (i.e., what is said, and what is left out) can be observed even in the first word combinations of 20- to 24-month-old children.

These findings do not seem so surprising if one again examines the structure of the languages in question. Compared with the same verb forms in English, Italian verbs are quite complex. To illustrate, take the following conjugation in English: "I eat, you eat, he eats, we eat, you all eat, they eat." Notice that there is only one contrasting inflection (third person singular "eats") in the entire present indicative conjugation. Now consider the same conjugation in Italian: "Io mangio, tu mangi, lui mangia, noi mangiamo, voi mangiate, loro mangiano." Where English provides only two forms of the verb, Italian provides six. Because the Italian verbs are even more difficult than their English equivalents, we cannot explain verb omission in terms of the avoidance of difficult morphemes. English children, with an easier task, are actually doing more verb avoidance! Because the pictures used in this experiment tapped verbs of equivalent semantic complexity in both languages, the cross-linguistic findings cannot be accounted for on semantic grounds.

The difference seems to be owing to the relative *informativeness* of verbs in the two languages. The various contrasts for person and number on the Italian verb provide a great deal of information about who did what to whom. That information proves to be essential for sentence understanding in Italian, for two further reasons. First, Italian (like the case-inflected languages described earlier) permits extensive variation of word order for highlighting and emphasis (e.g., people really can say things such as "The spaghetti ate Giovanni"). Second, Italians also omit the subject of the sentence in a very large proportion of their utterances (e.g., saying the equivalent of "Raining! Will take an umbrella" instead of the more typical English construction "It's raining! I'll take an umbrella."). Because of these instances of subject omission and variations in word order, Italian listeners *have* to rely on verb inflections. For the same reason, Italian speakers cannot afford to omit the verb as easily as English speakers. The resulting pressure to produce verbs is reflected in the behavior of Italian children before the age of two (1), and may even be reflected in the onset time and number of verbs that are observed in the one-word stage.

With this approach, we can also explain the other findings in the MacWhinney and Bates study (51). The tendency for Italian children to omit the subject is quite consonant with rates of subject omission in Italian adult speech (about 70% of the time in informal conversation) (1). Subject omission is not always possible in Hungarian because the subject-noun phrase carries a case inflection that marks the actor role, and, indeed, Hungarian children are not as likely to omit the subject as their Italian counterparts. Objects also carry case inflections in Hungarian, which should prevent their omission. However, Hungarian verbs often carry a marker that agrees with the object—offering enough redundancy to make object omission possible. Hungarian children seem to have understood this fact, at least at some unconscious level, resulting in greater rates of object omission in this language.

To summarize, we find at least three different patterns of omission in early child language: a bias toward verb omission, a bias toward subject omission, and a bias toward object omission. Universal #2 is clearly wrong, but again, there is a universal tendency underlying all of this variation: Children are sensitive to the informativeness of elements in their language and/or to the statistical distribution of those elements in adult speech. This predisposition may be attributable to a species-specific preparation for language; it might also reflect the operation of general learning principles within the language domain.

The next two proposed universals come from the domain of sentence comprehension.

Universal #3: Semantic cues to the comprehension of agent-object relations will be acquired before word-order cues.

Bever (12) proposed that three-year-old children rely primarily on semantic strategies in comprehending simple declarative sentences, whereas four-year-olds will make primary use of word order. Variations of this "semantics first" hypothesis have been proposed (23,78); however, the main idea is that some kind of semantic information will be used in advance of grammatical information (such as word order), by all children in all languages.

This "semantics first" hypothesis has not held up under cross-linguistic study; it does not even hold up in English. In one study, English and Italian children were given a series of simple active declarative sentences with two concrete nouns and an action verb (7). The stimuli were designed to test all three word orders (NVN: "the cow is hitting the horse"; NNV: "the horse the cow is hitting"; and VNN: "is hitting the cow the horse") in orthogonal combinations of animacy (first noun animate and second inanimate, first noun inanimate and second animate; and both nouns animate). Each sentence was read to the child, who then had to act out the sentence with toy animals and objects. The results were absolutely clear-cut: Word order was the first cue to have a significant effect on sentence interpretation for English children, starting at two years of age; animacy was the first cue to have a significant impact on Italians, again by two years of age. At no point in the English data did an animacy strategy dominate over word order; and at no point in the Italian data did word order dominate over animacy. Very similar findings, with appropriate language-specific variations, have also been reported for French (40), Hungarian (52), and Serbo-Croatian (S. Smith, *personal communication*).

We are forced to abandon Universal #3. It appears to have been based on two anglocentric notions: that semantic strategies are primitive or in some sense "pre-linguistic," and word order *ought* to dominate in the behavior of a sophisticated adult. This is not borne out by the facts. When given a sentence such as "The pencil kicked the cow," sophisticated Italian adults (e.g., graduate students in linguistics) choose the cow as the agent; when given the same sentence, English two-year-olds choose the pencil as the agent. Once again, however, there is a universal tendency underlying language-specific sequences of development: Children begin at a very early age to identify and utilize those clues to sentence meaning that are most informative for their language. This predisposition leads to word order in English, and to lexical semantics in Italian.

Universal #4:   Word-order cues to comprehension of agent-object relations will be acquired before grammatical morphology.

This proposed universal has been offered most recently by Pinker (65) in this form: "For case-inflected languages, children will utter sentences in the dominant word order and will use the dominant word order as a cue in comprehending sentences before they have mastered their language's morphology."

About the same time, however, Slobin and Bever (74) offered a rather clear counterexample to this claim, with data on sentence interpretation by Turkish children. As we noted earlier, the Turkish system of case inflections is perhaps the most regular, semantically transparent, and unambiguous system in the world. It then would not be surprising to find that case markings are a comprehension cue that children find relatively easy to identify and use. Indeed, Slobin and Bever showed that Turkish children have completely mastered the use of these case contrasts very early (by age two); however, they show little or no sensitivity to word-order contrasts until about the age of four, and even then, word-order never becomes an important source of information about sentence meaning.

Recent information on the acquisition of Hungarian (52,67) and Polish (83) suggests that this pattern of development also holds for these languages. In other words, these children seem to acquire case inflections (even though those morphological systems are not as regular as the Turkish counterpart) before they demonstrate systematic use of word-order patterns, in comprehension or production. However, word-order cues are used earlier and/or for a longer period by children acquiring the difficult inflectional systems of Russian (35) or Serbo-Croatian (68).

Putting together the evidence on comprehension, we find that children can begin to interpret sentences from at least three different starting points: word order, lexical semantics, or grammatical morphology (in particular, case inflections on nouns). Initial hypotheses and sequences of acquisition are predicted by the regularity, clarity, and informativeness of target structures in the language that the child is trying to acquire. This is a universal, but one that points to the operation of general biases about language learning, and/or about learning in general.

Summary

In order to construct a universalistic account of the acquisition of grammar, researchers have had to introduce concepts that extract universal patterns from what appear to be particularistic data. In recent work, Slobin (73) documented variations similar to these in the acquisition of grammar across a large range of typologically distinct languages, from American Sign Language to Hebrew to Samoan. According to Slobin, "It is only by detailed examination of patterns of children's verbal interaction with others that we can form a picture of the child's activity in constructing language. By observing repetitions of such patterns across individual children and languages we can begin to form hypotheses about the underlying capacities that may be responsible for language acquisition *in general*" [emphasis added] (73, p. 1158).

Slobin's (70,71,73) approach encompasses a lengthy list of "operating principles" that seem to govern the acquisition of every natural language. These include a tendency to avoid discontinuous morphemes (e.g., "call" and "up" in "Call the girl up"), a preference for locating morphemes at the end rather than the beginning or the middle of a word, a belief that some meanings are inherently "grammaticizable" (e.g., person, gender, tense) whereas other meanings are not likely to be coded in the grammar (e.g., color, time of day), and a host of other probabilistic biases about what a language should be. Because natural languages do vary a great deal (as shown by the cross-linguistic studies outlined here), which is compounded by variations in the individual child's language learning environment (e.g., whether s/he is learning primarily from parents or peers), children may indeed look quite different from one another at any given stage. However, in this view, the various hypotheses that children entertain in the course of grammatical development can all be explained with reference to a universal set of biases about the nature of language and more general characteristics of the child's mental equipment.

Bates and MacWhinney (6,48,49) handle the same cross-linguistic variation somewhat differently. In their Competition Model, frequency, perceivability, memory load, semantic transparency, validity of cues, and other statistical properties of the input play the major role in determining order of acquisition. The organism adapts to the shape of the input provided by the language, with a set of biases or predispositions that may not be specific to language at all. This emphasis on general cognitive and perceptual principles contrasts with Slobin's willingness to attribute language-specific biases to the child.

Although these two models differ in detail, they both illustrate a clear shift in focus from the search for *universal content* to *universal mechanisms* or *processes*. The simpler "universalism" of the past has been abandoned, and the notion of universals has been reformulated in a set of clues or hints about processing that help the child to discover the peculiarities of his/her own language. The modern approach is analogous in some respects to the child's first encounter with a kaleidoscope—from one end, there seems to be an infinite set of variations, but from the other side we can see that all of this diversity is produced by a constant set of prisms interacting with some unsystematic arrangements of colored glass.

INDIVIDUAL DIFFERENCES WITHIN ENGLISH

The new view of language universals permits much more variation across natural languages. However, Slobin's operating principles and the Competition Model of Bates and MacWhinney both predict highly regular and universal sequences *within* any one language. There may be variations in rate of development—either because a particular child is slow in attending to the input, or because the environment is so impoverished that it takes longer for the critical information to appear. In general, the sequence and nature of development should be determined primarily by the qualitative and/or quantitative structure of the target language.

Assumptions about universal patterns within language groups have been reflected in both the theory and methodology of child language research. Investigators in this field have made extensive use of longitudinal case studies, based on the assumption that findings from a small sample are valid for the language as a whole. Roger Brown's influential book *A First Language* (22) is a classic example of how much can be learned from detailed case descriptions [see also (14,15,19,57)]. Much of the descriptive research from other languages has followed Brown's methodology (73).

Nevertheless, the field has been forced to acknowledge some limitations in the case study approach, in view of new information showing that a single language (English) is not always acquired in the same way by every child (21,34,43,61,62). This discovery has forced us to adopt a new set methods and assumptions about the mechanisms that underlie language learning. In the following sections, we review evidence from our work and that of other investigators, demonstrating individual differences in lexical, grammatical, and phonological development. These studies clearly suggest that qualitative *styles* of language learning can be identified, in addition to the expected differences in rate of development. By looking at individual differences and variations in the *content* and *structure* of early language, we hope to achieve a better understanding of universal *mechanisms*. In the long run, this focus on variation will also provide important information about the biological substrate for language.

Before we proceed, it is important to point out that we describe the extreme ends of one or more developmental continua. Most children will fall somewhere in the middle, displaying a mixture of the patterns described below. The extremes are informative not because they give us a typology of children, but because they illustrate the amount of plasticity that is available in normal language development.

Lexical Development

Nelson (58) was the first to point out how much children can vary in the content and structure of early vocabularies during the production of their first words. She examined the first 50 words of 18 children, in maternal diary data and home recordings, and uncovered a dimension of individual variation from *referential style* (i.e., vocabularies with a high proportion of common object names) to *expressive style* (i.e., heterogeneous vocabularies containing items from various classes, including some frozen forms or routines, such as "hi," "stop it," and "I love you"). Referential style reflects the "universal" naming strategy described earlier; it tends to be associated with faster rates of language development overall, and with a more "object-oriented" approach to interacting with adults. Expressive style involves a mix of words and phrases that is difficult to place on the supposedly universal route from first words to grammar; this approach tends to be associated with a slower overall pace of development, and with a less object-oriented and more direct style of interacting with other human beings.

This discovery has been replicated many times. Bloom, Lightbown, and Hood (16) reported a similar range of variation at the stage of first word combinations [see also (26,37,38,63,77)]. The longitudinal study of Snyder, Bates, and Bretherton (76) of 27 children from 13 to 28 months of age showed that the referential/expressive dimension is already established by 13 months, in both comprehension and production. More recently, Goldfield (35) uncovered evidence suggesting that this contrast may actually begin prior to speech. In her longitudinal study, children who engaged in more giving, showing, and pointing during the preverbal stage were more likely to display a referential approach once language got underway. By contrast, children who engaged in less object-oriented communication prior to speech tended later on to have more heterogeneous vocabularies and more social formulae. This finding suggests that the referential/expressive dimension in lexical development may have its roots in processing variables that are operating weeks or even months before the child is able to utter his/her first words. As we shall see, a similar dimension of variation will persist through the acquisition of grammar.

Grammatical Development

In the first major empirical study of individual differences in early grammatical development, Bloom et al. (16) introduced a contrast between *nominal style* (i.e., multiword constructions composed primarily of nouns and other content words) and *pronominal style* (i.e., multiword constructions in which the same meanings are conveyed with nonspecific pronominal forms). Their "nominal style" children conformed to the notion of a telegraphic stage, hooking content words together in their least marked form, with little if any use of grammatical morphology. These children tended to refer to themselves and the listener by name (e.g., "Mommy sock," "Kathryn milk"). Their "pronominal style" children used grammatical function words from the beginning, referring to themselves and the listener in pronominal form, with variable use of bound morphology [see also (59)]. They also displayed a somewhat greater tendency toward unselective imitation of adult speech. This qualitative difference between children in productive output cannot be attributed to a difference in the underlying meanings that the children want to express, since nominal and pronominal children tended to express the same number and range of semantic relationships. For example, one child might insist on her right to play with a toy truck by saying "Katherine play"; whereas another in a similar circumstance might say "I do it."

Unlike the referential/expressive dimension, the pronominal/nominal contrast seemed to persist only until children reached the level at which they are using about 2.5 morphemes per utterance. It is, nevertheless, a robust finding that has now been reported in several studies (2,20,32,63,64). There is some evidence tying the nominal/pronominal dimension in grammatical development to the referential/expressive dimension in one-word speech. In addition, research by Horgan (39) suggests the nominal/pronominal dimension may continue into the later stages of grammatical development in a different form. She describes a range of variation in the means that children use to expand phrases—early "noun lovers" tend to concentrate on expansions and elaborations of the noun phrase (e.g., adjectival modifiers, prepositional phrases, relative clauses); early "noun leavers" remain uninterested in noun-phrase development, concentrating primarily on verb morphology. Taken together, these studies suggest moderate stability and/or continuity in grammatical style, from first word combinations (and perhaps lexical style in the one-word stage) through grammatical developments well into the third and fourth year of life.

Phonology

Several studies have reported that the speech of many normal children is difficult to understand and transcribe (20,28,29,38,39,46,60,63). Indeed, some frustrated investigators have been driven to use the term "mushmouth" to describe some of their young subjects. At first glance, such differences in intelligibility seem to reflect nothing more or less than rate of development. Researchers in the Stanford Child Phonology Project have tried to replace this notion of intelligibility with a more principled account—and in the process, they have learned still more about qualitative differences in language learning. For example, Vihman (80) reports that there is a reliable and continuous dimension of "phonological consistency," i.e., whether the child pronounces a given word type the same way across instances, that persists from the beginning of first words through three years of age. Interestingly, at three years of age this variability in phonology is also associated with greater variability or inconsistency in the child's grammatical rule system (81).

A child who is low in phonological consistency is not necessarily "bad" at phonology. Rather, children seem to vary in the extent to which they emphasize different *aspects* of phonology. Some children take a more global strategy; they concentrate on "suprasegmental" features such as prosody or intonation, sketching out the broad outlines of a word or sentence and working on the details later (20,27,29,63). Other children take a more local strategy, concentrating on the process of segmenting speech sounds into phonemic/syllabic units that are gradually built up into whole forms. This segmental/suprasegmental dimension can be detected even before meaningful speech begins. For example, some children under one year of age babble in short syllabic segments (e.g., "ba," "da"). Dore (27) calls these "word babies," because their babbling more closely approximates short words. Other infants babble in long streams of sounds with sentence-like intonation, with few clear phoneme or syllable boundaries (i.e., "learning the tune before the words"). Dore calls these children "intonation babies" because they seem to approximate adult intonation contours before producing recognizable words.

In the evidence reviewed so far, there seems to be remarkable continuity in style—from babbling in prelinguistic infants to a dimension of rule consistency that holds up in both the phonological and grammatical systems of three-year-olds. The relationship between phonological and grammatical style may help to explain why it took so long for individual differences to become apparent in studies of language acquisition. Bellugi (*personal communication*) has described the early phases of the Roger Brown research project, when children were selected for participation in their landmark longitudinal study. Although many were considered, the three that were chosen had one thing in common—they spoke clearly enough to facilitate transcription and coding of audiotapes. No one thought that individual differences in intelligibility would prove to be associated in any way with qualitative differences in early grammar.

Explaining Individual Differences

To summarize, at least two distinct "strands" of abilities related to how children break into and master their language have been identified in language acquisition. These styles or strands cut across traditional linguistic boundaries, appearing consistently in lexical, phonological, and grammatical development. Other studies suggest that they may also have concomitants outside the domain of language, including demographic/environmental factors, parental style and child temperament, and cognitive style in nonlinguistic domains such as drawing and symbolic play (10,61,84). The list of individual differences is still growing, and the list of candidate explanations for these differences has grown accordingly [see (2) for a more complete review]. We consider some of these proposed explanations briefly here, but first two caveats are in order.

First, the "two-strand" approach is probably much too simple. The variations that we have described so far are drawn from a host of separate studies, investigating a small subset of variables, usually in a small sample of children. To date no study has examined all these variables over time in a single sample of children. The most comprehensive study so far is reported by Bates, Bretherton, and Snyder (2), who used an array of multivariate techniques to investigate aspects of lexical and grammatical development from 10 to 28 months of age. Although the findings are too extensive to review here in detail, many of the dimensions of variability reported by other investigators were replicated, and further evidence was given for the stability of "styles" across development and content domains. However, even though the two-strand notion did receive partial support, the total picture turned out to be much more complex. At least *three* factors were required to account for the variability found in the longitudinal data: *comprehension*, *analyzed production*, and *rote production*. In short, we cannot account for all of this variation with a simple dichotomy.

The second caveat involves the difference between *clusters of variables* and *clusters of children*. The individual difference variables that we have examined so far are all continuous and normally distributed. Although children at the extreme ends of any distribution do look strikingly different from one another, it is difficult to find any child who is *always* expressive and *never* referential or vice versa. Instead, these clusters of abilities represent tendencies with most children demonstrating a mixture of both styles. With these thoughts in mind, here is a final, brief summary of the facts to be explained.

The referential approach to language begins with an orientation toward individual words or word-like sounds in the prespeech stage, together with a particularly marked interest in interactions that are mediated through objects. This orientation toward objects shows up in the single-word stage in a high proportion of object names, which is in turn associated with more rapid expansion of the vocabulary and higher levels of language comprehension. Pronunciation at this and subsequent stages seems to be relatively more "articulate" and "crisp"—an impression based on the greater consistency with which such children apply their limited set of phonological principles or rules. By the stage of first-word combinations, this style of language is associated with nominal constructions and a telegraphic avoidance of pronouns and other forms of grammatical morphology. By the time grammatical morphology comes under productive control, these children may also be more advanced in grammar—even though they seemed superficially to be less advanced early in the process. The initial orientation toward nouns may persist into later stages of development, with greater expansion of noun phrases through adjectives and other descriptive terms. With regard to nonlinguistic variables, referential children are (in some studies, but not in others) more likely to be first born, female, and/or upper class. They tend to engage in longer bouts of play with objects and are more likely to engage in play that involves object substitution (e.g., using a shoe or a wooden block for a baby in a game of putting baby to bed). They will imitate adult speech, especially new object names, but imitation is not one of their more striking characteristics.

The expressive style begins in the prespeech phase with an orientation toward the "intonational packaging" of language rather than individual word units. These children are less oriented toward interactions involving objects, and more likely to engage directly in social interaction. They may be more gregarious overall, and some are more prone to imitate sounds and gestures without understanding the nature or purpose of those activities. In the single-word stage, these children have fairly heterogeneous vocabularies, sometimes consisting of sentence-length formulae. It is difficult to locate the border between single- and multiword speech, as more and more frozen formulae and partially productive *frame* + *slot* sentences appear in the child's repertoire. When sentences are produced, they are likely to contain pronouns and other grammatical morphemes from the very beginning, so it is also difficult to determine when a given morpheme is being used productively. This style tends to be associated with a slower pace of development overall (although it is quite possible to find expressive-style children who are advancing rapidly in *all* dimensions, but are especially precocious in mimicking sophisticated adult speech). Pronunciation can be highly variable from one utterance to another; hence despite their efforts to sound like other people, these children may be harder to understand at the early stages. Also, because they are more prone to imitate whole forms without analysis, comprehension may actually appear to lag behind production at certain points. The "noun avoidance" evident at the earlier stages may continue into later stages of language, so that an expressive child who is matched in mean length of utterance (MLU) to a referential child may "buy" his/her MLU through the expansion of verb phrases rather than nouns and their modifiers. Nonlinguistic associates that are reported in some studies (but not others) include a more social orientation at every age, a more impulsive "leap before you look" approach to life. These children are somewhat more likely to be later born, male, and/or lower class—but because these demographic differences do not replicate in all studies, they clearly do not bear any necessary causal relation to the syndrome. Finally, expressive-style children seem to be somewhat more oriented toward reproduction of reality in their play and less interested in breaking down a symbolic array into its component parts.

Assuming that these two strands do hang together [which they do to a limited and rather complicated degree (2)], how can we explain them? Almost every conceivable kind of explanation has been offered, including the following:

1. differences in maternal style, with the parents of referential children using strategies that foster communication about objects;
2. differences in brain organization (including purported differences in rate of maturation between the analytic left hemisphere and the holistic right hemisphere, and/or differences in the development of Broca's area and Wernicke's area within the left hemisphere);
3. temperamental factors (i.e., referential children are reflective, inhibited, shy; expressive children are impulsive, gregarious, sociable);
4. differences in cognitive style (i.e., referential style is analytic, field independent; expressive style is holistic, gestalt oriented, field dependent);
5. differences in language modality (i.e., referential style is associated with greater emphasis on comprehension; expressive style is associated with greater emphasis on production).

At this point, it is not possible to choose among these accounts. They are not mutually exclusive, and there is some support for all of them. To organize these findings, Bates et al. (2) suggest that individual differences have to be explained at two levels. At the deeper level, strands of variation are made possible by the existence of two or more partially dissociable learning mechanisms, which presumably have a neurological base. These include an analytic "pattern-seeking" mechanism that operates primarily by breaking input down into recognizable components, and a rote "pattern-reproducing" mechanism whose primary function is to bring in whole patterns for further covert analysis and/or for global and relatively unanalyzed use in social situations. To acquire any natural language, a child has to have both of these mechanisms. However, at the second level of explanation, a range of environmental and/or organic factors can affect the extent to which a given child relies on one or the other. These might include differences in the quantity and nature of parental input, differences in the child's own temperament and proclivities for interaction, differences in the amount of short-term memory available at any given point in development (a factor that could favor a strategy of memorizing relatively long, unanalyzed strings of speech), and differences in acoustic sensitivity (which could affect the child's sensitivity to the existence of unstressed inflections and function words, leading to their reproduction without understanding at a relatively early point in development).

CONCLUSION

Cross-language research gave us our first insights into the fact that normal children do not all acquire language the same way. Research in the last decade has also established the parameters for variation across individuals within a single language. There are some more recent efforts to put these two lines of variation together. By examining cross-linguistic "variations in variation," we may soon be able to specify the full *range* of patterns that are possible in the passage from prespeech to grammar (75).

If this approach is correct, then it has implications for other areas of neurolinguistic research. Recent cross-linguistic studies of grammatical breakdown in aphasia have demonstrated that the "same" syndrome can look quite different from one language to another (9,56). For example, Italian and German Broca's aphasics retain much more control over grammatical morphology, in both comprehension and production, than their English counterparts. This finding, as the cross-linguistic studies of children reported above, makes sense when we consider the massive differences among these languages in the relative quantity and importance of grammatical inflections and function words. To offer another example, Turkish aphasics (e.g., Turkish children) experience few problems in the retrieval of the clear and salient case markers of their language (A. Talay and D.I. Slobin, *in progress*). By comparison, aphasic speakers of languages with more arbitrary and irregular case inflections are more prone to make morphological omissions and/or substitutions.

Such cross-linguistic parallels between language acquisition and language breakdown are not at all mysterious. We need not invoke some abstract principle of ontogenesis and pathogenesis. The parallels fall out in sensible ways from known differences in the perceptual and/or articulatory properties of grammatical morphology in different languages.

More recently, some investigators have argued that we also have to consider individual differences in cognitive style and temperament in accounting for differences in aphasic syndromes within a given language (44). Some patients take a cautious, strategic approach to their problems; they produce highly simplified and reduced syntactic structures, but they also commit a relatively small number of errors. Other patients take greater risks and "aim" at fluent speech, resulting in a higher proportion of morphosyntactic errors within somewhat more complex sentence frames (3). This does not mean that all the selective impairments observed in adult aphasia can be attributed to a matter of personal style, but the style factor does have to be taken into account if we want to capture those facts about language breakdown that have a straightforward neurological explanation.

This move away from universals is by no means an inherently antibiological view. Genetically determined events do not always result in universals, and universal outcomes are not always attributable to a direct genetic cause (36). Biological factors are clearly responsible for some forms of variation across individuals (e.g., blue versus brown eyes), and environmental constraints can be responsible for attributes that all of us share (e.g., we all have to learn ways to adjust to gravity, as long as we are bound to planet Earth). We need a more realistic, epigenetic account of the biological substrate for language in our species, an account that can handle the extraordinary plasticity that is possible in language acquisition and language breakdown.

ACKNOWLEDGMENTS

The cross-linguistic research discussed here was supported by grants from NSF and NICHD to Brian MacWhinney and Elizabeth Bates. The research on individual differences was supported by grants from NSF and the Spencer Foundation to Elizabeth Bates and Inge Bretherton, and by the John D. and Catherine T. MacArthur Foundation Research Network on the Transition from Infancy to Childhood. Parts of the discussion have been presented in Bates and MacWhinney (1987), Bates, O'Connell, and Shore (1987), and Bates, Bretherton, and Snyder (1987).

REFERENCES

1. Bates, E. (1976): *Language and Context: The Acquisition of Pragmatics*. Academic Press, New York.
2. Bates, E., Bretherton, I., and Snyder, L. (1987): *From First Words to Grammar: Individual Differences and Dissociable Mechanisms*. Cambridge University Press, New York.
3. Bates, E., Friederici, A., and Wulfeck, B. *Grammatical Morphology in Aphasia: Evidence from Three Languages*. University of California, San Diego, La Jolla (*in press*).

4. Bates, E., and MacWhinney, B. (1979): A functionalist approach to the acquisition of grammar. In: *Developmental Pragmatics*, edited by E. Ochs and B. Schieffelin. Academic Press, New York.

5. Bates, E., and MacWhinney, B. (1982): Functionalist approaches to grammar. In: *Language Acquisition: The State of the Art*, edited by E. Wanner and L. Gleitman. Cambridge University Press, New York.

6. Bates, E., and MacWhinney, B. (1987): Competition, variation and language learning. In: *Mechanisms of Language Acquisition*, edited by B. MacWhinney. Lawrence Erlbaum, Hillsdale, New Jersey.

7. Bates, E., MacWhinney, B., Caselli, C., Devescovi, A., Natale, F., and Venza, V. (1984): A cross-linguistic study of the development of sentence interpretation strategies. *Child Dev.*, 55:341–354.

8. Bates, E., O'Connell, B., and Shore, C. (1986): Language and communication in infancy. In: *Handbook of Infant Competence*, 2nd edition, edited by J. Osofsky. Wiley and Sons, New York.

9. Bates, E., and Wulfeck, B. Cross-linguistic studies of aphasia. In: *Cross-Linguistic Studies of Sentence Processing*, edited by B. MacWhinney and E. Bates. Cambridge University Press, New York (*in press*).

10. Bauer, P., and Shore, C. (1986): Stylistic differences in language and symbolic play. Paper presented at the International Conference on Infant Studies, Los Angeles, CA, April.

11. Berko, J. (1958): The child's learning of English morphology. *Word*, 14:150–177.

12. Bever, T. (1970): The cognitive basis for linguistic structures. In: *Cognition and the Development of Language*, edited by J. Hayes. Wiley, New York.

13. Bickerton, D. (1984): The language bioprogram hypothesis. *The Behavioral and Brain Sciences*, 7(2):173–187.

14. Bloom, L. (1970): *Language Development: Form and Function in Emerging Grammars*. MIT Press, Cambridge, MA.

15. Bloom, L. (1973): *One Word at a Time: The Use of Single Word Utterances Before Syntax*. Mouton, The Hague.

16. Bloom, L., Lightbown, P., and Hood, L. (1975): Structure and variation in child language. *Monogr. Soc. Res. Child Dev.*, 40, Serial No. 160.

17. Bowerman, M. (1973): *Early Syntactic Development: A Cross-Linguistic Study with Special Reference to Finnish*. Cambridge University Press, New York.

18. Bowerman, M. (1982): Reorganizational processes in lexical and syntactic development. In: *Language Acquisition: The State of the Art*, edited by E. Wanner and L. Gleitman. Cambridge University Press, New York.

19. Braine, M.D.S. (1976): Children's first word combinations. *Monogr. Soc. Res. Child Dev.*, 41(1), Serial No. 164.

20. Branigan, G. (1977): If this kid is in the one word stage, so how come he's saying whole sentences? Paper presented at the Second Annual Boston University Conference on Language Development. Boston, September.

21. Bretherton, I., McNew, S., Snyder, L., and Bates, E. (1983): Individual differences at 20 months: Analytic and holistic strategies in language acquisition. *Journal of Child Language*, 10:293–320.

22. Brown, R. (1973): *A First Language: The Early Stages*. Harvard University Press, Cambridge, MA.

23. Chapman, R., and Kohn, L. (1978): Comprehension strategies in two- and three-year-olds. Animate agents or probable events? *J. Speech Hear. Res.*, 21:746–761.

24. Chomsky, N. (1981): *Lectures on Government and Binding: The Pisa Lectures*. Foris, Dordrecht.

25. Dale, P. (1976): *Language Development*, 2nd ed. Holt, Rinehart and Winston, New York.

26. Dore, J. (1974): A pragmatic description of early language development. *J. Psycholinguist. Res.*, 4:423–430.

27. Dore, J. (1975): Holophrase, speech acts and language universals. *Journal of Child Language*, 2:21–40.

28. Ferguson, C. (1984): From babbling to speech. Invited address to the International Conference on Infant Studies, New York, April.

29. Ferguson, C., and Farwell, C. (1975): Words and sounds in early language acquisition. *Language*, 51:419–439.

30. Gardner, H. (1983): *Frames of Mind*. Basic Books, New York.

31. Gleitman, L.R., and Wanner, E. (1982): Language acquisition: The state of the art. In: *Language Acquisition: The State of the Art*, edited by E. Wanner and L. Gleitman, pp. 3–51. Cambridge University Press, New York.

32. Goldfield, B. (1982): Intra-individual variation: Patterns of nominal and pronominal combinations. Paper presented at the Seventh Annual Boston University Conference on Language Development, October.
33. Goldfield, B. (1985): The contribution of child and caregiver to referential and expressive language. Unpublished doctoral dissertation, Harvard University.
34. Goldfield, B., and Snow, C. (1985): Individual differences in language acquisition. In: *Language Development*, edited by J. Gleason. Merrill Publishing Co., Columbus.
35. Gvozdev, A.N. (1961): *Voprosy izucheniya detskoy rechi*. Akademija Pedagogika Nauk RSFSR, Moscow.
36. Hardy-Brown, K. (1983): Universals and individual differences: Disentangling two approaches to the study of language acquisition. *Development Psychology*, 19:610–624.
37. Horgan, D. (1978): How to answer questions when you've got nothing to say. *Journal of Child Language*, 5:159–165.
38. Horgan, D. (1979): Nouns: Love 'em or leave 'em. Address to the New York Academy of Sciences, May.
39. Horgan, D. (1981): Rate of language acquisition and noun emphasis. *J. Psycholinguist. Res.*, 10(6):629–640.
40. Kail, M., and Combier, C. (1983): Rôle des indices pragmatiques, lexico-sémantiques et syntaxiques dans la compréhension de phrases simples dans une perspective génétiques et interlangue. Master's degree, University René Descartes.
41. Karmiloff-Smith, A. (1979): *A Functional Approach to Child Language: A Study of Determiners and Reference*. Cambridge University Press, New York.
42. Karmiloff-Smith, A. (1979): Language as a formal problem space for children. Unpublished paper presented at the MPG/NIAS Conference on Beyond Description in Child Language Research, Nijmegen, June.
43. Kempler, D. (1980): Variation in language acquisition. *UCLA Working Papers in Cognitive Linguistics*. UCLA Linguistics Department, Los Angeles.
44. Kolk, H., and Heeschen, C. (1985): Agrammatism versus paragrammatism: A shift of behavioral control. Paper presented at the Academy of Aphasia 23rd Annual meeting, Pittsburgh, PA.
45. Lenneberg, E. (1967): *The Biological Foundations of Language*. Wiley, New York.
46. Leonard, L., Newhoff, M., and Mesalam, L. (1980): Individual differences in early childhood phonology. *Applied Psycholinguistics*, 1:7–30.
47. MacWhinney, B. (1978): The acquisition of morphophonology. *Monogr. Soc. Res. Child Dev.*, 43(174), Serial No. 174.
48. MacWhinney, B. (1987): The competition model. In: *Mechanisms of Language Acquisition*, edited by B. MacWhinney. Lawrence Erlbaum, Hillsdale, NJ.
49. MacWhinney, B. (1987): *Mechanisms of Language Acquisition*. Lawrence Erlbaum, Hillsdale, NJ.
50. MacWhinney, B., and Bates, E. (1978): Sentential devices for conveying givenness and newness. *Journal of Verbal Learning and Verbal Behavior*, 17:539–558.
51. MacWhinney, B., and Bates, E. (eds.) *Cross-Linguistic Studies of Sentence Processing*. Cambridge University Press, New York (*in press*).
52. MacWhinney, B., Pleh, C., and Bates, E. (1985): The development of sentence interpretation in Hungarian. *Cognitive Psychology*, 17:178–209.
53. McClelland, J., and Rumelhart, D. (1986): *Parallel Distributed Processing: Explorations in the Microstructure of Cognition*, Vol. 1. MIT Press/Bradford Books, Cambridge, MA.
54. Rumelhart, D.E., and McClelland, J.L. (1987): Learning the past tenses of English verbs: Implicit rules or parallel distributed processing. In: *Mechanisms of Language Acquisition*, edited by B. MacWhinney. Lawrence Erlbaum, Hillsdale, NJ.
55. McNeill, D. (1970): *The Acquisition of Language: The Study of Developmental Linguistics*. Harper and Row, New York.
56. Menn, L., and Obler, L.K. (eds.) *Agrammatic Aphasia: Cross-Language Narrative Sourcebook*. John Benjamin, Amsterdam (*in press*).
57. Miller, W., and Ervin, S. (1964): The development of grammar in child language. In: *The Acquisition of Language*, edited by U. Bellugi and R. Brown. University of Chicago Press, Chicago.
58. Nelson, K. (1973): Structure and strategy in learning to talk. *Monogr. Soc. Res. Child Dev.*, 38, Serial No. 149.
59. Nelson, K. (1975): The nominal shift in semantic-syntactic development. *Cognitive Psychology*, 7:461–479.

60. Nelson, K. (1977): The conceptual basis for naming. In: *Language Learning and Thought*, edited by J. Macnamara. Academic Press, New York.
61. Nelson, K. (1981): Individual differences in language development: Implications for development and language. *Developmental Psychology*, 17:170–187.
62. Nelson, K. (1985): *Making Sense: The Acquisition of Shared Meaning*. Academic Press, New York.
63. Peters, A. (1977): Language learning strategies: Does the whole equal the sum of the parts? *Language*, 53:560–573.
64. Peters, A. (1983): *The Units of Language Acquisition*. Cambridge University Press, New York.
65. Pinker, S. (1982): A theory of the acquisition of lexical-interpretive grammars. In: *The Mental Representation of Grammatical Relations*, edited by J. Bresnan, pp. 655–726. MIT Press, Cambridge, MA.
66. Pinker, S. (1987): Constraint satisfaction networks as implementation of nativist theories of language acquisition. In: *Mechanisms of Language Acquisition*, edited by B. MacWhinney. Lawrence Erlbaum, Hillsdale, NJ.
67. Pleh, C. (1981): The role of word order in the sentence interpretation of Hungarian children. *Folia Linguistica*, 15:331–343.
68. Radulovic, L. (1975): Acquisition of language: Studies of Dubrovnik children. Unpublished doctoral dissertation, University of California, Berkeley.
69. Slobin, D.I. (1970): Universals of grammatical development in children. In: *Advances in Psycholinguistic Research*, edited by W.J.M. Levelt and G.B. Flores d'Arcais. North-Holland, Amsterdam.
70. Slobin, D.I. (1973): Cognitive prerequisites in the development of grammar. In: *Studies of Child Language Development*, edited by C.A. Ferguson and D.I. Slobin. Holt, Rinehart & Winston, New York.
71. Slobin, D.I. (1979): *Psycholinguistics*, 2nd ed. Scott, Foresman, Glenview, IL.
72. Slobin, D.I. (1985): Universal and particular in the acquisition of language. In: *Language Acquisition: The State of the Art*, edited by E. Wanner and L. Gleitman. Cambridge University Press, New York.
73. Slobin, D.I. (1986): *The Cross-Linguistic Study of Language Acquisition*, Vols. 1 and 2. Lawrence Erlbaum, Hillsdale, NJ.
74. Slobin, D., and Bever, T.G. (1982): Children use canonical sentence schemas: A cross-linguistic study of word order and inflections. *Cognition*, 12:1–37.
75. Snow, C.E., and Bates, E. (1984): Individual differences: A cross-language approach. Workshop presented at the Stanford Child Language Research Forum, Stanford, April.
76. Snyder, L., Bates, E., and Bretherton, I. (1981): Content and context in early lexical development. *Journal of Child Language*, 8:565–582.
77. Starr, S. (1975): The relationship of single words to two-word sentences. *Child Dev.*, 46:701–708.
78. Strohner, H., and Nelson, K.E. (1974): The young child's development of sentence comprehension: Influence of event probability, nonverbal context, syntactic form, and their strategies. *Child Dev.*, 45:567–576.
79. Varma, T.L. (1979): Stage I speech of a Hindi-speaking child. *Journal of Child Language*, 6:167–173.
80. Vihman, M. (1981): Phonology and the development of the lexicon: Evidence from children's errors. *Journal of Child Language*, 8:239–264.
81. Vihman, M., and Carpenter, K. (1984): Linguistic advance and cognitive style in language acquisition. Manuscript, Stanford University Department of Linguistics.
82. Weist, R. (1983): The word order myth. *Journal of Child Language*, 10(1):97–107.
83. Weist, R., and Koniecanza, E. (1985): Affix processing strategies and linguistic systems. *Journal of Child Language*, 12:27–36.
84. Wolf, D., and Gardner, H. (1979): Style and sequence in symbolic play. In: *Early Symbolization*, edited by M. Franklin and N. Smith. Lawrence Erlbaum, Hillsdale, NJ.

Language, Communication, and
the Brain, edited by F. Plum.
Raven Press, New York © 1988.

Sign Language and the Brain

*Ursula Bellugi, †Edward S. Klima, and *Howard Poizner

*Laboratory for Language and Cognitive Studies,
The Salk Institute for Biological Studies, La Jolla, California 92037, and
†University of California, San Diego, La Jolla, California 92093

LANGUAGE IN A VISUOSPATIAL MODALITY

Until recently, nearly everything learned about the human capacity for language has come from the study of spoken languages. It has been assumed that the organizational properties of language are inseparably connected with the sounds of speech and that the fact that language is normally spoken and heard determined the basic structural principles of grammar (9). There is good evidence indeed that structures involved in breathing, chewing, and the ingestion of food have evolved into a versatile and more efficient system for producing sound. Studies of brain organization for language indicate that the left cerebral hemisphere is specialized for linguistic material in the vocal-auditory mode and that, indeed, the major language-mediating areas of the brain are intimately connected with the vocal-auditory channel. It has been argued that hearing and the development of speech are necessary precursors to this cerebral specialization for language (12). Thus, the link between biology and linguistic behavior has been identified with the particular modality in which language has naturally developed.

Sign languages clearly present test cases as communication systems that have developed in alternate transmission systems—in visual-gestural channels. In research during the past decade, we have been specifying the ways in which the formal properties of languages are shaped by their modalities of expression, sifting properties peculiar to a particular language mode from more general properties common to all languages. American Sign Language (ASL) exhibits formal structuring at the same levels as spoken languages and similar kinds of organizational principles (constrained systems of features, rules based on underlying forms, recursive grammatical processes). Nevertheless, our studies show that at all structural levels, the form of an utterance in a signed language is deeply influenced by the modality in which the language is cast.

ASL, a primary gestural system passed down from one generation of deaf people to the next, has been forged into an autonomous language with its own internal mechanism for relating visual form with meaning. ASL has evolved linguistic mechanisms that are not derived from those of English (or any spoken language).

thus offering a new perspective on the determinants of language form (5,7). ASL shares underlying principles of organization with spoken languages, but the instantiation of those principles occurs in formal devices arising out of the very different possibilities of the visual-gestural mode (1). We consider briefly the structure of ASL at different linguistic levels: "phonology" without sound, vertically arrayed morphology, and spatially organized syntax.

"Phonology" without sound. Research on the structure of lexical signs has shown that like the words of spoken languages, signs are fractionated into sublexical elements. The elements that distinguish signs (handshapes, movements, and places of articulation) are in contrasting spatial arrangements and co-occur throughout the sign.

Vertically arrayed morphology. The grammatical mechanisms of ASL elaborately exploit the spatial medium and the possibility of simultaneous and multidimensional articulation. As with spoken languages, ASL has developed grammatical markers that serve as inflectional and derivational morphemes; these are regular changes in form across syntactic classes of lexical items associated with systematic changes in meaning. In ASL, families of sign forms are related via an underlying stem: the forms share a handshape, a location, and a local movement shape. Inflectional and derivational processes represent the interaction of the stem with other features of movement in space (e.g., dynamics of movement, manner of movement, directions of movement, spatial array, and the like), all *layered* with the sign stem.

Spatially organized syntax. Languages have different ways of marking grammatical relations among their lexical items. In English, it is primarily the order of the lexical items that marks the basic grammatical relations among verbs and their arguments; in other languages, it is the morphology of case marking or verb agreement that signals these relations. ASL, by contrast, specifies relations among signs primarily through the manipulation of sign forms in space. Thus in sign language, space itself bears linguistic meaning. The most striking and distinctive use of space in ASL is in its role in syntax and discourse, especially in nominal assignment to spatial loci, pronominal reference, verb agreement, subsequent coreference to spatial loci, and the referential spatial framework for discourse. Nominals introduced into ASL discourse may be associated with specific points in a plane of signing space. In signed discourse, pointing again to a specific locus clearly "refers back" to a previously mentioned nominal, even with many other signs intervening.

The ASL system of verb agreement, as its pronominal system, is also in essence spatialized. Verb signs for a large class of verbs move between the abstract loci in signing space, bearing obligatory markers for person (and number) via spatial indices, thereby specifying subject and object of the verb, as shown in the top section of Fig. 1. This spatialized system thus allows explicit reference through pronominals and agreement markers to multiple, distinct, third-person referents. The same signs in the same order, but with a reversal in direction of the verb's movement, indicate a reversal of grammatical relations. Furthermore, sentences with signs in different temporal orders can still have the same meaning, since grammatical relations are signified spatially. Coreferential nominals are indexed to

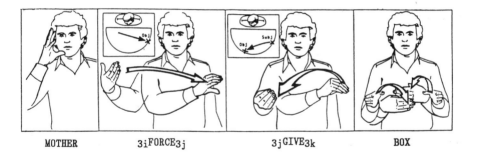

| MOTHER | 3iFORCE3j | 3jGIVE3k | BOX |

"Mother forced him to give her the box."

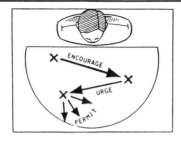

Spatial Reference for Multiclausal Sentence

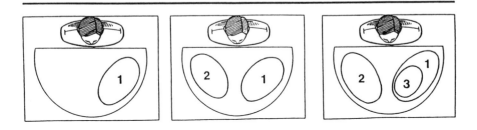

Embedded Spaces

FIG. 1. Syntactic spatial mechanisms in ASL.

the same locus, as is evident in complex embedded structures (Fig. 1, middle section). Different spaces may be used to contrast events, to indicate references to time preceding the utterance, or to express hypotheticals and counterfactuals, as schematically diagrammed at the bottom of Fig. 1. This use of spatial loci for referential indexing, verb agreement, and grammatical relations is clearly a unique property of visual-gestural systems.

The linguistic side of our studies focuses on the special nature of the grammatical processes in ASL, specifying organizational principles as well as interactions among structural layers. Our analysis has led us to view the organization of sign language as predominantly multilayered with respect to form—with differences in levels of grammatical function mirrored by differences in layers of form.

Acquiring linguistic structure in sign language is predicated upon the prior development of spatial representation. We have been investigating the acquisition of the spatial mechanisms of the language and the separable structural systems they embody in deaf children of deaf parents who are learning sign language as a primary linguistic system. The study of the acquisition of ASL in deaf children thus brings into focus some questions about the representation of language and the representation of space in the developing brain.

THE ACQUISITION OF A SPATIAL LANGUAGE

Studies of children's acquisition of spoken language have illuminated the nature of linguistic systems, the biological foundations for language, and the human capacity for language. Children learning a language analyze out grammatical rules, and their course of development can be revealing of the underlying linguistic structure. Because visual-gestural language is unlike spoken language in ways we have described, one might expect to find that sign language is acquired in radically different ways from spoken languages. The similarity in the acquisition of signed and spoken language, however, is remarkable. The differences that do appear reflect the spatial nature of sign language organization. We mention some developments in the acquisition of the spatial mechanisms of ASL by deaf children of deaf parents including pronominal reference, the morphological inflections associated with verb agreement, and the syntactic system of referential spatial indexing (1–3,10,14).

Pronominal Signs: The Transition from Gesture to Symbol

Deixis in spoken languages is considered a verbal surrogate for pointing; in ASL, however, it *is* pointing. The pronominal signs in ASL for "I" and "you" are the same pointing gestures used by hearing people as nonlinguistic gestures. Thus, we expected the acquisition in ASL of pronominal reference to self and addressee to be easy, early, and error free, even though in the development of spoken languages, pronoun reversal errors are found in young children. Instead, despite the identity of ASL pronouns with nonlinguistic gestures, the course of their acquisition is startlingly similar to that in spoken languages. Deaf infants between nine and eleven months point freely, to investigate, indicate, and draw attention to themselves and others, as do hearing children. During the second year, however, something dramatic happens. The deaf children stop pointing to themselves or their addressee; they seem to avoid such pointing. During this period, their language development evinces a steady growth in sign vocabulary, which they use stably in a variety of contexts and in multisign sentences. The next period displays the re-emergence of pointing to self and addressee, but now as part of a linguistic system. At this stage, surprising errors of reversal appear in the children's pronominal signing; children sign "you" when intending self, patently ignoring the transparency of the pointing gesture. These pronoun reversals are also found in hearing children of the same age. By about the age of 2½, such reversal errors are completely resolved, just as they are in hearing children of the same age. Since the form of the pronominal sign is the same as the pointing gesture, these errors and their resolution provide evidence for a *discontinuity* in the transition from prelinguistic gesture to a formal linguistic system (15).

Inflections: Spatial Verb Agreement

The ASL system of verb agreement functions is similar to that of spoken languages, but the form of verb agreement in ASL requires that the signer mark connections between spatial points. At about the age of two, deaf children begin using uninflected signs, even in imitating their mothers' inflected signs and even in cases in which the adult grammar requires marking for person and number. So even though they are perceiving complexly inflected forms, they begin, as hearing children do, by analyzing out the uninflected stems. By the age of three, deaf children have learned the basic aspects of verb morphology in ASL (e.g., inflections for person, for temporal aspect, and for number) (13). At this age, they make overgeneralizations to noninflecting verbs, analogous to overgeneralizations such as *eated* in the speech of hearing children. Such "errors" reveal the child's analysis of forms across the system (2,13). Despite the difference in the form of spatial marking, the development and the age of mastery of the spatial inflection for verb agreement are the same in ASL as for comparable processes in spoken languages.

Spatially Organized Syntax and Discourse

The integration of the pronominal reference and spatial verb agreement systems in the sentences and discourse of ASL is highly complex. When deaf children first attempt indexing verbs to arbitrary locus points in space, they may index all verbs for different referents to a single locus point. While telling the story of Rapunzel, for example, a child of 3½ (evidently using her early hypothesis about syntactic rules) indexed three verbs in space—see, ask, and push—but all at the same locus (see Fig. 2). She, in effect, "stacked up" the three referents (father, witch, Rapunzel) at a single locus point (11). In later developments, the loci for distinct referents are differentiated, although occasional discourse problems still interfere with the establishment and maintenance of the one-to-one mapping between referent and locus (10,11). Figure 2 gives a particularly complex example in which a deaf child was recounting an imaginary story in which she (Jane) had 10 children, and another woman arrived to claim them as her own. Jane (in the role of the other woman) signed, "(I) want my . . . your . . . Jane's children." One can understand why in this situation she finally resorted to the use of her own name sign to clarify the reference. By the age of five, however, children give the appropriate spatial

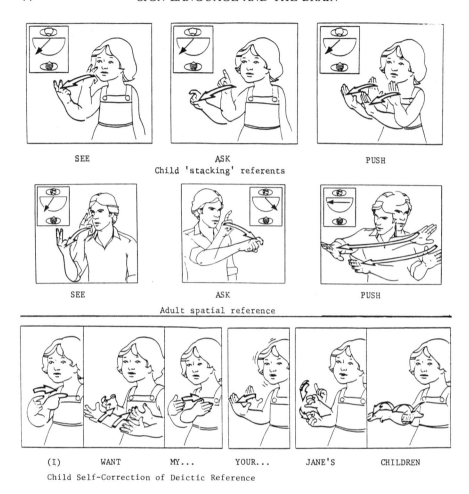

SEE   ASK   PUSH
Child 'stacking' referents

SEE   ASK   PUSH
Adult spatial reference

(I)   WANT   MY...   YOUR...   JANE'S   CHILDREN
Child Self-Correction of Deictic Reference

FIG. 2. Acquisition of spatialized syntax in ASL.

index to nearly every nominal and pronoun that requires one, and almost all verbs show the appropriate agreement.

Deaf children, as do their hearing counterparts, extract discrete components of the system presented to them. Furthermore, the evidence suggests that even when the modality and the language offer possibilities that seem intuitively obvious or transparent (e.g., pointing for pronominal reference), deaf children ignore this directness and analyze the language input as part of a formal linguistic system. The young deaf child is faced with the dual task in sign language of spatial perception, memory, and spatial transformations on the one hand, and processing grammatical structure on the other, all in the same visual event (18). Studies of the acquisition process have found that deaf and hearing children show a strikingly similar course of development if exposed to a natural language at the critical time. These data thus dramatically underscore the biological substrate of the human capacity for creating linguistic systems. These findings powerfully show how language, independent of its transmission mechanisms, emerges in children in a rapid, patterned, and—above all—linguistically driven manner.

BRAIN ORGANIZATION: CLUES FROM A VISUOSPATIAL LANGUAGE

ASL displays the complex linguistic structure found in spoken languages but conveys much of its structure by manipulating spatial relations, thus exhibiting properties for which each of the hemispheres of hearing people shows a different predominant functioning. The study of brain-damaged deaf signers offers a particularly revealing vantage point for understanding the organization of higher cognitive functions in the brain, and how modifiable that organization may be. We address questions such as the following: Is the development of hemispheric specialization dependent on auditory experience? How is language represented in the brain when it is expressed spatially? Does acquisition of a language with spatially expressed grammatical functions modify cerebral specialization for nonlanguage spatial functions?

We have investigated brain organization for sign language along several parallel tracks and developed a systematic program of studies that examines the effects of brain lesions on sign language processing and spatial cognition in deaf signers with either left or right hemisphere lesions. We have also studied functional asymmetries for sign language in the normal brain in a series of experimental investigations. Most recently we had the unique opportunity to extend these studies under conditions of chemical anesthesia to the brain. These lines of investigation provide converging evidence bearing on the basis for specialization of the two cerebral hemispheres in man.

Our broad aim is to investigate the relative contributions of the cerebral hemispheres with special reference to the interplay between linguistic functions and the spatial mechanisms that convey them. Subjects are administered a battery of tests specially designed to assess their capacities vis-à-vis each of the levels of ASL linguistic structure. We focus on the levels of the structure of ASL where there may be special processing requirements for a language whose form is perceived visually. We also investigate whether there is differential breakdown of two uses of space within sign language—a distinction between spatial syntax and spatial mapping.

Language Capacities of Left and Right Lesioned Signers

We have analyzed intensively six deaf signers with unilateral brain damage, three with damage to the left hemisphere, and three with damage to the right hemisphere.

Our general program includes an array of probes: (a) our adaptation, for ASL, of the Boston Diagnostic Aphasia Examination; (b) linguistic tests we designed to assess the processing of the structural levels of ASL (sublexical, semantic, morphological, and syntactic); (c) analysis of production of ASL at all linguistic levels; and (d) tests of nonlanguage spatial processing. The battery of language and non-language tasks was administered to deaf brain-lesioned subjects and to matched deaf controls (4,8,16,17).

The signers with left hemisphere damage showed frank sign language aphasias, as indicated by their results on our aphasia examination, on tests for processing the structural levels of ASL, and on a linguistic analysis of their signing. One left hemisphere damaged signer was agrammatic for ASL. Her signing was severely impaired, halting and effortful, reduced often to single sign utterances, and completely without the syntactic and morphological markings of ASL. Her lesion was typical of those that produce agrammatic aphasia for spoken language. The other two left hemisphere damaged signers had fluent sign aphasias. They differed, however, in the nature of their impairments. One made selection errors in the formational elements of signs, producing the equivalent of phonemic paraphasias in sign language. Her signing, however, was perfectly grammatical although vague, as she often omitted specifying to whom or what she was referring. The third left hemisphere damaged signer had many grammatical errors. He made selection errors and additions within ASL morphology, and erred in the spatialized syntax and discourse processes of ASL. Thus differential damage within the left hemisphere produced sign language impairments that were not uniform, but were ones that cleaved along lines of linguistically relevant components. Figure 3 presents characteristic errors of the three left lesioned patients.

The signers with right hemisphere damage presented special issues in testing for language impairments; sign language makes linguistic use of space and these signers showed nonlanguage spatial deficits. Left hemispatial neglect, for example, may introduce particular difficulties in signing, since the addressee must either view signs in his or her neglected visual field or shift his or her gaze away from the signer. Quite remarkably, the first three signers with right hemisphere damage we examined in depth were not aphasic for sign language. They exhibited fluent, grammatical, virtually error-free signing, with good range of grammatical forms, no agrammatism, and no signing deficits. Furthermore, only the right hemisphere damaged patients were unimpaired in our tests of ASL structures at different linguistic levels. Figure 4 shows results of one of the tests of ASL linguistic structure. Subjects were asked to indicate the two pictures that represented the sign equivalent of "rhyme" in ASL. In the figure, the correct answer would be "apple" and "key," since their associated signs are the same in two of the three major parameters (e.g., they have the same handshape and movement, but differ only in spatial location). Across the range of language tests given, the right hemisphere damaged signers were not impaired, whereas the left hemisphere damaged signers were generally impaired (8,17).

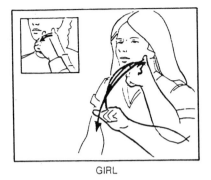

GIRL

a) Articulatory difficulty typical of Gail D.

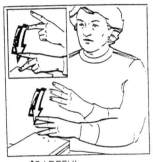 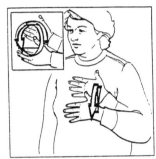

*CAREFUL
(Handshape substitution:
/W/ for /K/)

*ENJOY
(Movement substitution:
/N/ for /⊙/)

b) Sublexical substitutions of Karen L.

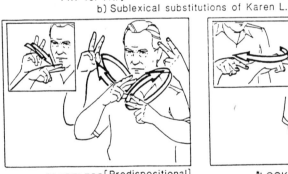 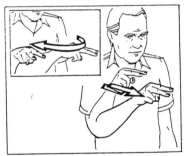

*CARELESS [Predispositional]
(addition of Inflected Form)

*LOOK [Habitual]
(Substitution of Habitual
Inflection for Multiple)

c) Paragrammatisms of Paul D.

FIG. 3. Typical errors of left hemisphere damaged signers. (Correct signs are shown in insets.) Note different levels of linguistic deficit across left hemisphere lesioned signers.

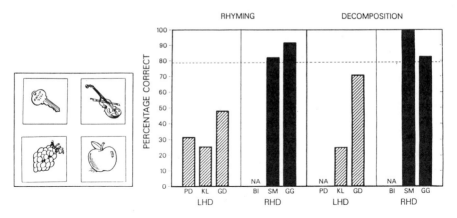

FIG. 4. Results of tests for processing sublexical structure in ASL. Rhyming and decomposition tests with left and right hemisphere lesioned deaf signers. Note that left hemisphere lesioned signers are impaired on these tests, in contrast to right hemisphere lesioned signers.

This preserved signing was in the face of marked deficits the right hemisphere damaged signers showed in processing nonlanguage spatial relations, which we describe below. Across a range of tests, these signers showed the classic visuospatial impairments found in hearing patients with right hemisphere damage. The right hemisphere damaged patients, then, had no impairment in the grammatical aspects of their signing, including in their spatially organized syntax; they even used the left side of signing space to represent syntactic relations, despite their neglect of left hemispace in nonlanguage tasks.

Spatial Cognition in Right and Left Hemisphere Lesioned Signers

We administered selected tests that are sensitive distinguishers of visuospatial performance in left versus right hemisphere damaged hearing patients; these tests included drawing, block design, selective attention, line orientation, facial recognition, and visual closure. As an example, results of a block design test given to deaf signers in which the subjects must assemble either four or nine three-dimensional blocks to match a two-dimensional model of the top surface are shown in Fig. 5. There were clear-cut differences in performance between the left hemisphere damaged patients (upper row) and the right hemisphere damaged patients (lower row). The left hemisphere damaged patients produced correct constructions on the simple block designs and made only internal featural errors on the more complex designs; in contrast, the right hemisphere damaged patients produced erratic and incorrect constructions and tended to break the overall configurations of the designs. The general difficulty of the right hemisphere damaged patients with this task reflects the classic visuospatial impairments found in hearing patients with right hemisphere

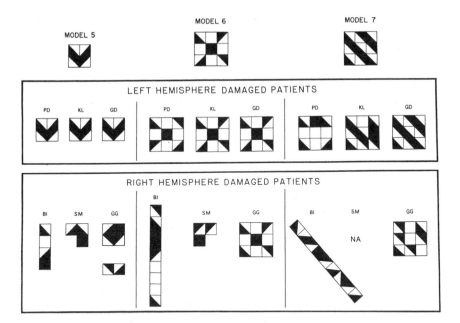

FIG. 5. Performance on block design task, a nonlanguage visuospatial task by left and right hemisphere lesioned deaf signers. Note the broken configurations and severe spatial disorganization of right hemisphere lesioned signers.

damage. The two groups of deaf signing patients differed across the range of visuospatial tasks administered, with right hemisphere damaged patients reflecting gross spatial disorganization. These nonlanguage data show that the right hemisphere in deaf signers can develop cerebral specialization for nonlanguage visuospatial functions (16). The drawings of the right hemisphere damaged patients also tended to show severe spatial disorganization, whereas those of the left hemisphere damaged patients did not. The right hemisphere damaged patients were not able to indicate perspective; several neglected the left side of space, and one right hemisphere damaged patient even added unprompted verbal labels on the drawings. The drawings of the left hemisphere damaged patients in general showed superiority, with overall spatial configurations preserved.

One right hemisphere damaged signer was an artist before her stroke, and showed severe spatial disorganization afterward, including neglect of left hemispace, inability to indicate perspective, and so forth, but her sign language (including spatially expressed syntax) was completely unimpaired. In light of her severe visuospatial deficit for nonlanguage tasks, correct use of the spatial mechanisms for signed syntax in these right lesioned patients may point to the abstract nature of these mechanisms in ASL. This shows how little effect right hemisphere damage can have on language function, even when expressed as a visuospatial language. In contrast, the left hemisphere damaged signer, who was most severely aphasic for sign language (completely agrammatic, without any morphology or syntax), showed normal nonlanguage visuospatial skills.

In summary, the right hemisphere lesioned patients in general showed severe left-sided neglect and were seriously impaired in nonlanguage visuospatial capacities, but their signing was still fluent and remarkably unimpaired. They showed virtually no impairment in any of the grammatical aspects of their signing; their impairments, however, were vividly apparent in spatial mapping, which we consider next. We investigated the breakdown of two uses of space within sign language, one for syntax, the other for mapping.

The Contrast Between Spatial Syntax and Spatial Mapping

Spatial contrasts and spatial manipulations act structurally at all linguistic levels in ASL. For *syntactic* functions, spatial loci and relations among those loci are actively manipulated as arbitrary points representing grammatical relations. As opposed to its syntactic use, space in ASL also functions in a *topographic* way: the space within which signs are articulated can be used to describe the layout of objects in space. In such mapping, spatial relations among signs correspond in a topographic manner to actual spatial relations among objects described.

The impairments in the use of space by the patients differ according to whether differentiated points in space are used syntactically or are used to give relative positions in space. Patients were asked to describe the spatial layout of their living quarters from memory; in this task, signing space is used to describe space and actual spatial relations are thus significant. The descriptions given by the right lesioned signers were grossly distorted spatially. These patients were able to enumerate all the items in the room, but displaced their locations and even grossly distorted the spatial relations among them. In contrast, the left hemisphere damaged patients' room descriptions sometimes were linguistically impaired (matching their linguistic breakdown in other domains) but without spatial distortions.

When space is used in the language to represent syntactic relations, however, the pattern was reversed. One left hemisphere damaged patient showed impairment of spatial syntax; he had a disproportionately high ratio of nouns to pronouns and tended to omit verb agreement (both pronouns and verb agreement involve spatial indexing in ASL). Furthermore, when he did use spatial syntactic mechanisms, he sometimes failed to maintain the correct agreement. For all three right lesioned signers, spatially organized syntax is correct and appropriate; indeed, all three even used the left side of signing space in syntax.

We found a disparity between spatial mapping and spatial syntax in right lesioned signers generally. This dissociation was most dramatically displayed in one right lesioned signer (see Fig. 6). In the description she gave of her room, the furniture was piled in helter-skelter fashion on the right, and the entire left side of the space was left bare, showing severe spatial disorganization. However, in her use of the spatial framework for syntax in ASL, she established spatial loci freely throughout

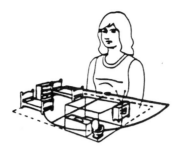

Correct Spatial Layout

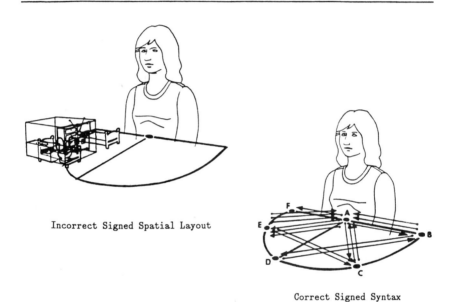

Incorrect Signed Spatial Layout

Correct Signed Syntax

FIG. 6. Contrast between spatial mapping and spatial syntax in a right hemisphere lesioned deaf signer.

the signing space (including on the left) and furthermore, she even maintained consistent coreference to spatial loci. Thus even within signing, the use of space to represent *syntactic* relations and the use of space to represent *spatial* relations may be differentially affected, with the former disrupted by left hemisphere damage and the latter by right hemisphere damage.

The Separation Between Apraxia and Sign Aphasia

In a long-standing controversy over the nature of aphasic disorders, some investigators have proposed a common underlying basis for disorders of gesture and disorders of language. Some attribute the specialization of the left hemisphere specifically to the control of changes in the position of both oral and manual articulators. In this view, disorders of language occur as a result of more primary disorders of movement control. A second position is that both apraxia and aphasia result from an underlying deficit in the capacity to express and comprehend symbols.

Since gesture and linguistic symbol are transmitted in the same modality in sign language, the breakdown of the two can be directly compared. In addition to an array of language tests, we administered a series of apraxia tests to our deaf patients, including tests of production and imitation of representational and nonrepresentational movements. The right hemisphere damaged patients so far examined were not apraxic; however, for the left hemisphere damaged patients, all of whom were aphasic for sign language, some strong dissociations emerged between their capacities for sign language and their nonlanguage gesture and motor capacities. The language deficits of these patients were on the whole related to specific linguistic components of sign language rather than to an underlying motor disorder, or to an underlying disorder in the capacity to express and comprehend symbols of any kind. This separation between linguistic and nonlinguistic functioning is all the more striking since sign language and gesture are transmitted in the same modality (17).

Converging Evidence from a Hearing Signer

We had the opportunity to analyze the sign language of a hearing signer proficient in ASL, during a left intracarotid injection of sodium amytal (Wada Test), and before and after a right temporal lobectomy. This study was carried out in collaboration with Drs. Antonio and Hanna Damasio. The subject was strongly right handed. Neuropsychological and anatomical asymmetries suggested left cerebral dominance for auditory-based language. Single photon emission tomography revealed lateralized activity of left Broca's and Wernicke's areas for spoken language. The Wada Test, during which all left language areas were rendered inoperative, caused a marked aphasia in both English and ASL. In the recovery period, correct English responses preceded those in ASL by 1½ minutes, a substantial amount of time in this procedure.

The patient's signing was markedly impaired, with many incorrect sign responses and sign neologisms. Since she was hearing and could sign and speak at the same time, we could compare her responses in two languages simultaneously—a unique possibility for languages in different modalities. This revealed a frequent mismatch between word and sign, the sign being frequently incorrect both in meaning and in form (see Fig. 7). The patient subsequently underwent brain surgery, and the anterior portion of her right temporal lobe was removed to relieve her epilepsy, documented by magnetic resonance imaging. Analysis of her signing after the surgery revealed no sign language deficit (e.g., there were no errors in her use of the spatially organized syntax of ASL before or after the surgery), indicating that

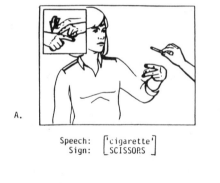

Speech: ⌜'cigarette'⌝
Sign: ⌊SCISSORS ⌋

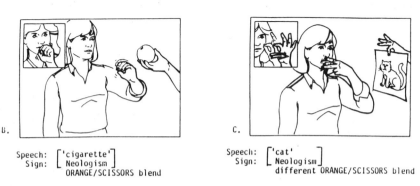

Speech: ⌜'cigarette'⌝
Sign: ⌊Neologism ⌋
ORANGE/SCISSORS blend

Speech: ⌜'cat' ⌝
Sign: ⌊Neologism⌋
different ORANGE/SCISSORS blend

FIG. 7. Left hemisphere impairment for sign and speech in a hearing signer.

effective production and comprehension of sign language can proceed normally without utilizing structures of the right temporal lobe. The abilities to sign and to understand signing were unchanged. These data add further support to the notion that anatomical structures of the left cerebral hemisphere subserve language in a visuospatial as well as an auditory mode (6).

These findings from a different domain provide remarkable converging evidence with our studies of sign aphasia produced by left hemisphere lesions in deaf signers, and the absence of sign aphasia in right lesioned signers. From these converging perspectives, it is becoming clear that the primary specialization of the left hemisphere rests not on the form of the signal but rather on the linguistic function it subserves.

SUMMARY

Analysis of the patterns of breakdown of a visuospatial language in deaf signers thus allows new perspectives on the nature and determinants of cerebral specialization for language. First, these data show that hearing and speech are not necessary for the development of hemispheric specialization—sound is *not* crucial. Second, the data show that in these deaf signers, it is the left hemisphere that is dominant for sign language. The patients with damage to the left hemisphere showed marked sign language deficits but relatively intact capacity for processing nonlanguage visuospatial relations. The patients with damage to the right hemisphere showed much the reverse pattern. Thus, not only is there left hemisphere specialization for language functioning, there is a complementary right hemisphere specialization for visuospatial functioning. The fact that much of the grammatical information is conveyed via spatial manipulation appears not to alter this complementary specialization. Furthermore, the finding that components of sign language (e.g., lexicon and grammar) can be selectively impaired suggests that the functional organization of the brain for sign language may turn out to be modular. Finally, patients with left and right hemisphere damage showed dissociations between two uses of space in the language—one to represent spatial relations and the other to represent syntactic relations. Right hemisphere damage disrupts the former but spares the latter; left hemisphere damage disrupts the use of space for syntactic relations but spares its use for spatial relations.

Taken together with studies of the processing of sign language "on line" by neurologically intact deaf signers, these data suggest that the left cerebral hemisphere in humans may have an innate predisposition for language, independent of language modality. Studies of the effects of brain damage on signing make it clear that accounts of hemispheric specialization are oversimplified if stated only in terms of a dichotomy between language and visuospatial functioning. Such studies may also permit us to come closer to the real principles underlying the specializations of the two cerebral hemispheres, since in sign language there is interplay between visuospatial and linguistic relations within the same system.

NOTATION

Notational conventions used in this chapter:

SIGN:
Words in capital letters represent English glosses for ASL signs. The gloss represents the meaning of the unmarked, unmodulated, basic form of a sign out of context.

SIGN['exhaustive']:
Morphological processes may be indicated by the specification of grammatical category of change or by the meaning of the inflected form.

ASL Spatialized Syntax:
As part of the spatialized syntax of ASL, a horizontal plane in signing space is used for abstract spatial loci. Nouns, indexible verbs, pronouns, classifiers, and size and shape specifiers can be associated with abstract spatial loci, and these are indicated by subscripts.

$_a$SIGN$_b$:

Subscripts from the beginning of the alphabet are used to indicate spatial loci. Nouns, pronouns, and verbs of location are marked with a subscript to indicate the locus at which they are signed (INDEX$_a$, BOY$_a$, AT-X$_a$) in planes of signing space. Inflected verbs are marked with an initial subscript to denote origin location, and/or a final subscript to indicate the endpoint location ($_a$GIVE$_b$).

$_i$SIGN$_j$:

Subscripts from the middle of the alphabet are used to indicate abstract indices, reference as well as coreference.

ACKNOWLEDGMENTS

This research was supported in part by the National Institutes of Health, grants #NS 15175, #NS 19096, and #HD 13249, as well as by National Science Foundation grant #BNS86-09085 to the Salk Institute for Biological Studies; and the John D. and Catherine MacArthur Foundation Research Network on "The Transition from Infancy to Early Childhood." We thank Robbin Battison, David Corina, Karen van Hoek, Diane Lillo-Martin, Maureen O'Grady, Lucinda O'Grady, Carol Padden, Dennis Schemenauer, and James Tucker for their help in these studies. We also thank the subjects and their families who participated. Illustration drawings by Frank A. Paul, copyright, Ursula Bellugi, The Salk Institute.

REFERENCES

1. Bellugi, U. The acquisition of a spatial language. In: *The Development of Language and Language Researchers, Essays in Honor of Roger Brown*, edited by F. Kessell. Lawrence Erlbaum, Hillsdale, NJ (*in press*).
2. Bellugi, U., and Klima, E.S. (1982): The acquisition of three morphological systems in American Sign Language. Keynote Address, Child Language Research Forum. *Papers and Reports on Child Language Development*. Stanford University, 21:K1–K35.
3. Bellugi, U., and Klima, E.S. (1982): From gesture to sign: Deixis in a visual-gestural language. In: *Speech, Place and Action: Studies of Language in Context*, edited by R.J. Jarvella and W. Klein, pp. 297–313. John Wiley, Sussex.
4. Bellugi, U., Poizner, H., and Klima, E.S. (1983): Brain organization for language: Clues from sign aphasia. *Hum. Neurobiol.*, 2:155–170.
5. Bellugi, U., and Studdert-Kennedy, M. (eds.) (1980): *Signed and Spoken Language: Biological Constraints on Linguistic Form*. Dahlem Konferenzen. Verlag Chemie, Weinheim/Deerfield Beach, FL.
6. Damasio, A., Bellugi, U., Damasio, H., Poizner, H., and Van Gilder, J. (1986): Sign language aphasia during left hemisphere amytal injection. *Nature*, 322:363–365.
7. Klima, E.S., and Bellugi, U. (1979): *The Signs of Language*. Harvard University Press, Cambridge, MA.
8. Klima, E.S., Bellugi, U., and Poizner, H. The neurolinguistic substrate for sign language. In: *Language, Speech and Mind; Festschrift for Victoria A. Fromkin*, edited by L.M. Hyman and C.N. Li. Croom Helm (*in press*).
9. Liberman, A.M. (1982): On finding that speech is special. *Am. Psychol.*, 37(2):148–167.
10. Lillo-Martin, D. (1986): Parameter setting: Evidence from use, acquisition, and breakdown in American Sign Language. Ph.D. dissertation, University of California, San Diego.

11. Loew, R.C. (1983): Roles and reference in American Sign Language: A developmental perspective. Ph.D. dissertation, University of Minnesota.

12. McKeever, W.F., Hoemann, H.W., Florian, V.A., and VanDeventer, A.D. (1976): Evidence of minimal cerebral asymmetries for the processing of English words and American Sign Language stimuli in the congenitally deaf. *Neuropsychologia*, 14:413–423.

13. Meier, R. (1981): Icons and morphemes: Models of the acquisition of verb agreement in ASL. *Papers and Reports on Child Language Development*, 20:92–99.

14. Newport, E., and Meier, R. Acquisition of American Sign Language. In: *The Crosslinguistic Study of Language Acquisition*, edited by D.I. Slobin. Lawrence Erlbaum, Hillsdale, NJ (*in press*).

15. Petitto, L.A. (1983): From gesture to symbol: The relation between form and meaning in the acquisition of ASL. *Papers and Reports on Child Language Development*, 22:100–107.

16. Poizner, H., Kaplan, E., Bellugi, U., and Padden, C. (1984): Visuospatial processing in deaf brain-damaged signers. *Brain and Cognition*, 3:281–306.

17. Poizner, H., Klima, E.S., and Bellugi, U. (1987): *What the Hands Reveal About the Brain*. MIT Press/Bradford Books, Cambridge, MA.

18. Stiles-Davis, J., Kritchevsky, M., and Bellugi, U. (eds.) *Spatial Cognition: Brain Bases and Development*. Lawrence Erlbaum, Hillsdale, NJ (*in press*).

Language, Communication, and
the Brain, edited by F. Plum.
Raven Press, New York © 1988.

Syndromes in Developmental Dysphasia and Adult Aphasia

Isabelle Rapin and Doris A. Allen

*Saul R. Korey Department of Neurology,
Department of Pediatrics, Division of Child Psychiatry, and
the Rose F. Kennedy Center for Research in Mental Retardation and Human
Development, Albert Einstein College of Medicine, Bronx, New York 10461*

The term developmental dysphasia refers to a variety of communication disorders of early childhood that are characterized by failure to acquire language normally and at the appropriate age, despite adequate hearing and normal nonverbal intelligence and the absence of major sensorimotor deficit or congenital malformation of the vocal tract (38,48,59,83). The dysphasias are assumed to reflect a variety of dysfunctions in brain systems required for the comprehension, elaboration, and production of language (65,72). The nature of these dysfunctions is unknown; they may arise genetically or as the result of very early insults to the immature brain.

For many years, developmental dysphasia was regularly ascribed to a lag in brain maturation. This maturational theory, coupled with the belief that an almost unlimited plasticity existed in the organization of young children's brains, led to a singular lack of speculation about the neurologic pathophysiology of developmental dysphasia. Since few dysphasic children have overt sensorimotor deficits and many dysphasic children learn to speak reasonably adequately by school age (8,82), there was little to suggest that permanent lesions might underlie dysphasia.

A number of recent developments have rekindled interest in the neurologic underpinnings of childhood dysphasia. One is the discovery of dysgenetic areas in the dominant perisylvian area in some dyslexic persons (32,34); another is the realization that the majority of dyslexic children have language deficits suggesting localized brain dysfunction on formal neuropsychologic testing (51) and that an unknown but significant proportion of dyslexics are the dysphasics of yesteryear (4,64,66,80).

If dysphasia is the result of permanent though subtle brain pathology rather than of a transient maturational lag, and if different dysphasic syndromes result from dysfunction at different stages of linguistic operations, different brain systems may be affected. New technologies for brain imaging (81) and for mapping electrical (26,61,89) and metabolic activity (47,52) of the brain while subjects are engaged in defined mental operations offer the prospect of addressing this issue. Judiciously choosing the tasks that subjects are to perform and having hypotheses as to which brain systems might be dysfunctional in particular dysphasia syndromes will greatly enhance the probability of success in identifying these systems. We propose looking to the adult aphasias for some guidelines.

Comparison of the dysphasias with the acquired aphasias of adults has usually been considered unwarranted because aphasia results from the breakdown of an overlearned cognitive skill whereas dysphasia reflects its faulty development. One must be cautious when making such comparisons; yet, in the near-absence of primary data on cerebral localization in dysphasia, such comparisons may provide useful clues to guide future biologic studies (20,53).

BRAIN LOCALIZATION IN APHASIA AND DYSPHASIA

The acquired aphasias have provided heuristic data concerning lateralization and localization of higher cortical functions. The concept of hemispheric dominance goes back to Broca's clinical studies of aphasic patients. The division of the aphasias into anterior (Broca or expressive) and posterior (Wernicke or receptive) types has prevailed for a century, even though aphasiologists have repeatedly stressed that most of the aphasias affect both expression and comprehension, albeit to different degrees. Geschwind (33) proposed dividing the aphasias into fluent and dysfluent types, pointing out that perisylvian pathology tends to be precentral in dysfluent patients and postcentral in fluent ones. Benson (16) stated that division along the fluency dimension is useful even though this division may apply to less than a third of aphasic patients. He indicated that repetition is another important dimension to consider: repetition is as impaired or more impaired than spontaneous speech in patients with perisylvian lesions, whereas repetition is superior to spontaneous speech in patients with pathology in the zones adjacent to the perisylvian language areas of the cortex.

The modern era in research on the localization of brain lesions in live aphasic patients was ushered in by radionucleide brain scanning, followed by computerized tomography (CT) (16,40,41), cerebral blood flow (46), and most recently by magnetic resonance imaging (MRI) and positron emission tomography (PET) (35). Classic concepts concerning cortical localization of pathology in the various aphasia syndromes received strong general confirmation from superposition of the images of aphasics' lesions, but it also became clear that there was considerable variation among individuals. Some of this variation is related to the freshness and type of pathological damage and some to such premorbid factors as hemispheric dominance (as indicated by handedness), asymmetries in the size of the anterior and posterior halves of the two hemispheres (14,34,76), and individual variations in brain organization (92) that no doubt have experiential as well as biologic roots (62,63). Recent work has started to focus on the contribution to language of subcortical structures, notably the thalamus (22,57), basal ganglia and subcortical fiber tracts (18,60). Investigators have progressed beyond oversimplified attempts to localize to particular gyri such complex behaviors as language, recognizing that language necessarily involves the integrated activity of widely distributed cortical and subcortical neuronal networks.

It is likely that cerebral dysfunction is bilateral in dysphasia, although direct evidence (44,47) is sparse. The most compelling indirect evidence is that either hemisphere is capable of sustaining language development, despite interhemispheric anatomic asymmetry (21,77,90) and the fact that the left hemisphere is genetically programmed to sustain language in most persons. Unilateral focal lesions of the dominant hemisphere acquired prenatally or in early life do not preclude the development of language (3). Furthermore, children who have undergone either left or right hemispherectomy learn to speak (12,25). Unilateral brain lesions acquired in childhood may produce a transient aphasia with discernible sequelae (5,6,36,96) but not a chronic language syndrome resembling the dysphasias. Whether language is organized in the left or the right hemisphere in patients with early unilateral brain lesions depends on the location of their pathology. Based on intracarotid injection of amobarbital in patients being considered for surgery to control childhood-onset intractable epilepsy, Milner (55) reported that if left-sided lesions are perisylvian, the right hemisphere is likely to be dominant for language, whereas if they are extrasylvian, dominance is on the left. The majority of these right-hemisphere-dominant epileptics can thus be assumed to be pathologically right brained, as opposed to the small number of normal, usually left-handed, individuals who are constitutionally right brained. Pathological lateralization of language testifies to functional plasticity in the organization of the young child's brain (28). [To what degree interhemispheric transfer of language representation and to what degree within-hemisphere reorganization are responsible for recovery from adult aphasia is rarely known (42,43).]

ETIOLOGY OF DYSPHASIA

It is extremely doubtful that any of the developmental disorders of early childhood has a single etiology or is due to a single pathogenetic mechanism (65). (These disorders include the dysphasias, dyslexias, and dyscalculias, the disorders of attention, developmental disorders of motor execution, some forms of mental deficiency, and the spectrum of autistic disorders.) Many of them, possibly most, are genetic, whereas others may result from a perinatal or intrauterine insult. Few are caused by defined postnatal encephalopathies. The marked predilection of all of these disorders for boys (4:1 or more for some of them) is consonant with the importance of constitutional factors and the relative rarity of acquired insults as etiologic factors.

One possibility that would account for the increased prevalence of dysphasia, dyslexia, and autism in boys is that they are inherited as X-linked traits. Although this may be true of some variants, e.g., autism associated with fragile-X syndrome (17,29), it does not seem to be the case for the majority. Another recently proposed possibility is that sex steroids affect intrauterine brain maturation (34,87). Intrauterine maturation of the cerebral hemispheres may be asymmetric and occur earlier on the right than the left. Testosterone may have a retardant effect on maturation. Geschwind and Galaburda (34) adduced these observations to explain earlier maturation of the brain in girls and greater vulnerability of left hemispheric function in boys. Exposure to testosterone may also explain the well-recognized superiority of boys for visual-spatial tasks, traditionally attributed to specialization of the right hemisphere, and of girls for verbal tasks controlled by the left hemisphere. Differences between the sexes in the cortical representation of language has received some support from studies in patients undergoing surgery for epilepsy; electrical stimulation was found to interfere with naming over a larger portion of the perisylvian cortex in males than females (50). This finding was felt to be consonant with the greater verbal proficiency of females than males since increased proficiency and discreteness of cortical representation seem to be correlated.

TAXONOMY OF APHASIA

There is no generally agreed upon taxonomy of the aphasias. Without going back to Marie's (40) and Head's (41) extreme position that there is but one aphasia, some aphasiologists recognize few aphasia syndromes. For example, Kertesz (40) stated that there are only four universally accepted syndromes: Broca's aphasia, Wernicke's aphasia, anomic aphasia, and global aphasia. However, when multivariate cluster analysis of the quantitative scores on his Western Aphasia Battery yielded a 10-syndrome solution, Kertesz stated that this statistical taxonomy was in the main congruent (with some exceptions) with clinically defined syndromes. Our comparisons of syndromes in aphasia and dysphasia are based on the more numerous aphasia syndromes so clearly delineated by Benson (16) (Table 1) since they are acceptable, at least in the main, to contemporary aphasiologists.

Benson's classification scheme rests on both anatomic and functional considerations. Differential impairment of repetition and spontaneous speech, as well as the

TABLE 1. *Aphasia syndromes according to Benson*[a]

A. Perisylvian
   Broca's aphasia
   Wernicke's aphasia
   Conduction aphasia

B. Borderzone
   Transcortical motor aphasia
   Transcortical sensory aphasia
   Mixed transcortical aphasia (isolation of the speech area)

C. Subcortical
   Aphasia with striatal pathology
   Aphasia with thalamic pathology
   Aphasia with striatal-capsular-thalamic pathology

D. Nonlocalizing
   Anomic aphasia
   Global aphasia

E. Modality-specific related
   Aphemia
   Pure word deafness

[a]Ref. 16.

location of lesions, serves to define the first two groups of patients. The first syndrome within groups A, B, and C (Broca's, transcortical motor, and striatal aphasias) is not only nonfluent but agrammatic; it is likely to denote pathology located in front of the central sulcus. The second syndrome in these three groups (Wernicke's, transcortical sensory, and thalamic aphasias) is fluent and impairs comprehension more severely than the first; it is usually attributable to pathology that lies behind the central sulcus. Conduction aphasia typically involves the connections between the frontal and temporal language areas, mixed transcortical aphasia diffuse damage to the dominant hemisphere sparing the perisylvian language areas, and striatal-capsular-thalamic aphasia a large subcortical lesion that undermines those areas. In group D, global aphasia usually denotes widespread destruction of perisylvian cortex and underlying subcortical structures due to a middle cerebral artery infarct.

Anomia is a feature of most aphasia syndromes and is likely to be a residual symptom after recovery from any of them (40). Luria (49) and Benson (16) pointed out that there are a number of different anomias. Patients with Broca's and transcortical motor aphasia have difficulty retrieving words (mostly nouns, less often adjectives and verbs) from the repository of word meanings (lexicon) but are helped by phonemic cueing. Patients with posterior aphasias have difficulty selecting words from the lexicon and are not helped by prompts; some are able to pick out the word they are seeking from several that are offered. They are also likely to produce circumlocutions and to make paraphasic errors that are semantically related to the target word they cannot produce. Other patients with posterior lesions lose word meanings altogether so that they are unable to pick out the correct word when it is offered. Anomia is worse for some of these patients when they have to insert words into sentences in spontaneous language than when asked to name an object to confrontation.

TAXONOMY OF DYSPHASIA

Although attempts to classify the acquired aphasias go back a century, it is only recently that investigators have paid enough attention to the considerable variability that exists among dysphasic children to consider developing a taxonomy of the dysphasias. Contemporary clinical (69), neuropsychologic (93,94), and formal language studies (7) of dysphasic children indicate that there are several types of developmental dysphasia and, therefore, that dysphasia is no more a single neurologic entity than is aphasia. A valid taxonomy of the dysphasias requires that behaviorally defined dysphasic subtypes be correlated with biologic measures such as those derived from neuroimaging and electrophysiologic studies (58).

Investigators from different disciplines have attended to different dimensions of language in their proposed taxonomies. Ingram (38), a child neurologist, distinguished on clinical grounds between primary dysphasia and disorders of speech and language secondary to mental deficiency, hearing loss, autism, social deprivation, structural defects of the vocal tract, dysarthria (neurogenic motor deficits of the orofacial musculature), and stuttering. Mellor (53), another child neurologist, compared the dysphasias with the adult aphasias on the basis of the characteristics of children's comprehension and production of language. Ajuriaguerra, a neuropsychologist and pediatric psychiatrist, and colleagues (1) divided dysphasic children along the fluency dimension and compared outcome in two groups: the fluent group had more severe comprehension deficits than the nonfluent group and had a worse outcome as far as the likelihood of their having learning disabilities and behavior problems on follow-up. Aram and Nation (7), speech pathologists, used Q-sort analysis to assign 47 preschool dysphasic children according to their scores on standardized tests of comprehension, production, and repetition of language at the levels of phonology, syntax, and semantics; they arrived at a six-syndrome solution. They found, in a follow-up study of 20 of these children, that few of them were entirely normal 5 and 10 years later (4,95), that 75% of them were variously learning disabled, and 20% of them were frankly mentally retarded. Wolfus et al. (94), neuropsychologists, used discriminant function analysis to divide 20 dysphasic children into an expressive group and an expressive-receptive group based on their scores on tests of language and verbal memory. They stated that their results did not support the thesis that an auditory-perceptual disorder was the singular cause of developmental dysphasia, as proposed by Tallal and colleagues (85,86). Wilson and Risucci (93), also neuropsychologists, used profile analysis based on scores from a neuropsychologic test battery to classify preschool dysphasic children. They arrived at a seven-syndrome solution that was reinforced by clinical data regarding the relative impairment of comprehension and production of language.

Rapin and Allen, a child neurologist and a developmental psycholinguist, proposed a six-syndrome clinical classification of dysphasic children (Table 2). This taxonomy is based on observation of the child's ability to use language communicatively in a play situation and to comprehend and produce language at the levels of phonology, syntax, semantics, and pragmatics (2,65,68–70,74).

There is considerable variability in the age at which children learn to express themselves intelligibly, fluently, and in sentences (13; E. Bates and V. A. Marchman, *this volume*). This greatly complicates the definition of dysphasic syndromes. Those defined by Rapin and Allen apply to preschool children. Subtyping children

TABLE 2. *Dysphasia syndromes according to Rapin and Allen*

A. Disorder of phonologic decoding
Verbal auditory agnosia
B. Disorders of phonologic encoding
Verbal dyspraxia
Phonologic programing deficit syndrome
C. Disorder of morphologic and syntactic decoding and encoding
Phonologic-syntactic deficit syndrome
D. Disorders of higher level processing
Semantic-pragmatic deficit syndrome
Lexical-syntactic deficit syndrome

during the very early stages of language acquisition is more difficult. For example, some children with the semantic-pragmatic deficit syndrome who are fluent chatterboxes in the preschool years may have spoken late or spoken only in fluent unintelligible jargon for many months. Other children with that syndrome may have spoken early and well, but in utterances consisting primarily of learned scripts. How could one have predicted, early on, that children with all these types of difficulty would look so much alike later on as to end up with the same syndrome? To the same point: when is defective phonologic output simply immature speech that persists for longer than usual and when is it the sign of a phonologic programing deficit? How can one assess the syntactic skills of children with verbal dyspraxia or verbal auditory agnosia who say very little or, at best, have learned some pigeon sign language? Only detailed and prospective studies of such children's language skills will provide answers to these questions.

The taxonomy of dysphasia of Rapin and Allen (Table 2) includes pragmatics as one of its classification variables, one that most adult aphasiologists do not use for classification. Pragmatics refers to the rules for the communicative use of language. Nonverbal pragmatics has to do with facial expression, mutual gaze, gestures, and body language. Verbal pragmatics refers to such aspects as turn taking, initiation of conversation, maintenance of topic, and ability to formulate and comprehend questions, commands, and comments. Pragmatics play a critical role for the development of meaningful communication. Infants begin to acquire both verbal and nonverbal pragmatic rules long before speech emerges: they learn in very few months to look and smile at their mother when she talks to them and to insert their responsive coos during the pauses of her talk (15,88).

Disordered pragmatics are a sign of nondominant, rather than dominant, hemispheric dysfunction in both adults and children (23,30,37,91). Perhaps it is because dysphasia reflects bilateral brain dysfunction that pragmatics are likely to be involved more prominently in dysphasia than in adult aphasia.

Dysphasic children with predominantly expressive deficits tend to have normal pragmatics except that the more dysphasic they are, the less likely they are to initiate communication. Pragmatics are regularly impaired in children with significant receptive deficits. Impaired pragmatics is one of the defining characteristics of autistic communication (10). Children with the semantic-pragmatic syndrome, a syndrome that is more common in autistic than nonautistic communication-disordered children, have dramatically impaired pragmatics. Such children, for example, may chatter to themselves rather than to others or fail to respond when addressed or to look at the person they are ostensibly addressing. They may use a questioning voice intonation when making an assertion or speak in a wooden manner with a poorly modulated voice.

PARALLELS BETWEEN SYNDROMES IN APHASIA AND DYSPHASIA

The comparisons of aphasia and dysphasia syndromes depicted in Tables 3–8 were motivated by the authors' need to formulate hypotheses for guiding future

TABLE 3. *Pure word deafness vs verbal auditory agnosia*

Aspects of language	Pure word deafness	Verbal auditory agnosia
Comprehension	Severely impaired	Severely impaired
Fluency	Unimpaired	Mute or impaired
Phonology	Unimpaired	Severely impaired[a]
Syntax	Unimpaired	—[a]
Semantics	Unimpaired	—[b]
Nonverbal pragmatics	Unimpaired	Variable[c]
Repetition	Cannot	Cannot
Echolalia	No	No
Word finding	?	?
Naming	?	?
Paraphasias		
Literal	Yes	Yes
Semantic	?	?
Reading		
Aloud	Unimpaired	Cannot
Silently	Unimpaired	Able to learn
Writing		
Spontaneously	Unimpaired	Able to learn
To dictation	Cannot	Cannot
Signing	?	Able to learn

?, insufficient data.
[a]Speech articulation and syntax always defective when they learn to speak.
[b]Semantics intact in written language and sign for concrete language only.
[c]Some children may be withdrawn and some frankly autistic; others are quite normal and try to communicate manually.

morphometric and electrophysiologic studies of dysphasic children. The tables, which systematically list deficits considered typical of corresponding syndromes, do some violence to the facts since these are not as neat as the tables indicate. Because of interindividual variability in brain organization and in type and extent of pathologies, syndromes necessarily have somewhat fuzzy edges. The tables should be viewed as heuristic hypotheses rather than established facts.

One dysphasia syndrome, *verbal auditory agnosia*, has an almost exact counterpart in an adult aphasia, pure word deafness. These correspondences are shown in Table 3.

Adults with pure word deafness are unable to comprehend speech but are able to read and write; in other words, their deficit is specific to the auditory modality (9,19). The same is true of children with verbal auditory agnosia who are able to understand gestures, can learn sign language and, with special instruction, reading and writing (71). The major difference between adults and children is that children are mute or extremely dysfluent whereas adults are able to speak either normally or with some literal paraphasic errors. This difference is readily accounted for by the fact that language is so overlearned in adults that they do not need auditory feedback to express themselves orally. Children with developmental verbal auditory agnosia have acquired no language as yet; toddlers or preschool children who develop this syndrome in the context of acquired epileptic aphasia cannot maintain what little language they have in the absence of comprehension. As children with this syndrome improve, they are generally dysfluent and have very defective phonology. There is evidence to suggest that their deficit, as seems to be the case in adults with pure word deafness, is at the level of phonologic decoding (31), the first step required for the comprehension of language.

Word deaf adults regularly have bilateral lesions affecting auditory association areas in the first temporal convolution or, if pathology affects the left side only, a lesion interupting fibers that connect the right auditory association areas with the damaged left. Benson (16) ascribed pure word deafness to bilateral involvement of Heschl's gyrus. Most investigators, however, indicate that this lesion produces cortical deafness, an auditory processing deficit for all sounds, not speech sounds selectively. Admittedly, there are very few case reports that are suitable for resolving this issue, and at least some patients may go through a phase of cortical deafness, followed by auditory agnosia for speech and nonspeech sounds, before being left with chronic word deafness (9,19,67). To our knowledge, the only child with dysphasia who came to autopsy probably suffered from verbal auditory agnosia; he had bilateral cystic temporal lesions that involved Heschl's gyrus and the entire first temporal convolution, with retrograde degeneration in the medial geniculate bodies (44). Cerebral blood flow, using the xenon inhalation method, was measured in a girl with verbal auditory agnosia (47); she had decreased blood flow over the posterior sylvian region bilaterally and verbal activation failed to produce the expected increase in blood flow in Broca's or Wernicke's areas.

Verbal auditory agnosia, which refers to a particular language decoding deficit, and epileptic aphasia—the so-called syndrome of Laudau and Kleffner (45)—are terms that are often erroneously considered synonymous. There are children with verbal auditory agnosia who have no clinical or electrographic signs of epilepsy and who were never able to decode phonology and, thus, to acquire speech normally (97). Although most children with acquired epileptic aphasia are severely deficient in their ability to comprehend language because of their inability to decode phonology (and thus have an acquired verbal auditory agnosia), a few children with epileptic aphasia have better comprehension than verbal expression. By definition, this latter group does not have verbal auditory agnosia. Making a distinction between verbal auditory agnosia acquired in the toddler and early preschool years and developmental verbal auditory agnosia is often difficult. The distinction, however, may not be very important as long as the pathogenesis of epileptic aphasia and of developmental verbal auditory agnosia remains unknown and the efficacy of the treatment of epileptic aphasia with anticonvulsant drugs is unpredictable.

A second dysphasic syndrome, *verbal dyspraxia*, has a close adult counterpart, aphemia (see Table 4). Adults with aphemia are mute but comprehend well and can read silently. Their writing does not contain the spelling and grammatical errors typical of patients with Broca's aphasia who make similar errors in speech and writing (39,78). Children with verbal dyspraxia are also mute or extremely dysfluent (27,98). Their comprehension is far superior to their expressive abilities. They are

TABLE 4. *Aphemia vs verbal dyspraxia*

Aspects of language	Aphemia	Verbal dyspraxia
Comprehension	Unimpaired	Unimpaired
Fluency	Mute	Mute or impaired
Phonology	Anarthric	Very poor
Syntax	—[a]	—[a]
Semantics	—[a]	—[a]
Nonverbal pragmatics	Unimpaired	Unimpaired
Repetition	Cannot	Cannot
Echolalia	No	No
Word finding	—[a]	—[a]
Naming	—[a]	—[a]
Paraphasias		
Literal	?	?
Semantic	?	?
Reading		
Aloud	Cannot	Cannot
Silently	Unimpaired	Able to learn
Writing		
Spontaneously	Unimpaired	Able to learn
To dictation	Unimpaired	Able to learn
Signing	?	Able to learn[b]

?, insufficient data.
[a]Preserved for written language.
[b]May have motor dyspraxia and difficulty learning sign language.

able to learn to read and write. In both aphemia and verbal dyspraxia the deficit seems to be at the stage of transforming word images into commands for the production of speech. Aphasiologists have debated for years whether this deficit should be considered a language disorder.

Some investigators make no clear distinction between aphemia, viewed as the most "distal" of the expressive language disorders, and dysarthria and oromotor apraxia, which are nonlinguistic motor disorders of the muscles of articulation. Aphemics and dysfluent adult aphasics, like children with verbal dyspraxia and those with the phonologic-syntactic deficit syndrome, often have oromotor dysfunction. These oromotor deficits are rarely severe enough to provide an adequate or convincing explanation for the patients' profoundly deficient verbal expression. Adults with pseudobulbar palsy are seldom mute and make every effort to speak, however unintelligibly; this contrasts with aphemic patients who may be essentially mute. Children with severe cerebral palsy and pseudobulbar palsy or athetosis may produce more speech, albeit incomprehensible, than children with verbal dyspraxia. The articulation errors made by dysarthric patients tend to be consistent whereas those of children with the phonologic-syntactic deficit syndrome and those of Broca's aphasics (79) depend on the position of phonemes in words. Affected children may misarticulate a speech sound in the middle or the end of a word that they are able to produce quite well in isolation or as an initial word sound; this pattern cannot readily be ascribed to a motor deficit. A speculative difference between dysfluent aphasic and dysphasic patients and those who are dysarthric as well as language impaired may be the location of their pathology, predominantly in the premotor cortex in the former whereas it may extend to sensorimotor or subcortical areas in the latter.

Pure aphemia is rare, compared to Broca's aphasia. According to Benson (16) and Schiff et al. (78), aphemia typically occurs in patients with a small lesion in or near Broca's area, in the lower part of the sensorimotor cortex, or in the connections between the supplementary motor area or Broca's area and the orofacial area of the sensorimotor cortex. A young patient of ours who is in his twenties and had persistent verbal dyspraxia and oromotor deficits has bilateral small atrophic lesions in his frontal operculum shown by CT. Lou and colleagues (47) demonstrated in three boys with verbal dyspraxia decreased perfusion of both frontal lobes at rest and failure of verbal activation to increase perfusion of Broca's area; one of the three also had left posterior perisylvian hypoperfusion. Ferry and colleagues (27) pointed out that patients with verbal dyspraxia have a much more guarded prognosis for the development of serviceable speech than those with other dysphasic syndromes.

There does not seem to be an adult aphasia syndrome that resembles the *phonologic programing deficit syndrome* (Table 5). These children have excellent comprehension and have a lot to say. They are fluent but speak unintelligibly in long, well modulated "sentences" that sound like jargon to strangers and even, to a lesser extent, to their parents. Normal children often go through a stage of producing language that has these characteristics. One is therefore tempted to state that this

TABLE 5. *Phonologic programing deficit syndrome*

Aspects of language	
Comprehension	Unimpaired
Fluency	Unimpaired
Phonology	Very impaired
Syntax	Unimpaired ?
Semantics	Unimpaired
Pragmatics	Unimpaired
Repetition	Like spontaneous speech
Echolalia	No
Word finding	Unimpaired ?
Naming	Unimpaired ?
Paraphasias	
Literal	Yes
Semantic	?
Reading	Able to learn
Writing	Able to learn
Signing	?

?, insufficient data.

syndrome may in fact represent a maturational lag. When unintelligibility persists, however, to age three, four, or even later, the hypothesis of a lag becomes unattractive. Also, not enough detail is available about the language of these children to be able to state categorically that their syntactic skills and repetition are normal and that they have no word-finding problem. In adult aphasics, fluency and impaired phonology do not seem to go together, with the possible exception of the florid paraphasias of patients with conduction aphasia. More study of this dysphasic syndrome is clearly needed.

There are many resemblances between patients with Broca's aphasia and those with the *phonologic-syntactic deficit syndrome* (Table 6). In both cases speech is dysfluent, poorly articulated, and lacks the "little words" (functors or closed-class words such as auxiliaries, articles, prepositions, and the like), as well as morphologic endings that mark tense, number, possession, and other syntactic relations (16,49). Patients with Broca's aphasia and children with the phonologic-syntactic syndrome are prone to making literal (phonemic) paraphasic errors. Comprehension is superior to production in both syndromes, although it is typically better in Broca's aphasia than in the phonologic-syntactic deficit syndrome. There are word finding deficits in both syndromes, but whether the children profit as much as the adults do from phonologic prompts has not been determined. Repetition is impaired in both and closely parallels spontaneous production. [Menyuk (54) pointed out that children repeat what they know about the rules of language, not what they hear.]

TABLE 6. *Broca's aphasia vs phonologic-syntactic deficit syndrome*

Aspects of language	Broca's aphasia	Phonologic-syntactic deficit syndrome
Comprehension	>> production[a]	> or = to production
Fluency	Very impaired	Mute or impaired
Phonology	Impaired	Impaired
Syntax	Telegraphic[b]	Telegraphic[b]
Semantics	Unimpaired	Variable[c]
Nonverbal pragmatics	Unimpaired	Impaired
Repetition	> spontaneous speech	Like spontaneous speech
Echolalia	No	No
Word finding	Impaired	Impaired
Naming	Impaired	Impaired
Paraphasias		
Literal	Many	Many
Semantic	?	Some
Reading		
Aloud	Impaired	Have trouble learning
Comprehension	May be normal	Limited
Writing spontaneously	Like spontaneous speech[b]	Worse than spontaneous speech[b]

?, insufficient data.
[a]Comprehension of syntactically complex utterances limited.
[b]Language (oral and written) lacks functors and morphemic markers; spelling poor.
[c]Dependent on severity of comprehension deficit.

Adults with lesions in the vicinity of the foot of the third frontal convolution (Broca's area), particularly if they also involve the lower part of the sensorimotor cortex, are those most likely to produce the clinical picture of Broca's aphasia (16,40,56). There is very little information regarding the location of the dysfunction responsible for the phonologic-syntactic deficit syndrome, whose severity varies greatly among children. Lou and colleagues (47) reported decreased anterior and posterior perisylvian perfusion bilaterally in four boys said to be suffering from this dysphasic syndrome; verbal activation in one of them did not increase left perisylvian perfusion.

The language of children with the *semantic-pragmatic deficit syndrome* has many similarities to transcortical sensory aphasia as Benson (16) described it (Table 7). The children are fluent, speak in phonologically and grammatically correct sentences, but have a serious comprehension deficit for the content of what they hear. Echolalia, both immediate and delayed, is often prominent. Much of what the children say is empty verbiage, although their "canned" and repetitive scripts may actually be related to what would have been appropriate for them to say; the scripts stand for utterances the children have difficulty formulating themselves or serve as fillers for turntaking in conversation. Immediate echolalia, e.g., repeating a question rather than answering it, provides another opportunity and extra time for processing. These children have superior verbal memories and can often repeat extremely long

TABLE 7. *Transcortical sensory aphasia vs semantic-pragmatic deficit syndrome*

Aspects of language	Transcortical sensory aphasia	Semantic-pragmatic deficit syndrome
Comprehension	Impaired	Impaired
Fluency	Increased	Increased
Phonology	Unimpaired	Unimpaired[a]
Syntax	Unimpaired	Unimpaired[a]
Semantics	Impaired	Impaired
Pragmatics	?	Impaired
Repetition	Unimpaired, echolalia	Unimpaired, echolalia
Echolalia		
Immediate	Yes	Yes
Delayed	?	Yes
Word finding	?	Impaired
Naming	Impaired	May be normal
Paraphasias		
Literal	No	No
Semantic	Yes	Yes
Reading		
Aloud	Paraphasic	Hyperlexia[b]
Comprehension	Impaired	Impaired
Writing spontaneously	Impaired	May be precocious

?, insufficient data.
[a]Speech may be delayed and jargon at first.
[b]Precocious reading with poor comprehension not universally present.

syntactically complex sentences that they neither comprehend nor could produce spontaneously. A number of them are preoccupied with letters and numbers, and some learn to read precociously but often with little understanding of what they are reading (75).

Pathology in transcortical sensory aphasia is posterior, usually temporo-parieto-occipital. The semantic-pragmatic deficit syndrome is seen particularly in two conditions. The first is congenital or early infantile hydrocephalus (24,84) in which ventricular enlargement tends to predominate in the atrium and occipital horns more than the frontal; white matter pathology in these children, although admittedly widespread, underlies the cortical regions implicated in the adult syndrome. This syndrome is also common in high-functioning verbal autistic children (11). What systems are implicated in the latter children is unknown.

The *lexical-syntactic deficit syndrome*, which occurs frequently in children, does not seem to have an exact counterpart among the aphasias. It shares features with both anomic aphasia and conduction aphasia (Table 8). The children have word-finding difficulty in discourse, and greater difficulty producing language within the constraints of conversational demands than in spontaneously generated utterances.

TABLE 8. *Lexical syntactic-deficit syndrome vs anomic and conduction aphasias*

Aspects of language	Aphasias		Lexical-syntactic deficit syndrome
	Anomic	Conduction	
Comprehension	Unimpaired	Unimpaired	Impaired[a]
Fluency	Normal save for anomic pauses	Normal save for anomic pauses	Normal save for anomic pauses
Phonology	Unimpaired	Unimpaired	Adequate for age
Syntax	Unimpaired	Unimpaired	Immature[b]
Semantics	Impaired	Unimpaired	Variable[c]
Pragmatics	Unimpaired	Unimpaired	Unimpaired
Repetition	Unimpaired	Cannot	Unimpaired
Echolalia	No	No	Some immediate[d]
Word finding	Very impaired	Paraphasic	Impaired
Naming	Very impaired	Paraphasic	Impaired
Paraphasias			
Literal	No	Many	Yes
Semantic	Yes, circumlocution	?	Yes
Reading			
Aloud	Unimpaired	Paraphasic	Difficulty learning
Silently	Unimpaired	Unimpaired	Difficulty learning
Writing			
Spontaneously	Unimpaired	Paraphasic	Difficulty learning
To dictation	?	?	?

?, insufficient data.
[a]Comprehension impaired except for the here and now.
[b]Syntax better in spontaneous speech than in elicited speech, immature rather than frankly deviant.
[c]Abstract language more impaired than concrete.
[d]Shorter echoes than in the semantic-pragmatic syndrome.

Benson (16) noted that patients with anomic aphasia have greater difficulty retrieving words in discourse than in naming to confrontation. Difficulty retrieving words in discourse may be severe enough in children with the lexical-syntactic deficit syndrome to produce the superficial impression of stuttering. These children would be fluent were it not for their anomia, a finding that is also noted in conduction aphasia. On the other hand, the children do not have the cardinal finding of conduction aphasia: impaired ability to repeat. In addition to semantic paraphasias, they produce some literal paraphasias, but not nearly as many as do adults with conduction aphasia. Further research is needed to determine whether this dysphasic syndrome has an adult aphasia counterpart.

SUMMARY AND CONCLUSION

We have attempted to draw some parallels between syndromes of adult acquired aphasia and of childhood developmental dysphasia. There appear to be two syndromes that are almost exact duplicates in the adults and the children: (a) pure word deafness and verbal auditory agnosia, and (b) aphemia and verbal dyspraxia. Two other syndromes seem to have rather close but not exact counterparts: Broca's aphasia and the phonologic-syntactic deficit syndrome, and transcortical sensory aphasia and the semantic-pragmatic deficit syndrome. There are two dysphasic syndromes, the phonologic production deficit syndrome and the lexical-syntactic deficit syndrome, that do not seem to have close adult counterparts. Neither of these dysphasic syndromes has been defined in adequate linguistic detail, and it is possible that their description may have to be modified when more data become available.

Whether these comparisons between dysphasias and aphasias have heuristic value for guiding external validation studies of the clinically defined dysphasic syndromes of preschool children remains to be determined. Our purpose was to formulate hypotheses as to which cerebral systems are likely to be dysfunctional in children with clinically defined dysphasic syndromes. We recognize that the disorders of language acquisition and those of overlearned adult language have fundamental differences, and that plasticity of the child's developing brain introduces further complexities. Nevertheless, it seems reasonable to think that there are constants in brain organization that span all ages. Looking for language deficits common to aphasic adults (whose lesions can usually be delineated with contemporary neuroimaging techniques) and to dysphasic children (in whom there are rarely any neurologic clues) may be a fruitful way to begin to define the cerebral correlates of the children's deficits.

ACKNOWLEDGMENT

This work was supported in part by grant NS 20489 from the National Institute of Neurological and Communicative Disorders and Stroke, U.S. Public Health Service.

REFERENCES

1. Ajuriaguerra, J.de, Jaeggi, A., Guignard, F., Kocher, F., Maquard, M., Roth, S., and Schmid, E. (1976): The development and prognosis of dysphasia in children. In: *Normal and Deficient Child Language*, edited by D.M. Morehead and A.E. Morehead, pp. 345–385. University Park Press, Baltimore.
2. Allen, D.A., Mendelson, L., and Rapin, I. Syndrome-specific remediation in preschool developmental dysphasia. In: *Contemporary Issues in Child Neurology and Developmental Disabilities*, edited by J.H. French et al. Paul H. Brooks, Philadelphia (*in press*).
3. Annett, M. (1973): Laterality of childhood hemiplegia and the growth of speech and intelligence. *Cortex*, 9:3–33.
4. Aram, D.M., Ekelman, B.L., and Nation, J.E. (1984): Preschoolers with language disorders: 10 years later. *J. Speech. Hear. Res.*, 27:232–244.
5. Aram, D.M., Ekelman, B.L., Rose, D.F., and Whitaker, H.A. (1985): Verbal and cognitive sequelae following unilateral lesions acquired in early childhood. *J. Clin. Exp. Neuropsychol.*, 7:55–78.
6. Aram, D.M., Ekelman, B.L., and Whitaker, H.A. (1986): Spoken syntax in children with acquired unilateral hemisphere lesions. *Brain Lang.*, 27:75–100.
7. Aram, D.M., and Nation, J.E. (1975): Patterns of language behavior in children with developmental language disorders. *J. Speech Hear. Res.*, 18:229–241.
8. Aram, D.M., and Nation, J.E. (1980): Preschool language disorders and subsequent language and academic difficulties. *J. Commun. Disord.*, 13:159–170.
9. Auerbach, S.H., Allard, T., Naeser, M., Alexander, M.P., and Albert, M.L. (1982): Pure word deafness: Analysis of a case with bilateral lesions and a defect at the prephonemic level. *Brain*, 105:271–300.
10. Baltaxe, C. (1977): Pragmatic deficits in the language of autistic adolescents. *J. Pediatr. Psychol.*, 2:176–180.
11. Baltaxe, C., and Simmons, J. (1975): Language in childhood psychosis: A review. *J. Speech Hear. Dis.*, 15:439–458.
12. Basser, L. (1962): Hemiplegia of early onset and the faculty of speech with special reference to the effects of hemispherectomy. *Brain*, 85:427–460.
13. Bates, E. (1979): *The Emergence of Symbols: Cognition and Communication in Infancy*. Academic Press, New York.
14. Bear, D., Schiff, D., Saver, J., Greenberg, M., and Freeman, R. (1986): Quantitative analysis of cerebral asymmetries: Fronto-occipital correlation, sexual dimorphism and association with handedness. *Arch. Neurol.*, 43:598–603.
15. Beebe, B., Stern, D., and Jaffe, J. (1979): The kinesic rhythm of mother-infant interactions. In: *Of Speech and Time: Temporal Patterns in Interpersonal Contexts*, edited by A.W. Siegman and E. Feldstein, pp. 23–34. Lawrence Erlbaum, Hillsdale, N. J.
16. Benson, D.F. (1979): *Aphasia, Alexia, and Agraphia*. Churchill Livingstone, New York.
17. Brown, W.T., Friedman, E., Jenkins, E.C., Brooks, J., Wisniewski, K., Raguthu, S., and French, J.H. (1981): Association of fragile X syndrome with autism. *Lancet*, 1:780.
18. Brunner, R.J., Kornhuber, H.H., Seemuller, E., Suger, G., and Wallesch, C.-W. (1982): Basal ganglia participation in language pathology. *Brain Lang.*, 16:281–299.
19. Buchman, A.S., Garron, D.C., Trost-Cardamone, J.E., Wichter, M.D., and Schwartz, M. (1986): Word deafness: One hundred years later. *J. Neurol. Neurosurg. Psychiatry*, 49:489–499.
20. Caramazza, A., and Zurif, E.B. (eds.) (1978): *Language Acquisition and Language Breakdown: Parallels and Divergencies*. The Johns Hopkins University Press, Baltimore.
21. Chi, J.G., Dooling, E.C., and Gilles, F.H. (1977): Gyral development of the human brain. *Ann. Neurol.*, 1:86–93.
22. Crosson, B. (1984): Role of the dominant thalamus in language: A review. *Psychol. Bull.*, 96:491–517.
23. Denckla, M.B. (1983): The neuropsychology of social-emotional learning disabilities. *Arch. Neurol.*, 40:461–462.
24. Dennis, M., Hendrick, E.B., Hoffman, H.J., and Humphreys, R.P. The language of hydrocephalic children and adolescents. *J. Clin. Exp. Neuropsychol.* (*in press*).
25. Dennis, M., and Kohn, B. (1975): Comprehension of syntax in infantile hemiplegics after hemidecortication: Left-hemispheric superiority. *Brain Lang.*, 2:472–482.

26. Duffy, F.H., Denckla, M.B., Bartels, P.H., and Sandini, G. (1980): Dyslexia: Regional differences in brain electrical activity by topographic mapping. *Ann. Neurol.*, 7:412–420.

27. Ferry, P.C., Hall, S.M., and Hicks, J.L. (1975): 'Dilapidated' speech: Developmental verbal dyspraxia. *Dev. Med. Child Neurol.*, 17:749–756.

28. Finger, S., and Stein, D.G. (1982): *Brain Damage and Recovery: Research and Clinical Perspectives.* Academic Press, New York.

29. Fisch, G.S., Cohen, I.L., Wolf, E.G., Brown, W.T., Jenkins, E.C., and Gross, A. (1986): Autism and the fragile X syndrome. *Am. J. Psychiatry*, 143:71–73.

30. Foldi, N.S., Cicone, M., and Gardner, H. (1983): Pragmatic aspects of communication in brain-damaged patients. In: *Language Functions and Brain Organization*, edited by S.J. Segalowitz, pp. 51–86. Academic Press, New York.

31. Frumkin, B., and Rapin, I. (1980): Perception of vowels and consonant-vowels of varying duration in language impaired children. *Neuropsychologia*, 18:443–454.

32. Galaburda, A.M., and Kemper, T.L. (1978): Cytoarchitectonic abnormalities in developmental dyslexia: A case study. *Ann. Neurol.*, 6:94–100.

33. Geschwind, N. (1971): Aphasia. *N. Engl. J. Med.*, 284:654–656.

34. Geschwind, N., and Galaburda, A.M. (1985): Cerebral lateralization. Biological mechanisms, associations, and pathology: A hypothesis and a program for research. *Arch. Neurol.*, 42:428–459,521–552,634–654.

35. Gonzalez, C.F., Grossman, C.B., and Masdeu, J.C. (1985): *Head and Spine Imaging.* John Wiley, New York.

36. Hécaen, H. (1976): Acquired aphasia in children and the ontogenesis of hemispheric functional specialization. *Brain Lang.*, 3:114–134.

37. Heilman, K.M., Bowers, D., Speedie, L., and Coslett, H.B. (1984): Comprehension of affective and nonaffective prosody. *Neurology*, 34:917–921.

38. Ingram, T.T.S. (1975): Speech disorders in childhood. In: *Foundations of Language Development*, edited by E.H. Lenneberg and E. Lenneberg, pp. 195–261. Academic Press, New York.

39. Johns, D.F., and LaPointe, L.L. (1976): Neurogenic disorders of output processing: Apraxia of speech. In: *Studies in Neurolinguistics*, Vol. 1, edited by H. Whitaker and H.A. Whitaker, pp. 161–199. Academic Press, New York.

40. Kertesz, A. (1979): *Aphasia and Associated Disorders: Taxonomy, Localization, and Recovery.* Grune and Stratton, New York.

41. Kertesz, A. (ed.) (1983): *Localization in Neuropsychology.* Academic Press, New York.

42. Kinsbourne, M. (1971): The minor hemisphere as a source of aphasic speech. *Arch. Neurol.*, 25:302–306.

43. Knopman, D.S., Rubens, A.B., Selnes, O.A., Klassen, A.C., and Meyer, M.W. (1984): Mechanisms of recovery from aphasia: Evidence from serial xenon 133 cerebral blood flow studies. *Ann. Neurol.*, 15:530–535.

44. Landau, W., Goldstein, R., and Kleffner, F. (1960): Congenital aphasia: A clinico-pathologic study. *Neurology*, 10:915–921.

45. Landau, W., and Kleffner, F. (1957): Syndrome of acquired aphasia with convulsive disorder in children. *Neurology*, 7:523–530.

46. Lassen, N.A., Ingvar, D.H., and Skinhøj, E. (1978): Brain function and blood flow. *Sci. Am.* (Oct.), 239:62–71.

47. Lou, H.C., Henrikson, L., and Bruhn, P. (1984): Focal cerebral hypoperfusion in children with dysphasia and/or attention deficit disorder. *Arch. Neurol.*, 41:825–829.

48. Ludlow, C. (1980): Children's language disorders: Recent research advances. *Ann. Neurol.*, 7:497–507.

49. Luria, A.R. (1966): *Higher Cortical Functions in Man.* Basic Books, New York.

50. Mateer, C.A. (1983): Localization of language and visuospatial functions by electrical stimulation. In: *Localization in Neuropsychology*, edited by A. Kertesz, pp. 153–183. Academic Press, New York.

51. Mattis, S., French, J.H., and Rapin, I. (1975): Dyslexia in children and young adults: Three independent neuropsychological syndromes. *Dev. Med. Child Neurol.*, 17:150–163.

52. Mazziotta, J.C., and Phelps, M.E. (1985): Human neuropsychological imaging studies of local brain metabolism: Strategies and results. In: *Brain Imaging and Brain Function*, edited by L. Sokoloff, pp. 121–137. Raven Press, New York.

53. Mellor, D.H. (1983): Developmental language disorders: Neurological and aetiological considerations. In: *Assessment and Remediation of Specific Language Disorders*, edited by P. Griffiths, pp. 4–17. Invalid Children's Aid Association, London.

54. Menyuk, P. (1969): *Sentences Children Use.* MIT Press, Cambridge, MA.
55. Milner, B. (1974): Hemispheric specialization: Scope and limits. In: *The Neurosciences: Third Study Program,* edited by F.O. Schmitt and F.G. Worden, pp. 75–89. MIT Press, Cambridge, MA.
56. Mohr, J.P. (1976): Broca's area and Broca's aphasia. In: *Studies in Neurolinguistics.* Vol. 1, edited by H. Whitaker and H.A. Whitaker, pp. 201–235. Academic Press, New York.
57. Mohr, J.P. (1983): Thalamic lesions and syndromes. In: *Localization in Neuropsychology,* edited by A. Kertesz, pp. 269–293. Academic Press, New York.
58. Morris, R., and Fletcher, J. Classification in neuropsychology: A theoretical framework and research paradigm. *J. Clin. Exp. Neuropsychol. (in press).*
59. Myklebust, H.R. (1971): Childhood aphasia: An evolving concept. In: *Handbook of Speech Pathology and Audiology,* edited by L.E. Travis, pp. 1181–1202. Appleton-Century-Crofts, New York.
60. Naeser, M.A., Alexander, M.P., Helm-Brooks, N., Levine, H.L., Laughlin, S.A., and Geschwind, N. (1982): Aphasia with predominantly subcortical lesion sites: Description of three capsular-putaminal aphasia syndromes. *Arch. Neurol.,* 39:2–14.
61. Novick, B., Lovrich, D., and Vaughan, H.G. (1985): Event-related potentials associated with the discrimination of acoustic and semantic aspects of speech. *Neuropsychologia,* 23:87–101.
62. Ojemann, G., and Mateer, C. (1979): Human language cortex: Localization of memory, syntax, and sequential motor-phoneme identification systems. *Science,* 205:1401–1403.
63. Ojemann, G.A., and Whitaker, H.A. (1978): The bilingual brain. *Arch. Neurol.,* 35:409–412.
64. Paul, R., and Cohen, D.J. (1984): Outcome of severe disorders of language acquisition. *J. Autism Dev. Disord.,* 14:405–421.
65. Rapin, I. (1982): *Children with Brain Dysfunction: Neurology, Cognition, Language, and Behavior.* Raven Press, New York.
66. Rapin, I. (1982): Developmental language disorders and brain dysfunction as precursors of reading disability. In: *Topics in Child Neurology,* Vol. II, edited by G.A. Wise, M.E. Blaw and P.G. Procopis, pp. 177–183. Spectrum Publications, New York.
67. Rapin, I. (1985): Cortical deafness, auditory agnosia, and word-deafness: How distinct are they? *Human Communic. Canada,* 9:29–37.
68. Rapin, I., and Allen, D.A. (1982): Progress toward a nosology of developmental dysphasia. In: *Child Neurology: IYDP Commemorative International Symposium on Developmental Disabilities (1981), Tokyo, Japan,* edited by Y. Fukuyama, M. Arima, K. Maekawa, and K. Yamaguchi, pp. 25–35. Excerpta Medica, Amsterdam.
69. Rapin, I., and Allen, D.A. (1983): Developmental language disorders: Nosological considerations. In: *Neuropsychology of Language, Reading, and Spelling,* edited by U. Kirk, pp. 155–184. Academic Press, New York.
70. Rapin, I., and Allen, D.A. (1986): The physician's assessment and management of young children with developmental language disorders. *Pädiatrische Fortbildungskurse für die Praxis,* 60:1–12.
71. Rapin, I., Mattis, S., Rowan, A.J., and Golden, G.S. (1977): Verbal auditory agnosia in children. *Dev. Med. Child Neurol.,* 19:192–207.
72. Rapin, I., and Wilson, B.C. (1978): Children with developmental language disability. In: *Developmental Dysphasia,* edited by M.A. Wyke, pp. 13–41. Academic Press, London.
73. Resnick, T.J., Allen, D.A., and Rapin, I. (1984): Disorders of language development: Diagnosis and intervention. *Pediatrics in Review,* 6:85–92.
74. Resnick, T.J., and Rapin, I. (1986): Normal and disordered acquisition of language. In: *Diseases of the Nervous System: Clinical Neurobiology,* edited by A.K. Asbury, G.M. McKhann, and W.I. McDonald, pp. 759–768. W.B. Saunders, Philadelphia.
75. Richman, L.C., and Kitchell, M.M. (1981): Hyperlexia as a variant of developmental language disorder. *Brain Lang.,* 12:203–212.
76. Rosenberger, P.B., and Hier, D.B. (1980): Cerebral asymmetry and verbal intellectual deficits. *Ann. Neurol.,* 8:300–304.
77. Scheibel, A.B. (1984): A dendritic correlate of human speech. In: *Cerebral Dominance: The Biological Foundations,* edited by N. Geschwind and A.M. Galaburda, pp. 43–52. Harvard University Press, Cambridge, MA.
78. Schiff, H.B., Alexander, M.P., Naeser, M.A., and Galaburda, A.M. (1983): Aphemia: Clinical-anatomic correlations. *Arch. Neurol.,* 40:720–727.
79. Shankweiler, D., and Harris, K.S. (1966): An experimental approach to the problem of articulation in aphasia. *Cortex,* 2:278–292.

80. Silva, P.A., McGee, R., and Williams, S.M. (1983): Developmental language delay from three to seven years and its significance for low intelligence and reading difficulties at age seven. *Dev. Med. Child Neurol.*, 25:783–793.

81. Sokoloff, L. (ed.) (1985): *Brain Imaging and Brain Function.* Raven Press, New York.

82. Stark, R.E., Bernstein, L.E., Condino, R., Bender, M., Tallal, P., and Catts, H. (1984): Four-year follow-up study of language impaired children. *Ann. Dyslex.*, 34:49–68.

83. Swisher, L. (1985): Language disorders in children. In: *Speech and Language Evaluation in Neurology—Pediatric Disorders*, edited by J. Darby, pp. 33–97. Grune and Stratton, New York.

84. Swisher, L.P., and Pinsker, E.J. (1971): The language characteristics of hyperverbal hydrocephalic children. *Dev. Med. Child Neurol.*, 13:746–755.

85. Tallal, P., and Piercy, M. (1978): Defects of auditory perception in children with developmental dysphasia. In: *Developmental Dysphasia*, edited by M. Wyke, pp. 63–84. Academic Press, London.

86. Tallal, P., Stark, R., and Mellits, D. (1985): The relationship between auditory temporal analysis and receptive language development: Evidence from studies of developmental language disorder. *Neuropsychologia*, 23:314–322.

87. Taylor, D.C. (1969): Differential rates of cerebral maturation between sexes and between hemispheres. *Lancet*, 2:140–142.

88. Trevarthen, C. (1983): Development of the cerebral mechanisms for language. In: *Neuropsychology of Language, Reading, and Spelling*, edited by U. Kirk, pp. 45–80. Academic Press, New York.

89. Vaughan, H.G.,Jr. (1987): Topographic analysis of brain electrical activity. In: *The London Symposia (EEG Suppl. 39)*, edited by R.J. Ellingson, N.M.F. Murray, and A.M. Halliday, pp. 137–142. Elsevier, Amsterdam.

90. Wada, J.A., Clarke, R., and Hamm, A. (1975): Cerebral hemispheric asymmetry in humans: Cortical speech zones on 100 adult and 100 infant brains. *Arch. Neurol.*, 32:239–246.

91. Weintraub, S., and Mesulam, M.-M. (1983): Developmental learning disabilities of the right hemisphere: Emotional, interpersonal, and cognitive components. *Arch. Neurol.*, 40:463–468.

92. Whitaker, H.A., and Selnes, O.A. (1976): Anatomic variations in the cortex: Individual differences and the problem of the localization of language functions. *Ann. NY Acad. Sci.*, 280:844–854.

93. Wilson, B.C., and Risucci, D.A. (1986): A model for clinical-quantitative classification. Generation I: Application to language-disordered preschool children. *Brain Lang.*, 27:281–309.

94. Wolfus, B., Moscovitch, M., and Kinsbourne, M. (1980): Subgroups of developmental language impairment. *Brain Lang.*, 10:152–171.

95. Wolpaw, T.M., Nation, J.E., and Aram, D.M. (1979): Developmental language disorder: A follow-up study. *Illinois Speech. Hear. J.*, 12:14–18.

96. Woods, B.T., and Carey, S. (1979): Language deficits after apparent clinical recovery from childhood aphasia. *Ann. Neurol.*, 6:405–409.

97. Worster-Drought, C., and Allen, I.M. (1930): Congenital auditory imperception (congenital word-deafness) and its relation to idioglossia and other speech defects. *J. Neurol. Psychopathol.*, 10:193–236.

98. Yoss, K.A., and Darley, F.L. (1974): Developmental apraxia of speech in children with defective articulation. *J. Speech Hear. Res.*, 17:399–416.

Language, Communication, and the Brain, edited by F. Plum
Raven Press, New York © 1988.

Language Development: A Sensory Development and Signal Processing Perspective

Kurt E. Hecox

Project Phoenix of Madison, Inc.,
Nicolet Audiodiagnostics, Madison, Wisconsin 53711

There is a tendency among behavioral and biological scientists to conceive of language comprehension as a continuous process that begins at the transducer surface, activates sensory-neuronal fibers (sensation), and ultimately culminates in a perceptual experience. This process is thought to consist of increasingly complex transformations, typically reflected in the distinctions made between sensations and perceptions. The task of defining the chain of events associated with or necessary for language development can be trivial or exceedingly complex. This chapter focuses on selected aspects of the question and presents an admittedly personal perspective. There is no attempt to be exhaustive or "evenhanded" in the treatment of the various perspectives.

The presence of highly developed language systems among the profoundly deaf argues that auditory sensory input is not critical to the process of language development. The descriptions and considerations put forth by Dr. Bellugi in this volume emphasize the need to carefully specify what we intend by the term language and what we assume are the sensory prerequisites for its development. The discussions put forth by Dr. Bates in this volume, on the other hand, sensibly urge that acoustic sensory information is important in the process of "normal" communication development. It is important to distinguish what is developmentally possible for a sensory handicapped individual from the developmental achievements and mechanisms of a person with an intact auditory system.

Normal language development and maintenance involve sensory information from multiple modalities, including vision, audition, and somesthesis. The relative importance of these sensory modalities varies with the particular aspect of verbal communication under consideration. For example, the speech production process and the speech comprehension process engage anatomically distinct neuronal regions. A general discussion of all the processes underlying communication behavior is beyond the scope of this chapter. Instead, the chapter focuses on sensory mechanisms that may be important in the development of verbal language comprehension.

For the sake of brevity, the distinction between speech perception and language comprehension has been ignored, although any detailed considerations of the role of sensory mechanisms must honor that distinction.

In general, the experimental territory separating sensory from language development is extremely wide with only isolated islands of understanding between the two. I cannot point to any substantial experimental bridge that has been made between sensory and language development. Thus, there are no successful models of how we might close this important gap. The absence of successful models or methods makes theoretical issues and empirical descriptions from related areas more important in selecting the approach.

EMPIRICAL FINDINGS ON AUDITORY DEVELOPMENT

The task of discriminating the multiple characteristics of speech sounds and establishing linguistically meaningful categories based on the acoustic characteristics is imposing—especially for an infant. The infant comes to recognize the invariant aspects of the speech acoustic signal despite enormous interspeaker acoustic variability. The achievement of this perceptual constancy is also one of the most fundamental requirements of building a language system from speech acoustic components.

One approach to characterizing the behavioral limits imposed by sensory immaturity on speech perception or language comprehension development is to define the limits of perceptual discrimination. This approach has been taken by a number of investigators with respect to many acoustic cues, e.g., frequency limens, intensity limens, and spatial resolution limens. [For an excellent review, see Aslin et. al. (1).] With the introduction of increasingly sophisticated methods of response analysis and dependent variables for infants, the documented difference between adult and infant capabilities is diminishing.

One shortcoming of characterizing the limits of sensory psychophysics and then expressing them in terms of limitations on language comprehension or speech perception is that we have little information on the minimal perceptual requirements for normal speech and language performance. For example, we know that measures of frequency resolution (e.g., tuning curves) can be abnormal in the hearing impaired without necessarily compromising speech perception—at least as reflected in speech discrimination scores. Similarly, alterations in sensitivity or threshold do not generally produce significant impairment of speech perception or language acquisition for losses of 25 to 30 dB or less in both ears. The impact of both of these impairments shows that the auditory system can be compromised in its resolving power or sensitivity without significantly altering speech discrimination or language comprehension. If so, sensitivity or discriminative performance differences between infants and adults may not affect speech or language development. It is not yet clear which aspects of the acoustic signal are necessary or sufficient for normal speech perception, nor is the range of acceptable sensory performances over which normal performance can be expected available. It seems likely that future research on this question will take into account findings from both the hearing impaired and the developmentally immature.

There is a second historical perspective from which these questions have been asked. For years, developmentalists have asked the extent to which development is determined by experiential factors versus genetic factors. One related question is, to what extent does the newborn enter the world with a nervous system "tuned" to its species-specific acoustic signals? Although the "genetics versus experience" discussions are less prominent and salient today than in the 1960s or 1970s, the characterization of the speech discrimination skills of the very young infant is still important.

The species-specific "genetic" capacity perspective is exemplified by the 1971 study of Eimas and colleagues, who investigated the existence of categorical perception of voicing cues. Results of these experiments and subsequent studies are consistent with the notion that infants are capable of discriminating virtually every type of phonetic contrast that has been tested. Infants are sensitive to place of articulation, differences between stop consonants (2,17,18), fricatives (12), glides (11), and nasals (P.D. Eimas and J.L. Miller, *unpublished observations*). In a series of important experiments, Lasky, Syrdal-Lasky, and Klein (15) and Streeter (23) found that the infant's ability to discriminate phonetic contrast did not depend on specific experiences with the sounds to be discriminated. In the case of Lasky et al. (15), comparisons were made for a voice onset time boundary for English among infants from a Spanish-speaking community, whereas Streeter's studies focused on the performance of infants from a Kikuyu-speaking culture. The time course over which the ability to perceive categorically noncommunity-specific distinctions is lost, secondary to exposure to a specific language community, is not yet known. In the literature, considerable skepticism has been expressed regarding the implication of categorical perception of phonetic contrasts by infants. The presence of categorical perception for human speech by nonhuman species and of categorical perception for nonspeech signals has tempered the original enthusiasm for interpreting the infant categorical perception studies as evidence for "genetic" feature detectors. [For a review of this area, see Jusczyk (10).]

Another important aspect of perceptual development is the ability to recognize speech acoustic cues despite transformations associated with different speakers, accents, or intonation patterns. Considerably less information is available on the development of perceptual constancy, but it appears that the very young infant is also capable of perceptual constancy with regard to speech acoustic cues (8,14).

These behavioral studies make several points clear: (a) infants (1–4 months of age) have nearly adult-like resolving capacities and sensitivity, and comparisons to data obtained from the hearing impaired suggest that the signal processing capabilities of the newborn are more than adequate to permit nearly adult-like speech or language comprehension; (b) categorical perception of acoustic phonetic continua exists in infants; (c) minimal, if any, experience is required with the specific acoustic phonetic distinction for categorical perception to be manifested; and (d) the young infant displays perceptual constancy. The perceptual literature suggests that by one month of age the perceptual capacities of the human infant are considerable and probably sufficient to allow adult-like performance with regard to much of speech perception and language comprehension. Although these studies are not exhaustive, the historical trend is toward ascribing greater and greater discriminative power to the very young infant. These findings leave three possibilities: (a) sensory development is sufficiently mature in the human infant so that it does not impose limitations on language or speech comprehension development; (b) the discriminative capacities sampled thus far do not adequately describe the immaturity of the human auditory system; or (c) sensory immaturity plays an important role in limiting the development of speech perception and language comprehension, but does so only at less than one month of age. Deciding among these three possibilities is extremely difficult. The first possibility would require accepting the null hypothesis. The second possibility has no clear "end-point" of investigation, although more will be said in that regard in the next section. The third possibility can be tested, although testing infants of less than four weeks of age presents special problems. It is especially difficult to devise behavioral methods applicable to the infant less than four weeks of age that can still be compared to results from older infants. One answer to this dilemma has been to use surface electrophysiologic probes, i.e., evoked potentials.

The human auditory evoked potential can be subdivided according to the latency of its components (19). The broadest distinction among auditory evoked potential components is between endogenous and exogenous responses. Exogenous responses are sensitive to the manipulation of physical acoustic parameters, but insensitive to changes in subjective state. Endogenous responses are those that faithfully reflect alterations in subjective state but are relatively insensitive to the absolute value of acoustic parameters.

The most commonly used probe among evoked potential measures for the investigation of auditory development is the brainstem auditory evoked response. This exogenous evoked potential is universally present regardless of age and reflects the activation of the peripheral auditory nerve and subsequent brainstem auditory nuclei. Using this response, a number of investigators have tracked the maturation of the peripheral auditory appartus and subsequent brainstem auditory nuclei and tracts. The degree of maturity interacts with the acoustic parameter under investigation. Abnormalities of development are easily and quantitatively detected using this probe. [For a review of the brainstem auditory evoked response manifestations of immaturity, see Hecox and Burkhard (6).] Essentially, all of those aspects of the brainstem and auditory nerve behavior are adult-like by one year of age. The more rostrally generated long latency components continue to mature several years thereafter.

Electrophysiologic data obtained from this and other laboratories suggest that the newborn human has no more than a 20-dB decrease in sensitivity to broadband signals, compared with the human adult. This difference is probably not large enough to diminish the speech processing capabilities of the newborn, unless there are unappreciated frequency dependencies to these sensitivity differences. The similarity between newborns and adults, regarding a variety of masking functions, also suggests that the frequency resolving power of the immature auditory system is sufficient to permit discrimination of the acoustic cues inherent in speech signals. More specifically, in our experience the magnitude of masking differences between the hearing-impaired and normal-hearing adult is substantially larger than that between the unimpaired adult and newborn. One must exercise caution in such respects, however, since the performance requirements for acquisition may not be the same as the performance requirements for maintenance of speech and language capabilities. Beyond the considerable descriptive material that has been collected concerning differences between adult and newborn brain electrical responses, many recent efforts in developmental human neurophysiology have focused on testing a hypothesis put forward by Dr. Rubel and colleagues (20).

Rubel hypothesized that a key aspect of auditory system maturation is the development of tonotopicity. Rubel's hypothesis is able to accommodate apparently contradictory anatomic and physiologic findings with regard to the frequency specificity of maturation (16,21). Whether correct or incorrect, this hypothesis has produced more empirical studies than any prior model of auditory development. Extension of Rubel's chick embryo work in both the gerbil and guinea pig are consistent with Rubel's hypothesis (4). Our own studies in the human newborn using low pass, high pass and broadband maskers are not consistent with Rubel's hypothesis. Either the human newborn is more mature at birth than the newborn chick, gerbil, and guinea pig, or the mechanisms involved in peripheral auditory development are species specific. Studies in human premature infants should help resolve this question.

Until the past decade, methods for the study of hair cell mechanics and the coupling of inner and outer hair cells have not been available. Over the past few years an increasing number of studies using intrahair cell electrodes have provided new and important information on hair cell physiology, particularly with respect to the linearity of basilar membrane behavior and the basilar membrane to hair cell coupling (22). The hypothesized "second filter" needed to explain the sharpness of tuning in eighth nerve data compared with the tuning basilar membrane motion needs significant revision on the basis of the intracellular hair cell recordings. The sharpness of tuning at the level of the hair cell appears adequate to explain virtually all results obtained from eighth nerve studies. Thus, sharpening of the mechanical tuning of the traveling wave has occurred prior to activation of the hair cell. These intracellular hair cell studies are extremely exciting and represent a true methodologic breakthrough in the auditory neurosciences. There have been no developmental studies thus far that examine the maturation of hair cell mechanics or the maturation of coupling between the hair cell and basilar membrane motion. Despite the technical difficulties in performing such studies, it seems likely that this information will be forthcoming in the next decade and will prove critical in testing the hypothesis that one important aspect of auditory development is the maturation of basilar membrane mechanics or the maturation of the coupling between basilar membrane mechanics and eighth nerve activation.

ALTERNATIVE PERSPECTIVES

There is a widespread awareness in auditory neurophysiology that there are a number of important nonlinearities operating at various anatomic levels of the auditory pathway. Although controversies continue regarding the magnitude, significance, and acoustic dependencies of these nonlinearities at the cochlear level, there is nearly universal acceptance of their operation at the hair cell/neuronal junction and at subsequent points along the central auditory neuraxis (13). These nonlinearities account for a variety of widely observed phenomena, including the nonadditivity of maskers, the sharpness of tuning curves, the presence and pattern of combination tones, and the presence of so-called ''suppression'' areas in single unit studies.

The maturational course for these nonlinearities is virtually unknown. One alternative perspective or model of auditory development is to hypothesize that the linear mechanism of auditory performance develops prior to the nonlinear mechanism and that the nonlinear aspects of auditory information processing unfold postnatally in the human infant. There is very little direct evidence supporting this hypothesis, largely because the question has gone unasked. There are, however, a number of indirect pieces of information supportive of this notion (8). For example, the broadened tuning curves, altered masking patterns, and diminished combination tone activity seen in the impaired ear have also been reported in the immature ear. Recent evidence suggests that one of the important aspects of auditory pathology is that the impaired auditory system performs more linearly than the unimpaired system. The loss of normal nonlinearities then is hypothesized to account for the above-described abnormalities in the hearing-impaired population. If true, this hypothesis has broad implications from the standpoint of the mechanisms involved in auditory development and has implications from the standpoint of the appropriate methods required to describe the underlying mechanism of development including stimulus selection. These notions run counter to the historical effort to use more sophisticated systems analysis techniques to characterize biological function.

Virtually all of these systems analysis techniques require the assumption of linearity. Generally speaking, no biologic system operates linearly, since virtually all physiologic systems display saturation behavior at the limits of their output. This problem is avoided by applying the linear systems analysis techniques over the normal operating range of input signals and by avoiding the output saturation behavior.

Most system analysis techniques have been successfully applied in a number of biologic areas, but the interpretation of their success is difficult. Does the ability to model using linear techniques imply that the underlying mechanisms are linear or only that the parameterization of the problem lends itself to a linear approximation? Perhaps one of the reasons that there are so few ''general models'' of auditory system behavior relates to the need to select very carefully stimulus parameters so as not to violate the assumptions required for the application of linear systems analysis. The concept that linear behavior is pathologic behavior strikes at the heart of this approach to studying auditory information processing.

Preliminary data collected in our laboratory using additivity-of-masking and adaptations paradigms show that, like the sensory impaired ear, the newborn auditory system is ''linearized'' compared with that of the normal-hearing adult (*unpublished data*).

One of the obstacles to the acceptance of the notion that the performance or behavior of the auditory system is normally nonlinear is that it leaves us without the very powerful methods of linear systems analysis. There are generally two alternatives to abandoning linear systems analysis. The first approach is to abandon systems analysis in general and to resort to less quantitative and general techniques from the signal processing perspective. The second alternative is to apply nonlinear systems analysis techniques. There is unfortunately little familiarity with nonlinear systems analysis techniques, both at the level of applications and at the theoretical level. Clearly, neither of these alternatives is particularly attractive to an investigator who has found the application of the linear techniques intellectually satisfying and quantitatively productive.

Acceptance of the presence and importance of nonlinear processing of auditory information also has corollaries with regard to stimulus selection. One of the tenets of linear systems analysis is that system characterization can be equivalently performed by the use of individual pure tones or broadband noise. This is especially emphasized in the single unit neurophysiology literature. In fact, as long as there is adequate energy within the frequency region of interest, the specific distribution of energies as a function of frequency is not critical to the outcome of the systems transfer function. This means that the generation of pure tone audiogram-like data, whether for a single unit cell or for a human observer, is formally equivalent to using broadband noise input in terms of providing a description of how the system operates.

For nonlinear systems the accuracy with which a system performance is characterized is directly related to the frequency/intensity composition of the stimulus used to test the system. For example, if a nonlinearity operates only above the 4,000-Hz frequency region and the input stimulus contains frequencies only below 2,000 Hz, then the nonlinearities above 4,000 Hz would not be reflected in the system's performance. Many forms of nonlinearities (e.g., static or transient intermodulation distortion, combination tones, and so forth) are elicited only when several tones are presented simultaneously.

Generally speaking, nonlinear biological systems show performance differences as a function of the input intensity. Thus, experiments in which a system's performance is characterized at a single intensity inaccurately represent the operation of any nonlinear mechanisms (3). From this perspective it is clearly inadvisable to evaluate the performance of a system using single frequency pure tone stimuli or single intensity probes. It is only with the use of more complex signals that one can hope to describe or approximate the underlying nonlinear mechanisms. Complexity of the stimulus provides control of the nonlinearities under study.

Traditionally, a major complaint of systems-oriented modelers and those interested in quantitative behavioral models has been that the complexities of the speech signal make it intractable from the standpoint of quantitative analysis. Not only is this no longer the case, but the "intractable" complexity of the speech stimulus may be necessary to represent accurately the performance of the human auditory system (9). It is interesting that this more sophisticated or complicated nonlinear systems analytic approach converges to the same position as the relatively non-quantitative theories espoused by ethologists (24). The best signal for accurately characterizing the information-processing capabilities of a biologic organism may be its species-specific call. Species-specific calls are generally highly complex, time-varying signals such as human speech.

SUMMARY

The relationship between the development of sensory mechanisms and the maturation of language behavior is poorly understood. From the outset it is important to distinguish between what is necessary for the development of any language system versus what is involved in the development of the verbal language system in the unimpaired child. The presence of highly sophisticated language systems among persons who communicate manually reminds us that no single source of sensory information is absolutely required for the development of at least some form of language system. Nevertheless, there persists a general belief that the availability of an accurate representation of the acoustic environment will facilitate at least the normal process of language acquisition.

A more tenable question is whether the completeness or accuracy of the sensory representation places limitations on the emergence of language comprehension and production. I think this is unlikely, unless the relatively untested area of the maturation of "nonlinear processing mechanisms" provides information different than that obtained from more traditional linear systems analysis approaches. The relative integrity of the language systems of the hearing impaired, despite very dramatic differences in auditory sensitivity and frequency-resolving power, argues strongly that whatever mechanisms account for language organization are relatively immune to significant alterations in sensory input. Caution must be exercised here, however, since these comments generally refer to the outcome of studies performed on persons with acquired hearing loss. Naturalistic or descriptive studies of patients with congenital hearing loss are always susceptible to the criticism that whatever agent or agents produced the sensory impairment may also have produced concomitant impairment of nonsensory mechanisms. Nevertheless, comparisons of young infants and hearing-impaired adults, with respect to behavioral studies, suggest that there is a sufficiently rich sensory representation of the acoustic environment to permit the development of language skills much earlier than they naturally emerge. Electrophysiologic comparisons of human newborns and adults also suggest that the diminished auditory sensitivity and alterations in the frequency contour of sensitivity are insufficient to explain age differences in language comprehension and production performance. It may well be that the brain mechanisms responsible for the establishment of language behavior are sufficiently flexible to accommodate even a greatly impoverished sensory representation. The inability of hair cells to regenerate following acoustic trauma or other peripheral auditory impairments and the absence of alternative transducer mechanisms in the inner ear are in sharp contrast to the well-described, although poorly understood, "plasticity" of the central nervous system. I think that any limitations imposed by sensory mechanisms on the acquisition or maintenance of language skills are unlikely to be described from a linear systems analysis perspective. It is only with the application of nonlinear systems techniques and input signals that specifically elicit nonlinear mechanisms that we may hope to discover any restrictive interactions between language and sensory development.

ACKNOWLEDGMENTS

The author thanks Jan Habich for her technical support and the many students and colleagues who have contributed to the laboratory's efforts over the years. Work was supported by NIH grant #RO1N16436 and Project Phoenix of Madison.

REFERENCES

1. Aslin, R.N., Pisoni, D.B., and Jusczyk, P.W. (1983): Auditory development and speech perception in infancy. In: *Infancy and the Biology of Development. Vol. II of Carmichael's Manual of Child Psychology (4th ed.)*, edited by M.M. Haith and J.J. Campos. Wiley, New York.
2. Eimas, P.D. (1974): Auditory and linguistic processing of cues for place of articulation by infants. *Perception and Psychophysics*, 16:513–521.
3. Hall, J.L. (1980): Cochlear models: Evidence in support of mechanical nonlinearity and a second filter (a review). *Hearing Research*, 2:455–464.
4. Harris, D.M., and Dallos, P. (1984): Ontogenetic changes in frequency mapping of a mammalian ear. *Science*, 225:741–743.
5. Hecox, K.E. (1975): Electrophysiological correlates of human auditory developement. In: *Infant Perception: From Sensation to Cognition*, vol. 11, edited by L.B. Cohen, and P. Salapatek. Academic Press, New York.
6. Hecox, K.E., and Burkhard, R. (1983): Developmental dependencies of the human BAER. *Ann. NY Acad. of Sci.*, 388:538–556.
7. Hecox, K., and Galambos, R. (1974): Brainstem auditory evoked responses in human infants and adults. *Arch. Otolaryngol.*, 99:30–33.
8. Holmberg, T.L., Morgan, K,A., and Kuhl, P.K. (1977): Speech perception in early infancy: Discrimination of fricative consonants. Paper presented at the 94th Meeting of the Acoustical Society of America, Miami Beach, FL, December 12–16.
9. Jesteadt, W., and Norton, S. (1985): The role of suppression in psychophysic measures of frequency selectivity. *JASA*, 78:365–374.
10. Jusczyk, P.W. (1986): Toward a model of the development of speech perception. In: *Invariance and Variability in Speech Processes*, edited by J.S. Perkell and D.H. Klatt. Lawrence Erlbaum, Hillside, NJ.
11. Jusczyk, P.W., Copan, H.C., and Thompson, E.J. (1978): Perception by two-month-olds of glide contrasts in multisyllabic utterances. *Perception and Psychophysics*, 24:515–520.
12. Jusczyk, P.W., Murray, J., and Bayly, J. (1979). Perception of place-of articulation in fricatives and stops by infants. Paper presented at the biennial meeting of the Society for Research in Child Development, San Francisco, CA, March.
13. Kim, D. (1986): Overview of nonlinear and active cochlear models. In: *Peripheral Auditory Mechanisms*, edited by J. Allen, J. Hall, A. Hubbard, S. Neely, and A. Tubis, pp. 298–305. Springer, New York.

14. Kuhl, P.K. (1983): Perception of auditory equivalence classes for speech in early infancy. *Infant Behavior and Development*, 6:263–285.
15. Lasky, R.E., Syrdal-Lasky, A., and Klein, R.E. (1975): VOT discrimination by four- to six-and-a-half month old infants from Spanish environments. *J. Exp. Child Psychol.*, 20:213–225.
16. Lippe, W., and Rubel, E.W. (1983): Development of the place principle: Tarotepic organization. *Science*, 219:514.
17. Miller, C.L., Morse, P.A., and Dorman, M. (1977): Cardiac indices of infant speech perception: Orienting and burst discrimination. *Q. J. Exp. Psychol.*, 29:533–545.
18. Moffit, A.R. (1971): Consonant cue perception by twenty- to twenty-four-week-old infants. *Child Dev.*, 42:717–731.
19. Picton, T.W., Hillyard, S.H., Krauz, H.J., et al. (1974): Human auditory evoked potentials. I. Evaluation of components. *Electroencephalogr. Clin. Neurophysiol.*, 36:179–190.
20. Rubel, E.W. (1976): In: *Handbook of Sensory Physiology, Vol. 9, Development of Sensory Systems*, edited by M. Jacobson. Springer-Verlag, Berlin.
21. Rubel, E.W., and Ryals, B.M. (1983): Development of the place principle: Acoustic trauma. *Science*, 219:512.
22. Sellick, P.M., Patuzzi, R., and Johnstone, B.M. (1983): Comparison between the tuning properties of inner hair cells and basilar membrane motion. *Hear. Res.*, 10(1):93–100.
23. Streeter, L.A. (1976): Language perception of 2-month-old infants shows effects of both innate mechanisms and experience. *Nature*, 259:39–41.
24. Worden, F.G. (1972): Auditory processing of biologically significant sounds. *Neurosciences Research Program Bulletin*, NRP Work Session, vol. 10.

*Language, Communication, and
the Brain*, edited by F. Plum.
Raven Press, New York © 1988.

Contextual Effects in Language Comprehension: Studies Using Event-Related Brain Potentials

Marta Kutas and Steven A. Hillyard

*Department of Neurosciences, University of California, San Diego,
La Jolla, California 92093*

In natural spoken or written language, the individual words of a message are understood in relation to the context built up by previous words. A coherent interpretation is achieved by integrating the meanings of successive words within the evolving context. One aspect of this interpretive system is the formation of expectancies for words that are about to occur in the message. In many cases, the subsequent words in a sentence can be predicted accurately after hearing the first few words. These word expectancy effects are readily observable in everyday life when our friends helpfully finish our sentences with an annoying degree of precision. In the more dispassionate setting of the laboratory, it has been shown that word expectancies play an important role in language comprehension (e.g., 6,17,28,33,35–37).

Most studies of context and word expectancy effects have measured verbal or manual reaction times to the stimuli of interest. An alternative approach that we have taken is to record the electrical responses of the brain (event-related potentials or ERPs) that are associated with the processing of individual words in sentences. The ERPs triggered by sensory stimuli represent summated field potentials arising from the neuronal circuits engaged in processing of stimulus information (14). ERPs can be recorded noninvasively from the scalp in the form of voltage-time waveforms that include a number of peaks or ''components'' at specific latencies.

There are two principal advantages of the ERP technique in studies of language processing. First, the method is nonintrusive, in that the subjects need not perform a secondary behavioral task (such as making a speeded motor response) that might interfere with the reading or listening process under investigation. Second, the ERP latencies give a measure of processing differences that are more closely coupled in time with the relevant cerebral events rather than being delayed by several hundred msec, as are reaction time (RT) measures. In general, ERP recordings and behavioral measures provide converging and mutually complementary data for isolating and defining the processes underlying language comprehension.

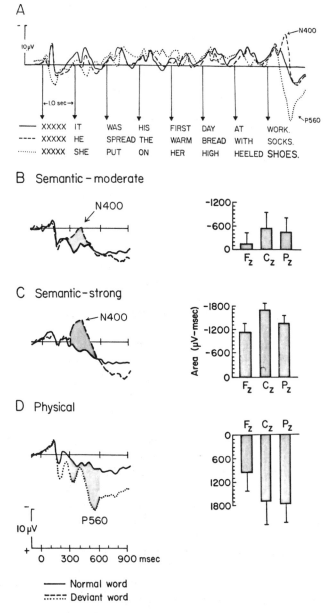

FIG. 1. Event-related potentials elicited by semantically and physically incongruous words occurring unpredictably at the ends of visually presented sentences. **A:** timing of word presentations for three sample sentences and typical ERP waveforms elicited by each sentence type. Note the N400 wave following semantically anomalous ending "socks." **B–D:** In each comparison, grand average ERPs for congruous (*solid line*) and deviant (semantic, *dashed line*; physical, *dotted line*) terminal words are superimposed. The 300-msec area that was quantified is indicated by shading. The means and S.E. of these difference areas (for deviant minus normal endings) are shown in bar graphs at right. From Kutas and Hillyard (19).

The experimental design that we have used in a number of ERP studies of contextual effects is illustrated at the top of Fig. 1 (20). A series of sentences (160 or more) was presented to the subjects, one word at a time, on a video monitor. The only instruction was to read the sentences, with the understanding that questions may be asked about their contents at the end of the experiment. The sentences differed in the degree to which the terminal words fit the context established by the initial words. Some of the sentences were terminated by expected, congruous words, and others ended with semantically anomalous words and still others with physically incongruous words in bold-face type. Sentences having these various types of endings were presented in unpredictable order.

The ERP averaged over the semantically incongruous endings was characterized by a broad negative deflection that had its onset at about 200 msec and peaked at 400 msec; this negative peak was not evident in the ERPs to semantically acceptable endings. The amplitude of this "N400" was larger for those terminal words that were the most highly discrepant from the sentence context. In contrast, the unpredictable occurrence of physically deviant words in bold-face type elicited a late positive complex of waves rather than a negativity.

Subsequent experiments demonstrated that other types of nonsemantic deviations in sentence contexts similarly failed to elicit an N400 wave. Grammatical errors of various types appearing unpredictably in a text elicited only small and inconsistent late waves (Fig. 2) that did not have the posterior, right-sided scalp distribution

SEMANTIC DEVIATION

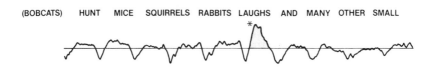

GRAMMATICAL DEVIATION

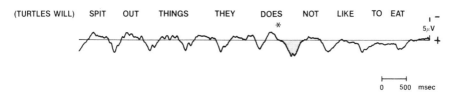

FIG. 2. Comparison of ERPs to semantically and grammatically deviant words presented unpredictably in prose passages. ERPs shown are averaged over several dozen different deviant words of each class for each subject. Note that semantic anomalies elicit an N400 wave, whereas grammatical deviations (incorrect noun number, verb tense, or verb number) do not. Based on data from Kutas and Hillyard (20).

characteristic of the N400 elicited by semantic anomalies (Fig. 3), nor did the occasional appearance of exotic, colored ("modern art") slides in place of words in a text elicit an N400 wave, but rather a late ERP complex consisting of a frontal N300 and a parietal P450 wave (21). Deviant events within a patterned physical sequence or deviant notes within a musical passage also appear to trigger a late parietal positivity that resembles the well-known P300 wave rather than a late negativity (2).

On the other hand, semantic anomalies in linguistic communications were found to elicit N400 waves whether the modality of presentation was auditory, visual, or

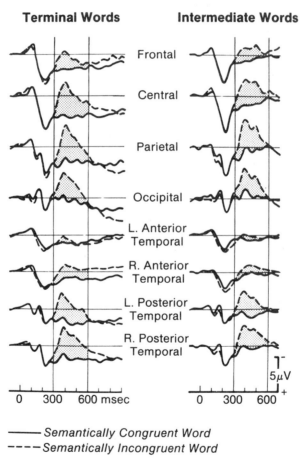

Terminal Words   **Intermediate Words**

Frontal

Central

Parietal

Occipital

L. Anterior Temporal

R. Anterior Temporal

L. Posterior Temporal

R. Posterior Temporal

0   300   600 msec   0   300   600

5μV

———— *Semantically Congruent Word*
---- *Semantically Incongruent Word*

FIG. 3. Grand average ERPs from eight scalp sites elicited by semantically anomalous (*dashed lines*) and semantically congruous (*solid lines*) words in a prose passage. Note N400 component to anomalous words is largest over parietal and posterior temporal areas, with a slight right hemispheric preponderance. N400 waves are elicited equally well by anomalous words at the ends of sentences (left column) and at intermediate positions in the sentences (right column). From Kutas and Hillyard (20).

American Sign Language (15,24,27,29). In each modality the anomalous word or sign triggered an N400 having the typical, posterior scalp distribution, suggesting that a common mode of processing was activated by the semantic discrepancies. These observations narrow the possible interpretations that may be given to the processes underlying the N400. The elicitation of N400 waves by anomalies in spoken language indicates that this ERP does not depend on the transformation of orthographic into phonological representations (i.e., phonemic recoding), since this step is not required when listening to speech, nor does the N400 reflect the accessing of a word's meaning through phonology (i.e., its sound), since this process is obviously absent in congenitally deaf users of sign language. Evidently, the N400 wave is independent of the surface structure and modality of the language in which the anomalies are presented.

A number of studies have demonstrated that semantic anomaly is not a prerequisite for eliciting the N400 wave (7,8,22,23). Instead, the N400 amplitude appears to grow systematically as a function of how unexpected a word is in a given context, with anomalies representing one end of the continuum of expectedness. In one experiment (22), for example, subjects were presented with 320 sentences that all had semantically acceptable endings but varied in the degree to which the terminal word was predictable (expected), as established by the Cloze procedure (3). Sentences varied from those with highly constrained and predictable endings ("He mailed the letter without a *stamp*.") to more open-ended sentences with less predictable endings ("He was soothed by the gentle *wind*."). Recordings of ERPs to the terminal words showed that N400 amplitude was an inverse function of word expectancy (Fig. 4). The correlation between N400 amplitude and Cloze probability was above 0.9 at posterior electrode sites.

The finding that N400 amplitudes were systematically reduced for more expected words suggested that this ERP might be a manifestation of a semantic priming process (22). Semantic priming is generally conceived as a process whereby specific representations in semantic memory are partially activated by the presentation of a prior stimulus or context. Memory representations of words and their associated meanings are activated according to their semantic or associative relationship to the priming stimulus. Words that have had their representations primed by a prior context can be accessed and recognized faster and more reliably than can unprimed words [for a review see (9)]. Since N400 amplitude varied in a manner similar to behavioral measures of priming, we suggested that the N400 elicited by a word was a graded, inverse measure of the extent to which that word had been primed by the prior context (22).

A number of experimental observations have lent support to the hypothesis linking semantic priming and N400. Fischler and colleagues (8) found that the N400 to terminal words in sentences of the form "A robin is a *bird*" and "A sparrow is not a *vehicle*" did not depend on the truth or falsity of the proposition but rather on the degree of semantic association between the principal noun arguments in the sentence. Thus the word "vehicle" would elicit a large N400 by virtue of not having been primed by "sparrow," even though the sentence is perfectly acceptable

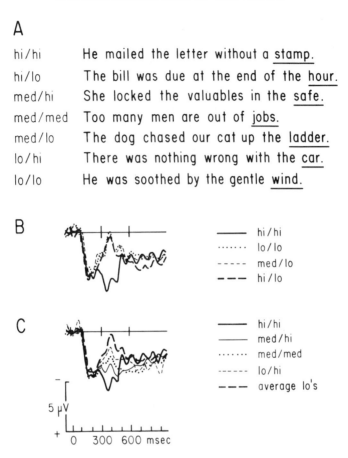

A

hi/hi	He mailed the letter without a <u>stamp</u>.
hi/lo	The bill was due at the end of the <u>hour</u>.
med/hi	She locked the valuables in the <u>safe</u>.
med/med	Too many men are out of <u>jobs</u>.
med/lo	The dog chased our cat up the <u>ladder</u>.
lo/hi	There was nothing wrong with the <u>car</u>.
lo/lo	He was soothed by the gentle <u>wind</u>.

B

—— hi/hi
········ lo/lo
- - - - med/lo
— — hi/lo

C

—— hi/hi
—— med/hi
········ med/med
------ lo/hi
— — average lo's

5 μV

0   300   600 msec

FIG. 4. A: Examples of seven sentences that varied both in degree of contextual constraint and in Cloze probability of the terminal word. On the left are shown the degree of contextual constraint/cloze probability for each sentence class. **B:** Comparison of grand average ERP to words having a high Cloze probability (*solid line*) with ERPs to words of low Cloze probability (*dotted* and *dashed lines*). All low Cloze probability words elicited on N400, regardless of the degree of contextual constraint. **C:** Grand average ERPs to low, medium, and high Cloze probability words terminating sentences of medium contextual constraint. From Kutas and Hillyard (22).

grammatically and semantically. A similar effect of semantic association was found when anomalous or low probability sentence endings were segregated according to whether they were semantically related to the most expected endings (22,23). Terminal words that were related to the most expected and, hence, the most primed endings elicited a smaller N400 than did unrelated endings, even though both types of endings were nonsensical. In the sample sentences shown in Fig. 5, for example, the terminal word "drink," which is a semantic associate of the most expected ending "eat," elicited a smaller N400 than did the completely unrelated ending

THE PIZZA WAS TOO HOT TO

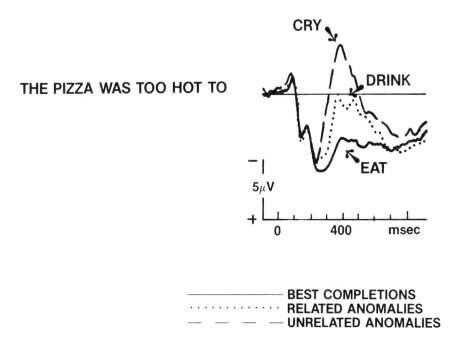

——————— BEST COMPLETIONS
· · · · · · · · · · · · RELATED ANOMALIES
— — — — UNRELATED ANOMALIES

FIG. 5. Grand average ERPs to the most expected terminal words (best completions) and to semantically anomalous words that were either related or unrelated to the best completion. Note that N400 is reduced when anomalous endings are related to the most expected ending. Sample endings are for illustrative purposes only, since the same sentence frames were never repeated in this experiment. Data from Kutas et al. (23).

"cry." Such results were interpreted in terms of a partial priming of the related but incongruous ending.

If the N400 amplitude indeed reflects the amount of semantic priming a word has received from prior context, one would also expect to find N400 waves elicited by all the words in a sentence, varying in amplitude to the extent that each had been semantically primed by prior words. Such N400s can be observed by making across-sentence averages on a longer time base (Fig. 6) (26). These averages highlighted the lateral asymmetry of the N400 component (right hemisphere more negative than left), an asymmetry that was reduced in subjects having a family history of left-handedness. The N400 was found to be larger to the open class (i.e., content) words in the sentences than to the closed class (i.e., function) words; this may reflect a difference in memory organization for these two types of words although other factors such as frequency of usage, concreteness, and word length could not be ruled out in this experiment. In accordance with the priming hypothesis, N400 amplitudes were reduced for the last few content words in a sentence, presumably because they had received more extensive priming from the earlier words.

ERPs that appear equivalent to the N400 have also been observed in studies in which sequences of content words rather than sentences were presented. When the

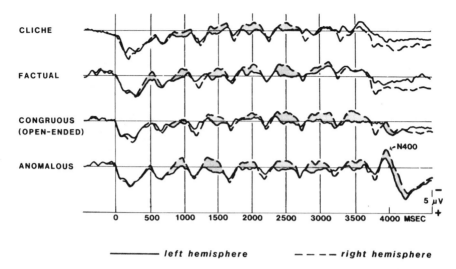

CLICHE

FACTUAL

CONGRUOUS
(OPEN-ENDED)

ANOMALOUS

N400

5 μV

0   500   1000 1500 2000 2500 3000 3500 4000 MSEC

———————— *left hemisphere*   — — — — *right hemisphere*

FIG. 6. Grand average ERPs to warning stimuli at time zero (xxxxx) and subsequent seven word sentences, recorded from left and right posterior temporal sites. ERPs to three different types of congruous sentences and to semantically anomalous sentences are shown. Note N400 to terminal word in latter case. From Kutas et al. (26).

first few words of a sequence belonged to one semantic class (e.g., names of cities, birds, and the like), the final word elicited a smaller late negativity at 300 to 400 msec when it was from the same semantic class than when it belonged to a different class (5,13,30). Bentin et al. (1) presented subjects with sequences of words and pseudowords and asked them to make a lexical decision on each item. Again, it was found that words preceded by semantically related words elicited a smaller late negativity than words preceded by unrelated words. The authors related this reduction of N400 to a facilitation of RT for the lexical decision when a word was preceded by semantic associates. Such facilitation is frequently interpreted as an index of semantic priming.

The N400 also behaves as an index of semantic priming in studies in which ERPs were recorded to pairs of words that varied in their degree of semantic association (4,16,18,32). In the study of Kutas (18), for example, each trial consisted of two words separated by a stimulus onset asynchrony (SOA) of 700 msec, followed by a single letter probe. The subject's task was to indicate whether the probe letter was contained in either of the two prior words. Even though this task was designed not to draw the subject's attention to the semantic relationship between the two words it was clear that related word pairs had smaller N400 amplitudes than did unrelated pairs (Fig. 7, left). This suggests that the N400 differences in this task may have reflected an automatic component of semantic priming. In another condition (Fig. 7, right), the subject's attention was actively directed to the semantic relationship between the two words by requiring them to rate the strength of the semantic association between them. This manipulation did not appear to alter the

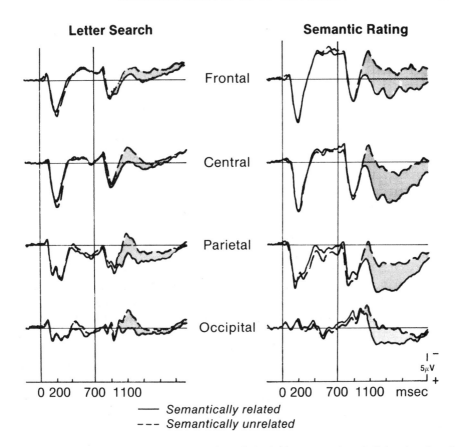

Letter Search   **Semantic Rating**

Frontal

Central

Parietal

Occipital

$5\mu V$

0 200 700 1100   0 200 700 1100 msec

—— *Semantically related*
--- *Semantically unrelated*

FIG. 7. Grand average ERPs to pairs of words in the letter search task (left column) and semantic rating task (right column). Note larger N400 when second member of word pair is semantically unrelated to the first word. From Kutas and Van Petten (25).

N400 difference between related and unrelated word pairs prior to about 400 msec; after 400 msec the related words elicited an enhanced late positivity. These results suggest that both automatic and attentional components of priming may be reflected in the ERP.

All the evidence reviewed above appears consistent with the view that the N400 wave is closely related to semantic priming processes. Although there are indications that N400 amplitudes may be sensitive to other forms of priming based on phonology and orthography (25,31), it is clear that semantic associations and context exert the strongest influence over this ERP. This finding suggests that the N400 should be useful in the diagnosis and clinical evaluation both of psychopathological conditions in which word associations are made abnormally and of language disorders in which word meanings are not accesssed and related to contexts in the normal manner. Although we are not aware of any studies that employed the N400 measure to evaluate such clinical conditions, we have used this approach to study a cerebral system that reportedly has its own peculiar language organization— the right cerebral hemisphere of split-brain (cerebral commissurotomy) patients.

The interest in studying commissurotomy patients with ERPs stems from a controversy that has emerged from behavioral studies of right hemisphere language in these patients. On the one hand, Zaidel (38–40) has reported that the surgically separated right hemispheres of two West Coast patients (L.B. and N.G.) possess lexical semantics together with a rudimentary syntactic capability and an impoverished phonological system; this pattern suggested that right hemisphere language has different operating principles from those of left hemisphere language. On the other hand, Gazzaniga and associates (11,12,34) described a marked individual variation in right hemisphere language in a separate group of split-brain patients. This variability was taken as evidence against there being general qualitative differences between the language systems of the left and right hemispheres that would be applicable to all cases (10).

We (M. Kutas, S.A. Hillyard, and M.S. Gazzaniga, *in preparation*) compared the properties of left and right hemisphere language in five commissurotomy patients using a combination of behavioral and ERP methods. The main focus of interest was to determine whether the separated hemispheres were each capable of producing an N400 wave to semantic anomalies presented in a lateralized manner to one hemisphere at a time. Using this ERP index of semantic processing, we addressed the question of whether qualitatively similar neural systems are engaged when the right and left hemispheres are confronted with semantic anomalies.

Subjects were presented with 200 to 300 seven-word sentences in blocks of 20 each. The first six words were presented auditorily, at intervals of about 600 msec, and each sentence was completed by a 180-msec exposure of two words on a video terminal screen, one in the left visual field (LVF) and one in the right visual field (RVF). For 60% of the sentences, the words in the two visual fields were identical and semantically appropriate for the preceding context. The remaining 40% of the terminal word pairs contained anomalies: some had an anomalous word in one visual field (RVF or LVF, on a random basis) and a congruous word in the opposite field, and other sentences had inappropriate endings in both fields. On occasion, the subject was asked to name or write the terminal words that they had recently been shown. The order of normal and anomalous endings was randomized.

The ERPs were averaged separately according to whether semantically anomalous terminal words occurred in the RVF, LVF, both fields simultaneously, or neither field. "Difference waves" were then formed to reveal the N400 component by subtracting the ERP to the bilateral congruous word pairs from each of the ERPs to the word pairs containing unilateral or bilateral anomalies. The shaded areas in the difference waves in Fig. 8 represent the N400 effect associated with the differential processing of the anomaly.

Normal control subjects showed large N400 waves to either LVF or RVF anomalies (Fig. 8, left column). However, the split-brain subjects differed markedly in the amplitude of the N400 to LVF anomalies. Two of the patients (P.S. and

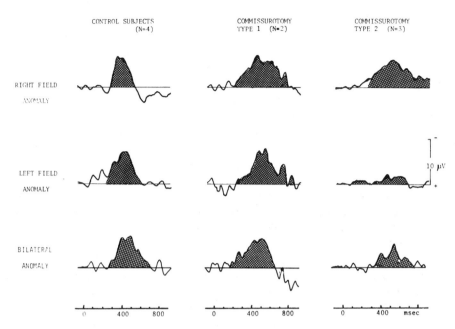

FIG. 8. Difference waves showing the N400 effect (*shaded area*) as a function of whether the anomalous word was presented to the RVF, LVF, or to both fields at once. Each difference wave was formed by subtracting the ERP to bilateral congruous endings from the ERP to the indicated type of anomaly. ERPs are shown averaged over normal control subjects (left), split-brain subjects who showed N400 waves to RVF anomalies (center), and split-brain subjects who did not (right). ERPs were recorded from a midline parietal electrode. Preliminary data from Kutas, Hillyard, and Gazzaniga, *in preparation*.

V.P.—whose data are averaged in the middle column) displayed large N400 waves to LVF anomalies, whereas three others (J.W., N.G., and L.B., right column) showed little or no N400 activity to LVF anomalies.

Although there was considerable intersubject variability in the amplitude of the N400 to bilateral anomalies, for no patient was the bilateral N400 appreciably larger than those elicited by either unilateral anomaly. This finding that the amplitude of the N400 elicited by bilateral anomalies does not approximate the linear sum of the amplitudes engendered by the unilateral LVF and RVF anomalies is inconsistent with the hypothesis that each hemisphere generates its own N400 wave independently of the other.

The large N400 amplitudes elicited by anomalous LVF words in patients P.S. and V.P. correspond with behavioral evidence that these two patients possess more highly developed right hemispheric language systems than do the other three patients. From the time of their surgery P.S. and V.P. were more advanced in syntactic competence, response to commands, and word rhyming judgments than the other patients; most significantly, both P.S. and V.P. have shown evidence for expressive language (overt speech) under the control of the right hemisphere (11,12,34). Thus, there seems to be a general association between the "generative capacity" of the right hemisphere in these patients and the production of an N400 to semantic anomaly. The ERP evidence is thus consistent with findings of considerable variability in the organization of language in the right hemisphere.

The interpretation of these N400 differences among the patients is aided by behavioral tests that were made in conjunction with the ERP studies. In separate sessions, subjects were shown congruous and incongruous sentence endings lateralized to the LVF and were asked to judge them as "sense" or "nonsense" by pointing to written response choices with the left hand. It was found that all patients, even those who did not produce an N400 to LVF semantic anomalies, could nonetheless make the semantic judgment of sense versus nonsense at an above-chance level. In particular, the right hemispheres of patients J.W., N.G., and L.B. were able to judge whether a word fit a semantic context, but they apparently did so by a mechanism that did not engender the N400 that characterizes the left hemisphere's response to semantic anomaly.

In light of the hypothesis that N400 is a sign of a semantic priming process, it might be expected that the right hemispheres of patients J.W., N.G., and L.B. would show less behavioral evidence of priming than would those of patients P.S. and V.P. Insofar as data are available, this appears to be the case (K.M. Baynes and M.S. Gazzaniga, this volume; 41). Thus, the right hemispheric language systems of the split-brain patients show marked interindividual variability along a number of dimensions that appear to include qualitative differences in the mechanisms by which semantic memory is organized, primed, and accessed.

ACKNOWLEDGMENTS

The work reported in this chapter has been supported by grants from NSF (BNS 83-09243), NINCDS (NS 17778), and NICHD (HD 22614). M. Kutas is supported by an RCDA Award from NIMH (MH 00322).

REFERENCES

1. Bentin, S., McCarthy, G., and Wood, C.C. (1985): Event-related potentials, lexical decision and semantic priming. *Electroencephalogr. Clin. Neurophysiol.*, 60:343–355.
2. Besson, M., Macar, F., and Pynte, J. (1984): Is N400 specifically related to the processing of semantic mismatch? *Soc. Neurosci. Abstr.*, 10:847.
3. Bloom, P.A., and Fischer, I. (1980): Completion norms for 329 sentence contexts. *Mem. Cognition*, 8:631–642.
4. Boddy, J. (1986): Event-related potentials in chronometric analysis of primed word recognition with different stimulus onset asynchronies. *Psychophysiology*, 23:232–245.
5. Boddy, J., and Weinberg, H. (1981): Brain potentials, perceptual mechanisms and semantic categorization. *Biol. Psychol.*, 12:43–61.
6. Fischler, I., and Bloom, P.A. (1979): Automatic and attentional processes in the effects of sentence contexts on word recognition. *J. Verb. Learn. Verb. Behav.*, 18:1–20.
7. Fischler, I., Bloom, P.A., Childers, D.G., Arroyo, A.A., and Perry, N.W. (1984): Brain potentials during sentence verification: Late negativity and long-term memory strength. *Neuropsychologia*, 22:559–568.

8. Fischler, I., Bloom, P.A., Childers, D.G., Roucos, S.E., and Perry, N.W., Jr. (1983): Brain potentials related to stages of sentence verification. *Psychophysiology*, 20:400–409.

9. Foss, D.J. (1982): A discourse on semantic priming. *Cognitive Psychol.*, 14:590–607.

10. Gazzaniga, M.S. (1983): Right hemisphere language following brain bisection: A twenty year perspective. *Am. Psychol.*, 38:525–537.

11. Gazzaniga, M.S., Smylie, C.S., Baynes, K., Hirst, W., and McCleary, C.A. (1984): Profiles of right hemisphere language and speech following brain bisection. *Brain Lang.*, 22:206–220.

12. Gazzaniga, M.S., Volpe, B.T., Smylie, C.S., Wilson, D.H., and LeDoux, J.E. (1979): Plasticity in speech organization following commissurotomy. *Brain*, 102:805–815.

13. Harbin, T.J., Marsh, G.R., and Harvey, M.T. (1984): Differences in the late components of the event-related potential due to age and to semantic and non-semantic tasks. *Electroencephalogr. Clin. Neurophysiol.*, 59:489–496.

14. Hillyard, S.A., and Kutas, M. (1983): Electrophysiology of cognitive processing. *Annu. Rev. Psychol.*, 34:33–61.

15. Holcomb, P.J. (1985): Unimodal and multimodal models of lexical memory: An ERP analysis. *Psychophysiology*, 22:576.

16. Holcomb, P.J. (1986): ERP correlates of semantic facilitation. *Electroencephalogr. Clin. Neurophysiol.*, 38(suppl.):320–322.

17. Kleiman, G.M. (1980): Sentence frames, context, and lexical decisions: Sentence compatibility and word-relatedness effects. *Mem. Cognition*, 8:336–344.

18. Kutas, M. (1985): ERP comparisons of the effects of single word and sentence contexts on word processing. *Psychophysiology*, 22:575–576 (Abstr.).

19. Kutas, M., and Hillyard, S.A. (1980): Reading senseless sentences: Brain potentials reflect semantic incongruity. *Science*, 207:203–205.

20. Kutas, M., and Hillyard, S.A. (1983): Event-related brain potentials to grammatical errors and semantic anomalies. *Mem. Cognition*, 11:539–550.

21. Kutas, M., and Hillyard, S.A. (1984): Event-related brain potentials (ERPs) elicited by "novel" stimuli during sentence processing. *Ann. NY Acad. Sci.*, 425:236–241.

22. Kutas, M., and Hillyard, S.A. (1984): Brain potentials during reading reflext word expectancy and semantic association. *Nature*, 307:161–163.

23. Kutas, M., Lindamood, T.E., and Hillyard, S.A. (1984): Word expectancy and event-related brain potentials during sentence processing. In: *Preparatory States and Processes*, edited by S. Kornblum and J. Requin, pp. 217–237. Lawrence Erlbaum, Hillsdale, NJ.

24. Kutas, M., Neville, H.J., and Holcomb, P.J. A preliminary comparison of the N400 response to semantic anomalies during reading, listening and signing. *Electroencephalogr. Clin. Neurophysiol.* [Suppl]. (in press).

25. Kutas, M., and Van Petten, C. Event related brain potential studies of language. In: *Advances in Psychophysiology*, edited by P.K. Ackles, J.R. Jennings, and M.G.H. Coles. JAI Press, Greenwich, CT (in press).

26. Kutas, M., Van Petten, C., and Besson, M. Event-related potential asymmetries during the reading of sentences. *Electroencephalogr. Clin. Neurophysiol.* (in press).

27. McCallum, W.C., Farmer, S.F., and Pocock, P.V. (1984): The effects of physical and semantic incongruities on auditory event-related potentials. *Electroencephalogr. Clin. Neurophysiol.*, 59:477–488.

28. Morton, J., and Long, J. (1976): Effect of transitional probability on phoneme identification. *J. Verb. Learn. Verb. Behav.*, 15:43–51.

29. Neville, H.J. (1985): Biological constraints on semantic processing: A comparison of spoken and signed languages. *Psychophysiology*, 22:576.

30. Polich, J. (1985): Semantic categorization and event-related potentials. *Brain Lang.*, 24:304–321.

31. Rugg, M.D. (1984): Event-related potentials and the phonological processing of words and non-words. *Neuropsychologia*, 22:435–443.

32. Sanquist, T.F., Rohrbaugh, J.W., Syndulko, K., and Lindsley, D.B. (1980): Electrocortical signs of levels of processing: Perceptual analysis and recognition memory. *Psychophysiology*, 17:568–576.

33. Schuberth, R.E., and Eimas, P.D. (1977): Effects of context on the classification of words and nonwords. *J. Exp. Psychol. [Hum. Percept]*, 3:27–36.

34. Sidtis, J.J., Volpe, B.T., Wilson, D.H., Rayport, M., and Gazzaniga, M.S. (1981): Variability in right hemisphere language function after callosal section: Evidence for a continuum of generative capacity. *J. Neurosci.*, 1:323–331.

35. Tyler, L. K., and Marslen-Wilson, W. D. (1977): The on-line effects of semantic context on syntactic processing. *J. Verb. Learn. Verb. Behav.*, 16:683–692.
36. Underwood, G., and Bargh, K. (1982): Word shape, orthographic regularity and contextual interactions in a reading task. *Cognition*, 12:197–209.
37. West, R. F., and Stanovich, K. E. (1982): Source of inhibition in experiments on the effect of sentence context on word recognition. *J. Exp. Psychol. [Learn. Mem. Cogn.]*, 8:385–389.
38. Zaidel, E. (1978): Auditory language comprehension in the right hemisphere following cerebral commissurotomy and hemispherectomy: A comparison with child language and aphasia. In: *Language Acquisition and Language Breakdown: Parallels and Divergencies*, edited by A. Caramazza and E. B. Zurif, pp. 229–275. The Johns Hopkins University Press, Baltimore.
39. Zaidel, E. (1978): Lexical organization in the right hemisphere. In: *Cerebral Correlates of Conscious Experience*, edited by A. Buser and A. Rougeul-Buser, pp. 177–197. INSERM Symposium No. 6. Elsevier, Amsterdam.
40. Zaidel, E. (1979): The split and half brains as models of congenital language disability. In: *The Neurological Bases of Language Disorders in Children: Methods and Directions for Research*, edited by C. L. Ludlow and M. E. Doran-Quine, pp. 55–89. NINCDS Monograph No. 22. U.S. Government Printing Office, Washington, DC.
41. Zaidel, E. (1983): Disconnection syndrome as a model for laterality effects in the normal brain. In: *Cerebral Hemisphere Asymmetry: Method, Theory, and Applications*, edited by J. B. Hellige, pp. 95–151. Praeger, New York.

Language, Communication, and
the Brain, edited by F. Plum.
Raven Press, New York © 1988.

Effect of Cortical and Subcortical Stimulation on Human Language and Verbal Memory

George A. Ojemann

*Department of Neurological Surgery,
University of Washington School of Medicine,
Seattle, Washington 98195*

This chapter reviews the brain mechanisms that underlie human language and memory from the perspective provided by effects of electrical stimulation during neurosurgical operations under local anesthesia. This perspective provides a model for those brain mechanisms that differs in a number of ways from the traditional models derived from pooling the location of lesions, particularly strokes, associated with various types of aphasias and memory deficits.

The application of an electrical current to a local area of brain has a variety of physiological effects (40). Neurons or fibers, with either excitatory or inhibitory effects locally or at a distance, may be activated by a current, or the same current may block function in some or all of these elements, through depolarization. Thus, the predominant effect of the current cannot be predicted physiologically, but must be determined empirically. On that basis, local application of a train of 60 Hz, 1 msec duration biphasic pulses delivered in a bipolar manner through electrodes separated by 5 mm, at a current level below the threshold needed to evoke an afterdischarge, generally evokes effects only from primary motor or sensory systems in the brain of a quiet patient. These responses are usually of a "positive" nature, evoked movements or sensations, that likely represent a predominance of excitatory stimulation effects. Application of this current to many brain areas outside these systems, including almost all of association cortex, has *no* detectable effect in the quiet patient.

However, if the patient is engaged in a language task, application of the same current to some, but not all of these same areas will now disturb performance on that task. Presumably the predominant effect of stimulation there is a blocking of function in a brain area that is essential for performance of the language task. In that case, stimulation and lesions would be expected to relate the same brain areas to a language function, as both make the link between a particular behavior and brain area when failure of function in the brain area is associated with a failure in the behavior. This relationship between the effects of stimulation and lesions has been examined in the anterior temporal lobe of the language-dominant hemisphere, for two language behaviors, naming of simple objects and performance on a recent verbal memory measure. Deficits on a standard aphasia battery were significantly more likely following an anterior temporal resection that encroached on a site where stimulation had repeatedly disturbed object naming than when the resection did not encroach on such sites (22). Deficits on a measure of recent verbal memory were more likely when such a resection included or encroached on sites related to recent verbal memory by stimulation (27). Both studies, then, suggested that stimulation and lesions related the same brain areas to a particular language function. Thus, this type of stimulation effect seems to represent a temporary lesion.

There are several other effects of stimulation during language and verbal memory measures that seem to reflect a predominance of excitatory processes. One effect is an acceleration of the rate of memory retrieval with left ventrolateral thalamic stimulation, an effect considered to be part of an evoked alerting response for verbal material [see "subcortical stimulation" section and (25)]. These subcortical alerting circuits, then, may be another brain system that, like motor and sensory systems, responds to stimulation with predominantly excitatory effects. Another stimulation effect that seems to represent excitatory processes is the acceleration of the production of the speech sound /s/ evoked from selected sites in lateral association cortex (46).

The different perspective on the brain organization of language provided by stimulation techniques is attributable to a number of special features of that technique compared with more traditional lesion-based techniques. Stimulation can be applied to many sites in an individual patient, limited only by the available surgical exposure. Thus a map of the sites essential for one or more language function in an *individual* subject can be obtained. By contrast, when examining the effects of a lesion, only the one damaged area can be related to behavioral changes in an individual subject. In addition, stimulation effects can be turned on and off, and thus used as a probe to separate the relationship of a site to such potentially overlapping processes as memory input, storage or retrieval, or speech production and perception. However, stimulation techniques have generally been applied only to special populations, i.e, those with the indications for neurosurgical procedures under local anesthesia. Most often patients undergoing cortical exposures under local anesthesia have had medically intractable epilepsy, whereas those with subcortical procedures have had dyskinesias, such as Parkinson's disease or pain problems. The generalization of findings in these special populations is uncertain. However, this problem also applies to investigations of language organization with traditional lesion-based approaches, for the largest group of patients studied with these techniques, the elderly with strokes, also constitute a special population (15). Generalization of findings depends on corroborative evidence from multiple special populations.

CORTICAL STIMULATION

Effects on Naming

Naming of objects was the function used in the initial studies of the brain organization for language using stimulation techniques, conducted by Penfield and his associates (39). Findings in a large series of patients were pooled; in those data, an arrest of all language output was evoked widely in the language-dominant hemisphere, and from Rolandic cortex in the nondominant hemisphere. Anomia, the inability to correctly name in the presence of intact speech, was the change in object naming evoked from the most restricted portion of lateral cortex. It was evoked only from the dominant hemisphere. However, even that type of naming error was evoked from a wider area than the traditional language areas derived from lesion studies. Subsequently, Van Buren, Fedio, and Frederick (49) also noted that anomia could be evoked widely in lateral cortex of the dominant hemisphere, including sites as far posterior as the parieto-occipital junction.

The effects of stimulation of lateral perisylvian cortex in the dominant hemisphere on object naming were extensively investigated by Ojemann and his associates (20,21,35). In individual patients, sites where stimulation repeatedly altered object naming were often localized to lateral cortical areas of about 1 cm^2. These areas had sharp boundaries (Fig. 1). Surrounding cortex was not related to naming: Latencies of naming were unchanged with stimulation there, and naming changes were not evoked by stimulation there through more widely spaced electrodes (J. Chen and G. Ojemann, *unpublished observations*). In each patient, one or more such discrete areas related to naming were usually present in posterior inferior frontal cortex, and in one or more separate areas in posterior temporal or parietal lobes. Recent observations in a four-year-old child just acquiring language have shown a similar discrete localization of a temporal area essential for naming (G. Ojemann, *unpublished observation*). Thus stimulation mapping suggests that sites essential for naming in an individual patient are organized in "mosaics," a more localized pattern for the brain organization of language than the much larger Broca and Wernicke language areas of traditional lesion-based aphasiology. That discrete localization is present early in the development of language, probably reflecting discrete anatomic specializations for language. These specializations are usually smaller than any of the cytoarchitectonic divisions described in human lateral perisylvian cortex.

Temporal or parietal lateral cortical sites where surface stimulation evoked repeated errors in naming were identified in 90% of 67 patients with dominant-hemisphere perisylvian stimulation (J. Ojemann and G. Ojemann, *unpublished observations*). Since more than half of lateral temporal cortex is buried in sulci, this finding suggests that there is something special about the surface of gyri in the role in language. The extent of involvement of the buried cortex in language

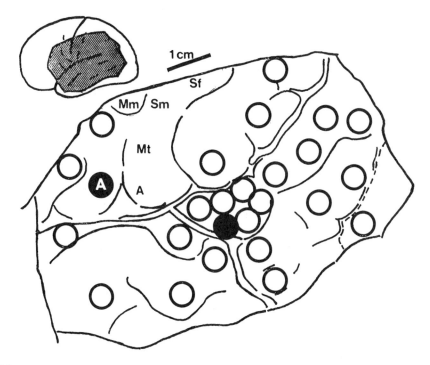

FIG. 1. Location of sites where stimulation altered naming in left fronto-temporo-parietal cortex of left-dominant hemisphere of a 36-year-old female with an adult onset seizure disorder and posterior-temporal focus (*dashed lines*). *Circles* represent the sites of stimulation during naming, using a train of 60 Hz 2.5 msec total duration biphasic square wave pulses at a current of 4 mA, between pulse peaks, delivered in a bipolar manner through electrodes separated by 5 mm. *Filled circles* indicate sites of repeated naming errors, *open circles*, no errors. "A" within circles indicates that the evoked naming errors were predominantly arrests of speech; naming errors at the temporal site were anomia. Letters indicate locations of evoked motor (M, A) and sensory (S) responses identifying Rolandic cortex. *Shaded area* in the insert indicates the location of the cortical exposure. Note the localized site of repeated naming errors in superior-temporal gyrus, and the lack of errors at immediately surrounding sites.

functions in unknown, but the observation that surface stimulation is adequate to identify the areas that must be spared to preserve language in a resection that includes buried cortex (20,21,39) indicates that areas essential for language are never only in buried cortex, and do not angle sharply away from the surface sites identified by stimulation. Perhaps this localization of areas essential for language to the cortical surface and at most the immediately adjacent buried cortex is an indication of a more general principle of organization of association cortex, into bands perpendicular to the long axis of the gyri.

Substantial variability in the location of these discrete areas identified by stimulation as essential for naming was evident in a series of 21 patients reported by Ojemann (20,21). Nearly all of these patients showed a site essential for naming in the portion of posterior frontal lobe immediately in front of face motor cortex. The predominant type of error in naming evoked from this area was an arrest of all speech, suggesting that this was a final motor pathway for speech production. Presumably this area is the true "Broca's area." Elsewhere in perisylvian cortex, including the remainder of posterior inferior frontal lobe, and all of inferior parietal and temporal lobes, there was substantial individual variability in the location of sites essential for naming. *No* area, including the traditional Wernicke area, showed naming changes in more than two-thirds of the sample. In addition, sites essential for naming were rather frequently identified in areas *outside* the traditional Broca and Wernicke language zones; e.g., one-fifth of the sample had such sites in superior temporal gyrus anterior to the level of motor cortex. This functional variability in perisylvian language cortex has a parallel in morphologic variability, in the gyral patterns at the end of the sylvian fissure (43) and in the extent of cytoarchitectonic divisions there (5). The implications of this substantial functional and morphologic variability for the evolution of human language have been discussed elsewhere (31).

Some of this variability was related to differences between males and females, and between verbally more or less intelligent patients. Males showed significantly more frontal sites with evoked naming changes compared with females (12). No differences were evident in temporal sites. The preoperative verbal IQ (VIQ) was used as a measure of verbal performance. Dividing the patients into higher and lower halves, based on VIQ, there were no differences in the overall extent of areas with evoked naming changes. However, the two groups differed in that sites in parietal lobe related to naming by stimulation were significantly more frequent in patients with the lower VIQ scores (21). This is further evidence that biologic differences in the organization of language cortex are present in some patients with less facile language.

Somewhat different types of naming errors have been evoked from different areas of lateral perisylvian cortex (22). Arrest of all speech output was confined to frontal and parietal sites, indicating the motor role of these cortical areas. Phonological errors ("bamp" for "lamp") were also evoked only from frontal and parietal sites. Errors involving semantic paraphasias, or unrelated or visually similar words, were evoked only from temporal sites. These findings were interpreted as suggesting fronto-parietal roles in phonological aspects of language, and a temporal role in storage of the word and its meaning.

Disturbances in naming have also been evoked with stimulation of the fusiform gyrus on the under surface of temporal lobe (8). This basal language area also seems to be discretely localized and shows substantial individual variability in its presence and exact location.

Effects on Naming in Different Languages

When the same cortical sites were stimulated during naming of the same object pictures in two different languages, some sites were identified where naming in one, but not the other language, was altered (36). In the initial report of this finding in two cases (36), and a subsequent third case (21), sites were identified for each of the two languages of patients who were considerably more competent in one of their two languages. In those cases, the area related to the language in which the patient was less competent was larger than the area related to the other language. More recently, some differences in the sites where stimulation altered naming in each language were reported for three Chinese-English true bilinguals (41). Similar findings were present in two additional cases (P. Black, *unpublished observations*; 38). Although this is a small sample, no case has so far been reported in which stimulation during naming in two languages evoked errors from only exactly the same cortical sites. These findings suggest that subtly different areas of cortex are essential for the same linguistic task, naming, in different languages. This could explain some of the unusual cases of polyglot aphasia, in which the preserved language follows none of the ''rules,'' of the language of the environment, most used tongue or mother tongue (37). Presumably in those cases only the cortex essential for the unusual language has been spared by the lesion.

Similarly, when the effects of stimulation on performance in an oral and manual communication system have been compared, sites have been identified where only one of the two systems was disturbed. In a hearing patient, anterior temporal lobe sites were identified where only performance on the manual communication system, finger spelling, was altered; oral language remained intact (11). Resection of those sites was followed by deficits in finger spelling but not oral language. In a second hearing patient, stimulation of an inferior parietal site altered the manual communication system, American Sign Language, while oral language was intact (13). In both these patients there were other sites where stimulation altered both oral and manual communication systems.

Effects on Multiple Language-Related Functions Including Verbal Memory

The studies discussed in the previous sections suggest that there are both *discrete localization* of sites essential for a language function and *differential localization* of sites related to the same linguistic function in different languages. Investigation of the effects of stimulation of the same cortical sites on a number of different language-related functions provides confirmatory evidence for this differential localization. Stimulation effects on measures of naming, sentence reading, recent verbal memory, orofacial motor control for speech gestures, and speech sound identification were determined by Ojemann and his associates, at 118 sites in 14 patients (21–23,32). At 23% of these sites, no changes in any function were evoked whereas 44% of the sites showed changes in only one of the measured functions. Naming, reading, and especially recent verbal memory were the functions most often altered alone. Sites with only changes in these functions were present both frontally and temporo-parietally. This type of organization for language cortex, with different mosaics related to different language functions, differs substantially from the type of organization derived from lesion studies, in which several language-related functions such as naming and reading are usually related to the same cortical area, because all are disturbed by a lesion damaging that area.

When the patterns of stimulation effects on the five different language-related functions in the 14 patients were pooled, a model for the organization of language in lateral perisylvian cortex was derived (Fig. 2) (21–23,32). This model has three major components. The first component is related to motor aspects of language and has two subdivisions. The first subdivision is a final motor pathway for all speech, involving the portion of posterior inferior frontal gyrus just anterior to face motor cortex. This is the same area identified as a final motor pathway in the investigations of naming discussed above, and it is characterized by an evoked arrest of all

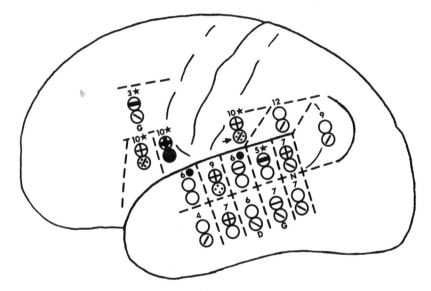

FIG. 2. Location of major components of the model of lateral-cortical organization of language-related functions described in the text. This model was derived from stimulation mapping during naming, reading, and short-term memory measures at 118 sites in 14 patients, and stimulation effects on measures of single and sequential orofacial/speech gesture movements and speech sound identification at 80% of these sites. The number of patients with sites sampled in each zone delineated by *dash lines* is indicated by the upper number. The *upper circle* in each zone indicates the proportion of those patients with evoked changes in naming (*vertical line*) or reading (*horizontal line*). *Narrow lines* indicate changes in 50% of sample; *wider lines*, changes in ≥ 70% of sample. *Lower circle* assigns each zone to one or more of the components of the model described in the text, based on the predominant effect of stimulation there. Motor component, *filled circles and dots*, the former identifying the final motor pathway. Sites specialized for single language functions, the second component of the model, *slashes to right*, N, only naming; G, only reading; D, only speech sound identification or orofacial movement. Memory component, *slash to left*. In two zones, including the one identified by the *arrow*, changes related to both motor and memory components were evoked, but at entirely separate sites within those zones. From (22). Details of patients, tests, stimulation parameters, and control error rates are included in that reference. Maps of stimulation effect on those language-related functions in several of these individual patients have also been published (21,32).

speech—naming, reading, or output from memory—and an inability to mimic even single orofacial speech gestures. The area is distinguished from face motor cortex by the absence of evoked movement.

The second subdivision of the motor component includes portions of inferior frontal, inferior parietal, and superior temporal lobes. At these sites, stimulation altered naming and/or reading, and the ability to mimic sequences of orofacial speech gesture movements, but not single movements. Stimulation of these sites generally did not alter performance on the recent verbal memory measure, providing evidence that alterations in perception of the test items did not account for any of the observed evoked changes. The area related to sequential motor speech functions in this model is substantially larger than the motor area of the traditional model of cortical language organization, but is very close to the extent of the ischemic lesions required to produce a permanent motor aphasia, as reported by Mohr (14). Those lesions involved the entire distribution of the upper division of the middle cerebral artery, which includes the inferior frontal, inferior parietal, and anterior temporal areas that constitute the motor component of the stimulation-derived model.

The area included in this motor component of the stimulation-derived model of language cortex also is important for the identification of speech sounds. The speech sound identification measure was constructed so that stimulation occurred only at the time the sound was heard, followed by a response period without stimulation. Thus, in this measure, effects of stimulation on the perception of the speech sound were separated from any motor effects of stimulation of that cortical area. Despite this, at 74% of the sites with evoked changes in orofacial motor control, speech sound identification was also disturbed. This identified a fronto-parieto-superior temporal perisylvian cortical area related to both the motor and auditory aspects of language production and perception. This finding is difficult to relate to the fronto-temporal, motor-receptive separation of the traditional lesion-based model of cortical language organization, because in the stimulation data there seem to be cortical areas in both frontal and temporal lobes that are essential for both motor and receptive language functions. On the other hand, this finding provides a potential anatomic basis for the psycholinguistically derived motor theory of speech perception (7). That theory suggests that the perception of speech sounds involves creation of an internal motor representation of the sound. The stimulation finding indicates an area of cortex related to both those functions. However, the stimulation finding that both speech gestures and identification of speech sounds are often altered at the same cortical site may also represent an evoked change in some other function common to both processes. Precise timing has been suggested as such a function common to both motor and receptive aspects of language (47).

The second component of the stimulation-derived model for cortical language organization includes frontal and temporal areas related only to single language functions—naming or reading. These sites are immediately anterior frontally, and immediately posterior temporally to the sites related to the motor component of this model. Sites related only to naming or to reading are present both frontally and temporo-parietally. Once again, the stimulation-derived model does not identify major fronto-temporal differences. (Indeed, in the stimulation data, only the final motor pathway subdivision of the motor component is unique to the frontal, as compared with the temporo-parietal, area.) In a separate study measuring stimulation effects on naming, word reading, and identification of word meaning in a different series of patients, sites related only to each of these functions, including only to identification of word meaning, were also identified frontally and temporo-parietally (H. Whitaker and G. Ojemann, *unpublished observations*). The nature of the reading errors evoked at these sites related only to reading was unique, involving omissions or errors in only the syntactic aspects of the sentences, in contrast to reading errors at sites related to the motor component, where the errors involved slow, effortful production of all aspects of the sentence. Thus these specialized areas for reading more probably represent specializations for grammatical aspects of language. The nature of the errors at the temporal sites related only to naming suggest a role in word storage, as noted above.

The third component of the stimulation-derived model of cortical language organization is related to recent verbal memory. This component surrounds the components related to motor function and specializations for naming and reading frontally and temporo-parietally. Sites where stimulation disturbed recent verbal memory seldom showed changes in other language functions. Outside of the final motor pathway, sites with evoked changes in other language functions rarely showed changes on the recent verbal memory measure. This includes correct retrieval during stimulation of words that could not be correctly named during stimulation of the same site with the same current. Thus separation of cortical sites related to language, and its generalized word memory, from sites related to recent, episodic memory using words seems to be a principle of cortical organization from the perspective of stimulation mapping.

The recent verbal memory measure used in the stimulation studies allowed separate assessment of stimulation effects at the time information entered memory, from those during the time the memory was stored, or from stimulation effects at the time of retrieval. At frontal sites, the maximum effect in disturbing memory occurred when the current was applied at the time of retrieval; at temporo-parietal sites the maximum effect occurred when the current was applied during the entry of information into memory or during its storage (21). This finding suggests that temporal sites related to recent verbal memory might be the location of the active storage processes of that type of memory. The recent identification of single neuronal activity in lateral temporal cortex with increased firing statistically related to memory input and the early phases of memory storage (26) is additional evidence of this memory role for lateral temporal cortex.

The importance of this lateral cortical recent verbal memory component to memory deficits with dominant-hemisphere temporal lobe resections was demonstrated by Ojemann and Dodrill (27). In those resections, medial temporal structures were spared if memory was dependent on that dominant hemisphere, based on preoperative intracarotid amytal assessment. Nevertheless, a post-resection verbal memory deficit was still present in half the patients. This residual memory deficit correlated with the lateral but not medial extent of the resection, and was predicted by the presence in the area of the resection or its margin of lateral cortical sites related by stimulation to memory. These findings, along with the presence of neurons in lateral temporal cortex with changes in firing related to memory, provide strong evidence that stimulation effects on memory are attributable to a local effect on lateral cortex and not propagation of the current to some distant structure such as the hippocampus. These findings also indicate that the model of brain organization for recent verbal memory must be revised based on stimulation findings. Lesion data suggested that verbal memory depended on structures around the third ventricle and in medial temporal lobe, particularly the hippocampus. The findings presented here require the addition of cortex surrounding perisylvian language areas to that model.

Several speculations have been derived from the findings summarized above. The fronto-temporo-parietal separation of sites related to memory into those areas important to retrieval or input-storage may be a more general phenomenon, accounting for different roles of other specialized sites found in both frontal and temporo-parietal lobes. Thus frontal sites specialized for naming may be important to word retrieval, those in temporal lobe to word storage. Frontal sites related to the syntactic aspects of reading may be important to retrieval of syntax, and such temporal sites to storage of syntax. This hypothesis awaits the design of appropriate behavior measures so that it can be directly tested. A second speculation derived from the stimulation model of language cortex is that the phylogenetic basis of language may involve the appearance of a lateralized orofacial motor control system and a surrounding lateralized recent memory system, with the specializations for language developing at the interface between these two components. The presence of a lateralized orofacial motor control system and a lateralized recent memory system have been described in primates (3,48).

SUBCORTICAL STIMULATION

Most of the investigations of the effects of subcortical stimulation on language and memory involve electrodes placed in lateral thalamic targets for the treatment of dyskinesias. In those patients, alterations in naming of objects were evoked from portions of lateral thalamus of the dominant (but not nondominant) hemisphere: anterior-superior-lateral pulvinar, medial-central ventrolateral nucleus, and the anterior-lateral portion of lateral thalamus (18,29,34). The types of evoked errors in naming differed among these lateral thalamic locations. In anterior-superior-lateral pulvinar, errors were largely omissions of the correct object name but with retained ability to speak, a pattern very similar to the naming changes evoked with cortical stimulation. Stimulation of medial-central ventrolateral nucleus evoked perseveration on the first syllable of correct or incorrect object names, a type of error not seen with cortical stimulation. Stimulation of the anterior-lateral pole of lateral thalamus during naming also evoked a unique type of error, production of a specific incorrect word each time naming was required during stimulation with a current above a particular threshold. In several patients. that wrong word was the last object correctly named during stimulation at a subthreshold current. Stimulation of the anterior-lateral pole of lateral thalamus has also evoked spontaneous speech (44).

Different mechanisms seem to be involved in the changes in naming evoked from different parts of lateral thalamus. The mechanisms altered by anterior-superior-lateral pulvinar stimulation and stimulation of the anterior-lateral pole of lateral thalamus are involved in both language and recent verbal memory, which again is in contrast to cortex, where language and recent verbal memory were generally related to different sites. Stimulation of the anterior-lateral pole of lateral thalamus during a recent verbal memory measure had different effects, depending on whether the current was applied at the time of entry of information into memory or at retrieval (17,25). Stimulation at the time of entry of information increased the accuracy of subsequent recall of that information, compared with recall of information presented in the absence of stimulation. This increased accuracy of recall with items presented during stimulation could be detected at least a week later. However, stimulation of the same lateral thalamic sites at the same currents, but at the time of retrieval, accelerated the rate of retrieval, but also increased the error rate. These effects of lateral-thalamic stimulation were considered to represent a "specific alerting response." When that response was driven by stimulation, attention was directed to incoming verbal information, increasing the likelihood of its subsequent recall, whereas, retrieval of already internalized information was blocked. Thus the intensity of the specific alerting response acted as a gate determining the ease of retrieval from recent verbal memory. The increase in accuracy of later recall for information presented during lateral-thalamic stimulation has also been shown for purely auditory material in a dichotic listening paradigm (24). A similar effect, but specific to visuospatial material rather than verbal material, has been shown with right-lateral-thalamic stimulation (19).

The importance of this specific alerting response in thalamic language mechanisms was indicated by the substantial negative correlation between the magnitude of this response and the appearance of anomia after a subsequent lateral-thalamic lesion (17). The specific alerting response mechanism also explains the unusual type of naming errors evoked from the anterior-lateral pole of lateral thalamus. The inability to produce the correct object name represents the failure of retrieval during stimulation, now from long-term word memory as well as short-term, recent verbal memory. The only word item available for retrieval is the word whose likelihood of retrieval was enhanced by previous stimulation at the time it entered the memory as the last word correctly named at the subthreshold current. Compared with anterior-lateral thalamus, anterior-superior-lateral pulvinar stimulation during recent verbal memory measures demonstrated less effect of stimulation during entry of information increasing the likelihood of subsequent recall, but more effect of stimulation at the time of retrieval blocking recall (16,28). The common naming error evoked with stimulation of that part of pulvinar, omission of the object name likely reflects this evoked failure in retrieval from both long-term and short-term verbal memory.

Language deficits after spontaneous thalamic lesions have also been related to defects in specific alerting-attending mechanisms (9,42).

Different mechanisms seem to be involved in the perseverative naming errors evoked from medial-central ventrolateral thalamic nucleus. Stimulation there also inhibits respiration in expiration, the appropriate respiratory substrate for speech (33). This effect has a lower threshold in left compared with right thalamus. The rate of articulation is also slowed with left-ventrolateral thalamic stimulation (10). Together these findings suggest that medial-central ventrolateral thalamus integrates motor and respiratory aspects of speech.

Stimulation of electrodes in more medial portions of thalamus has had little effect on object naming or recent verbal memory performance. Disturbances in recent memory have been described with stimulation of the head of the caudate nucleus (1).

EVIDENCE FOR AN INTERRELATIONSHIP BETWEEN CORTICAL AND THALAMIC LANGUAGE MECHANISMS

In an investigation of changes in the electrocorticogram (ECoG) recorded during naming, Fried, Ojemann, and Fetz (4) sought changes that were localized to cortical sites that stimulation had independently related to naming. Two changes localized to naming sites, compared with the surrounding sites not related to naming by stimulation, were identified in the ECoG averaged to presentation of the items to be named. These changes were slow potentials, of about 1 sec duration recorded from frontal sites related to naming, and local desynchronization, of the same onset and duration, recorded at temporal sites related to naming by stimulation. The relation of the desynchronization recorded during naming to temporal naming sites was subsequently confirmed quantitatively by spectral density analysis of single trials (30). In that analysis, desynchronization represented the loss of spectral density in the 7 to 12 Hz frequencies. During naming, naming sites demonstrated a significantly greater loss of spectral density in those frequencies in the 700 to 1,200 msec epoch after presentation of the item to be named, compared with surrounding sites not related to naming. Of interest is the finding that the changes in the ECoG recorded during naming that were localized to frontal and temporal naming sites occurred simultaneously; this study did not provide any evidence for serial processes between frontal and temporal language areas.

This study also contained several behavioral control measures. Overt output of the object name was delayed to a cue, to dissociate ECoG changes related to silent naming from those associated with motor speech functions. The same visual items used for silent naming were also presented in a spatial-matching task. The spatial-matching task used has been related to function of the nondominant hemisphere (2), so that any ECoG changes at naming sites that were specific to naming should not be present at those sites during the spatial-matching task. This was the case for the quantitative spectral density measures of desynchronization in some patients.

Thus local desynchronization seems to be a process that is both anatomically and behaviorally specific to naming, localized to naming sites only during naming and not present there during the behavioral control. Some mechanisms that produce local desynchronization in the ECoG have been identified in animals. The thalamocortical-activating system is one such mechanism (6,45). The thalamocortical-activating system is also a potential anatomic substrate for the changes in language and memory evoked by lateral-thalamic stimulation. Lateral-thalamic stimulation might alter function in *en passage* fibers of the thalamocortical-activating system passing across lateral thalamus from interlaminar nucleus, or by direct physiologic interactions between lateral thalamus and interlaminar nucleus. Lateral thalamus, then, may mediate effects on language (and likely memory) through the thalamocortical-activating system, producing local desynchronization in the cortical mosaic(s) essential to that language function.

ACKNOWLEDGMENTS

The author's research reported here was supported by NIH grants NS 21724, NS 17111, and NS 20482.

REFERENCES

1. Bechtereva, N., Genkin, A, Morsseva, N., and Smirnov, V. (1967): Electrographic evidence of participation of deep structures of the human brain in certain mental processes. *Electroencephalogr. Clin. Neurophysiol.*, 25:153–166.
2. Benton, A., Hannay, H., and Varney, N. (1975): Visual perception of line direction in patients with unilateral brain disease. *Neurology*, 25:907–910.
3. Dewson, J.H., III (1977): Preliminary evidence of hemispheric asymmetry of auditory function in monkeys. In: *Lateralization in the Nervous System*, edited by S. Harnard, R. Doty, L. Goldstein, J. Saynes, and G. Krauthamer, pp. 63–71. Academic Press, New York.
4. Fried, I., Ojemann, G., and Fetz, E. (1981): Language related potentials specific to human language cortex. *Science*, 212:353–356.
5. Galaburda, A., Sanides, F., and Geschwind, N. (1978): Human brain: Cytoarchitectonic left-right asymmetries in the temporal speech region. *Arch. Neurol.*, 35:812–817.
6. Jasper, H. (1960): Unspecific thalamocortical relations. In: *Handbook of Physiology*, vol. 2, edited by J. Fields, H. Magoun, and V. Hall, pp. 1307–1321. Williams and Wilkins, Baltimore.
7. Liberman, A.M., Cooper, F.S., Shankweiler, D.P., and Studdert-Kennedy, M. (1967): Perception of the speech code. *Psychol. Rev.*, 74:431–461.
8. Luders, H., Lesser, R., Hahn, J., Dinner, D., Morris, H., and Harrison, M. (1985): Global aphasia elicited by stimulation of the dominant fusiform gyrus. *J. Neurol.*, 232(Suppl.):212.
9. Luria, A.R. (1977): On quasiaphasic speech disturbance in lesions of the deep structures in the brain. *Brain Lang.*, 4:359–432.
10. Mateer, C. (1978): Asymmetric effects of thalamic stimulation on rate of speech. *Neuropsychologia*, 16:497–499.
11. Mateer, C., Polen, S., Ojemann, G., and Wyler, A. (1982): Localization of finger spelling and oral language: A case study. *Brain Lang.*, 17:46–57.
12. Mateer, C., Polen, S., and Ojemann, G. (1982): Sexual variation in cortical localization of naming as determined by stimulation mapping. Commentary on McGlone 1980. *Behavioral and Brain Sciences*, 5:310–311.
13. Mateer, C., Rapport, R., and Kettrick, C. (1984): Cerebral organization of oral and signed language responses: Case study evidence from amytal and cortical stimulation studies. *Brain Lang.*, 21:123–135.

14. Mohr, J. (1976): Broca's area and Broca's aphasia. *Studies in Neurolinguistics*, 1:201–236.
15. Obler, L., Albert M., Goodglass, H., and Benson, D. (1978): Aphasia type and aging. *Brain Lang.*, 6:318–327.
16. Ojemann, G. (1974): Speech and short-term verbal memory alterations evoked from stimulation in pulvinar. In: *Pulvinar-LP Complex*, edited by I. Cooper, M. Riklan, and P. Rakic, pp. 173–184. Charles C. Thomas, Springfield, IL.
17. Ojemann, G. (1975): Language and the thalamus: Object naming and recall during and after thalamic stimulation. *Brain Lang.*, 2:101–120.
18. Ojemann, G. (1977): Asymmetric function of the thalamus in man. *Ann. NY Acad. Sci.*, 299:380–396.
19. Ojemann, G. (1979): Altering memory with human ventrolateral thalamic stimulation. In: *Modern Concepts in Psychiatric Surgery*, edited by H. Ballantine and B. Myerson, pp. 103–109. Elsevier, New York.
20. Ojemann, G. (1979): Individual variability in cortical localization of language. *J. Neurosurg.*, 50:164–169.
21. Ojemann, G. (1983): Brain organization for language from the perspective of electrical stimulation mapping. *Behavioral and Brain Sciences*, 6:189–206.
22. Ojemann, G., (1983): Electrical stimulation and the neurobiology of language. *Behavioral and Brain Sciences*, 6:221–230.
23. Ojemann, G. (1983): The intrahemispheric organization of language derived with electrical stimulation techniques. *Trends in the Neurosciences*, 6:184–189.
24. Ojemann, G. (1985): Enhancement of memory with human ventrolateral thalamic stimulation: Effect evident on a dichotic listening task. *Appl. Neurophysiol.*, 48:212–215.
25. Ojemann, G., Blick, K., and Ward, A.A., Jr. (1971): Improvement and disturbance of short-term verbal memory during human ventrolateral thalamic stimulation. *Brain*, 94:225–240.
26. Ojemann, G., Creutzfeldt, O., and Lettich, E. (1985): Single neuron activity in the human temporal lobe: II. Naming, reading, memory, face and figure matching. *Soc. Neurosci. Abst.*, 11:879.
27. Ojemann, G., and Dodrill, C. (1985): Verbal memory deficits after left temporal lobectomy for epilepsy. *J. Neurosurg.*, 62:101–107.
28. Ojemann, G., and Fedio, P. (1968): The effects of stimulation of human thalamus and parietal and temporal white matter on short-term memory. *J. Neurosurg.*, 29:51–59.
29. Ojemann, G., Fedio, P., and Van Buren, J. (1968): Anomia from pulvinar and subcortical parietal stimulation. *Brain*, 91:99–116.
30. Ojemann, G., and Lettich, E. (1985): Electrocorticographic correlates of naming and verbal memory. *Electroencephalogr. Clin. Neurophysiol.*, 61:832.
31. Ojemann, G., and Mateer, C. (1979): Cortical and subcortical organization of human communication: Evidence from stimulation studies. In: *Neurobiology of Social Communication in Primates*, edited by H. Steklis and M. Raleigh, pp. 111–132. Academic Press, New York.
32. Ojemann, G., and Mateer, C. (1979): Human language cortex: Localization of memory, syntax and sequential motor phoneme identification systems. *Science*, 205:1401–1403.
33. Ojemann, G., and Van Buren, J. (1967): Respiratory, heart rate and GSR responses from human diencephalon. *Arch. Neurol.*, 16:74–88.
34. Ojemann, G., and Ward, A.A., Jr. (1971): Speech representation in ventrolateral thalamus. *Brain*, 94:669–680.
35. Ojemann, G., and Whitaker, H. (1978): Language localization and variability. *Brain Lang.*, 6:239–260.
36. Ojemann, G., and Whitaker, H. (1978): The bilingual brain. *Arch. Neurol.*, 35:409–412.
37. Paradis, M. (1977): Bilingualism and aphasia. *Studies in Neurolinguistics*, 3:65–122.
38. Penfield, W., and Jasper, H. (1954): *Epilepsy and the Functional Anatomy of the Human Brain*. Little, Brown, Boston.
39. Penfield, W., and Roberts, L. (1959): *Speech and Brain Mechanisms*. Princeton University Press, Princeton, NJ.
40. Ranck, J., Jr. (1975): Which elements are excited in electrical stimulation of mammalian central nervous system: A review. *Brain Res.*, 98:417–440.
41. Rapport, R., Tan, C., and Whitaker, H. (1983): Language function and dysfunction among Chinese and English-speaking polyglots: Cortical stimulation, Wada testing and clinical studies. *Brain Lang.*, 18:342–366.

42. Reynolds, A., Turner, P., Harris, A., Ojemann, G., and Davis, L. (1979): Left thalamic hemorrhage with dysphasia: A report of five cases. *Brain Lang.*, 7:62–73.
43. Rubens, A., Mahowald, M., and Hutton, J. (1976): Asymmetry of the lateral (Sylvian) fissures in man. *Neurology*, 26:620–624.
44. Schaltenbrand, G. (1965): The effects of stereotaxis electrical stimulation in the depth of the brain. *Brain*, 88:835–840.
45. Skinner, J., and Yingling, C. (1977): Central gating mechanism that regulate event-related potentials and behavior: A neural model for attention. *Prog. Clin. Neurophysiol.*, 1:30–69.
46. Smith, B. (1980): Cortical stimulation and speech timing: A preliminary observation. *Brain Lang.*, 10:89–97.
47. Tallal, P. (1983): A precise timing mechanism may underlie a common speech perception and production area in the perisylvian cortex of the dominant hemisphere. *Behavioral and Brain Sciences*, 6:219–220.
48. Trevarthan, C. (1974): Functional relations of disconnected hemispheres with the brain stem, and with each other: Monkey and man. In: *Hemispheric Disconnection and Cerebral Function*, edited by M. Kinsbourne and W.L. Smith., pp. 187–207. Charles C. Thomas, Springfield, IL.
49. Van Buren, J., Fedio, P., and Frederick, G. (1978): Mechanism and localization of speech in the parietotemporal cortex. *Neurosurgery*, 2:233–239.

*Language, Communication, and
the Brain*, edited by F. Plum.
Raven Press, New York © 1988.

Right Hemisphere Language: Insights into Normal Language Mechanisms?

*Kathleen Baynes and †Michael S. Gazzaniga

*Burke Rehabilitation Center, Cornell University Medical College,
White Plains, New York 10605, and †Division of Cognitive Neuroscience,
Cornell University Medical College, New York, New York 10021*

Neurolinguistic research has focused on language disruption in aphasia as a laboratory for modeling normal language processes (1,3,5). The presence of language in the right hemisphere of some patients after section of the corpus callosum offers another neurological perspective on language processing (8,9,12). This linguistic ability is particularly interesting in light of the right hemisphere's extremely limited intellectual functioning (11). The right hemisphere cannot, for instance, correctly infer "fire" if shown a match and a pile of wood even though it can identify a picture depicting the referents of "wood," "match," and "fire"(11). Thus, in the case of semantics, a lexicon rich enough to accomplish straightforward referential naming tasks does not depend on a conceptual system developed enough to accomplish inferences similar to the match-wood-fire problem.

This chapter considers syntactic knowledge accompanying right hemisphere language. As with semantics, the relation between syntactic competence and more general intellectual competence is not fully understood. The study of right hemisphere language could shed some light on this issue. When exploring the level of syntactic competence of the right hemisphere, we search for those grammatical tasks the right hemisphere can accomplish and those with which it experiences difficulty. For us, any dissociation is particularly interesting because it may indicate which aspects of the linguistic system depend on a rich intellectual capacity. We admit, however, that such observations are correlational without any claim for causality.

This chapter reviews the extant literature on right hemisphere language before reporting our work on its syntactic competence.

J.W., V.P., AND THEIR ESTABLISHED LINGUISTIC COMPETENCE

The differences in right hemisphere representation of language skills among commissurotomy patients has been striking, ranging from an absence of any response to language tasks to a sophisticated vocabulary with limited production skills (8).

In this chapter we focus on two split-brain patients, V.P. and J.W., who have well-established right hemisphere lexical skills. V.P. appears to have language skills in her right hemisphere that often parallel those in her left hemisphere, whereas J.W.'s right hemisphere language has a more unusual profile.

V.P. is a right-handed female who began to experience recurrent major seizures after a febrile illness at age 9. These seizures were controlled with anticonvulsants, but by 1976 she was experiencing episodes of blank staring lasting for several seconds several times a day. In 1979, V.P. was referred to the Medical College of Ohio. The initial surgery was undertaken in April 1979, and the second stage carried out six weeks later. Following both surgeries, V.P. showed immediate evidence of language comprehension in the right hemisphere. She showed evidence of right hemisphere control of speech within one year. An MRI scan demonstrated some intact fibers in the splenium and the rostrum of an otherwise completely sectioned corpus callosum (10).

J.W. is a right-handed male who has had intractable epilepsy since age 19. He sustained a closed head injury at age 13 resulting in brief, infrequent absence attacks. These were not treated. At 19, he had his first major motor seizure. During the next seven years, J.W. was frequently hospitalized with seizures despite adequate serum anticonvulsant levels. In 1979 he was referred to Dartmouth Medical Center where the corpus callosum was sectioned in a two-stage operation. An MRI scan demonstrated a complete section of the corpus callosum but an otherwise normal brain (10).

Both V.P. and J.W. have a right hemispheric auditory vocabulary, which would seem to imply some phonological skill. However, in formal testing of phoneme discrimination in a standard categorical perception paradigm, Sidtis et al. (19) demonstrated poor right hemisphere performance on phoneme identification for both subjects, although V.P.'s right hemisphere performed above chance. When V.P. and J.W. were asked to select words that rhymed with targets presented tachistoscopically to their left hemisphere, V.P.'s right hemisphere again remained above chance, but J.W.'s did not. Sidtis et al. (19) argued that V.P. showed phonological competence with her right hemisphere, albeit at an impoverished level. They also cautioned that the negative results from J.W. cannot be used as evidence of a qualitatively different method of analysis of auditory input in his right hemisphere, but may demonstrate only a failure to respond in this paradigm.

It should be noted that the conclusions of Sidtis et al. differ from those of Zaidel (22,23) and of Levy and Trevarthen (14), who worked with different split-brain subjects. Zaidel (24) found a well-developed auditory lexicon in the right hemispheres of these patients. When Levy and Trevarthen (14) used a rhyming task to investigate their phonological skills, their results were uniformly negative. They concluded that ''the right hemisphere lacks a phonetic analyzer that can generate phonetic images'' and that ''its verbal capacities depend on special right hemisphere processes.'' Clearly, better understanding of the difference between the two experimental groups is needed.

Semantic information appears to be available to the right hemisphere of J.W. and V.P. J.W. has demonstrated comparable vocabularies in his right and left hemispheres on the Peabody Picture Vocabulary Test (12). Moreover, both V.P. and J.W. have demonstrated a right hemisphere ability to identify synonyms, antonyms, functional relations among words, superordinates, and subordinates, although V.P. responds more accurately (19). These results have been replicated for superordinate and subordinate relations and extended to include the identification of same-class items and attributes (12). Using a lexical decision paradigm with a very short rate of presentation (150 msec), V.P. shows semantic priming in both hemispheres over a variety of relations. J.W.'s results are less consistent, but indicate that whereas his left hemisphere can demonstrate normal facilitation for targets preceded by related words, there is no trace of this effect in his silent right hemisphere. This result is of particular interest because it corresponds with the presence of an N-400 in response to semantic incongruity in both hemispheres of V.P., but only in the left hemisphere of J.W. (M. Kutas and S. A. Hillyard, *this volume*).

Gazzaniga and Hillyard (9) found some indication that verbs were less represented in the right hemisphere lexicon, although Zaidel (21) found controlling for word frequency makes comprehension of verbs and nouns more similar. Both J.W. and V.P. were able to carry out commands (necessarily verbs) lateralized to their right hemisphere at greater-than-chance levels (19). It appears that both hemispheres have a lexicon that can be accessed to make a variety of semantic judgments. Both have some capacity to understand nouns and verbs, but J.W. has no demonstrated skill with function words. V.P.'s performance is generally better than J.W.'s, but a qualitative difference between these patients has yet to emerge.

The skills of J.W. and V.P. may reflect a pattern similar to that reported by Caramazza, Berndt, and Basili for some aphasics (4), i.e., relatively intact lexical semantics in the face of impaired phonology and (consequently) syntax. Little work, however, has been done on the right hemisphere's syntactic competence, although there is one relevant study.

The experiment (12) turned on the ambiguity of phrases such as "flying planes," which could mean either (a) "the act of flying planes" or (b) "planes that are flying." This ambiguity disappears with the addition of the article "the," so that "flying the planes" can only mean (a) and "the flying planes" can only mean (b). J.W.'s right hemisphere was unable to use the information carried by the article to distinguish these two meanings, whereas V.P.'s right hemisphere performed much like her left hemisphere. This result was interpreted to indicate that V.P. had access to some syntactic information in her right hemisphere, but J.W.'s right hemisphere gave no indication of such sensitivity. We follow up on this observation in the experiments in the next section.

FURTHER EXPERIMENTAL ANALYSIS OF SYNTACTIC COMPETENCE OF THE RIGHT HEMISPHERE

In the aphasia literature, different methods have been used to measure sensitivity to syntax. Although each task purportedly tapped syntactic competence, performance of aphasic subjects differed from task to task. For example, Schwartz, Saffran, and Marin (18) used a two-choice–picture-pointing paradigm to test the ability of agrammatic aphasics to understand semantically reversible active and passive sentences (e.g., the boy hit the girl; the boy was hit by the girl). Agrammatic aphasics were *unable* to choose correctly the picture that matched the sentence they heard. In other words, they could not use the syntactic constraints in the sentences to determine who hit whom. In contrast, Linebarger, Schwartz, and Saffran (15) found that aphasics who were unable to interpret correct active and passive sentences were able to judge accurately whether sentences were grammatical.

The Linebarger et al. result is important because it suggests that even though a patient may not be able to use a grammatical constraint in a comprehension task, he or she may still *know* something about grammar and be able to use this knowledge in other tasks, such as a grammaticality judgment task. Linebarger et al. (15), for instance, pointed out that agrammatics' grammaticality judgments indicate that they possess knowledge of a number of grammar rules or constraints, such as subcategorization requirements, sensitivity to functors, and an ability to keep track of syntactic dependencies across words and even clauses.

Thus, in assessing right hemisphere language, a variety of syntactic probes should be used. In this chapter we adapted both the Schwartz comprehension task and the Linebarger grammaticality task. Because V.P.'s right hemisphere had demonstrated some minimal capacity for speech production and syntax-dependent comprehension, we expected that she might perform well on both tasks. J.W.'s right hemisphere had demonstrated only semantic knowledge previously. Consequently, we expected poor performance on the comprehension task. We were uncertain whether J.W.'s isolated right hemisphere lexicon would include in it enough grammar to distinguish grammatical from ungrammatical sentences.

Comprehension of Active and Passive Sentences

We adapted the stimuli used by Schwartz et al. to tachistoscopic presentation by first pairing each sentence with, in one case, a picture that illustrated it, and in another, one that illustrated the opposite relation; that is, the sentence "The boy is touched by the girl." was paired both with a picture of a girl touching a boy and a picture of a boy touching a girl. There were 48 pairings, based on 24 sentences.

J.W. and V.P. were presented with a single picture. They then heard a sentence binaurally over earphones and were instructed to decide whether the sentence matched the picture. J.W. and V.P. were instructed to fixate on an asterisk displayed in the center of a CRT and the responses "YES" and "NO" appeared for 150 msec in different quadrants of the screen. Both were in either the right or left visual field, with their horizontal position randomly alternated. J.W. and V.P. had to point to the quadrant where the correct answer appeared. Responses were always with the left hand to maximize right hemisphere accuracy.

This task requires a large memory load, as subjects have to remember not only the correct answer, but the quadrant in which that answer was displayed in order to respond correctly. Nonetheless, both V.P. and J.W. performed well above chance with their left hemispheres (Table 1). V.P. fell to chance with her right hemisphere on both active and passive sentences. On the other hand, J.W.'s right hemisphere response pattern demonstrated a surprising sensitivity to word order. Bever (2) has suggested that in the absence of a functioning grammatical system people may adopt the strategy of making the noun phrase before the verb the subject of the sentence and the noun phrase following the verb its object. If this strategy is used on active and passive sentences, active sentences would be interpreted correctly, but passive sentences would have just the opposite meaning. This pattern corresponds to that of J.W.'s right hemisphere responses.

Thus, J.W.'s performance suggests that the right hemisphere may in some instance represent and analyze the grammatical function of lexical items. V.P.'s inability to perform this task was surprising as prior work (10) indicated that she possessed some ability to use syntactic information to guide processing; however, differences in mode of presentation and in time span over which the elements must be processed may have contributed to her better performance in the prior work than in the present work. In the prior work, the three crucial lexical items were presented visually. In the present task, an entire sentence was presented aurally.

Grammaticality Judgments

We adapted a study done by Linebarger, Schwartz, and Saffran (15) with aphasics to the demands of split-brain research. Linebarger et al. showed that agrammatic

TABLE 1. *Semantically reversible active and passive sentences*

	RVF % (no.)	LVF % (no.)
V.P.		
Active	100 (24)[a]	46 (11)
Passive	88 (21)[a]	50 (12)
Combined	94 (45)[a]	48 (23)
J.W.		
Active	79 (19)[a]	75 (18)[a]
Passive	100 (24)[a]	38 (9)[b]
Combined	90 (43)[a]	56 (27)

RVF, right visual field; LVF, left visual field. Percent correct obtained matching binaurally presented sentences with pictures when the response choice is lateralized. Numbers in parentheses represent the number correct out of 24 for active and passive scores and out of 48 for combined scores.
[a]Binomial $p < 0.05$, better-than-chance performance.
[b]Binomial $p < 0.05$, less-than-chance performance.

aphasics can make judgments of grammaticality across a variety of sentence types, even though they cannot use grammatical constraints in the interpretation of sentences. Pilot work with J.W. indicated that not only could his right hemisphere make similar judgments, but his errors appeared to be on just those sentence types that Linebarger et al. (15) reported as difficult for the agrammatics. We decided to replicate these preliminary results on V.P. and retest J.W. We obtained copies of the original tapes used by Linebarger et al. (15). The two patients listened to each sentence individually as they were played back through earphones. As in the comprehension study, "yes" and "no" were presented tachistoscopically in four quadrants and V.P. and J.W. had to point with their left hand to a "yes" if the sentence was grammatical, "no" if it was ungrammatical. There were 10 different sentence types, and for each type, there were grammatical and ungrammatical examples. For instance, the grammatical rule known as subject-auxiliary inversion is correctly applied in the sentence, "Are you going to the store?", but violated in the sentence, "Are going you to the store?"

The results in Figs. 1 and 2 represent the response pattern for J.W. and V.P. for all 10 sentence types. Performance is measured following Linebarger et al. (15) using A', which corrects for guessing. A' varies from 0 to 1, with the larger the number the more accurate performance. The 10 different conditions represent grammaticality tests for the 10 different sentence types. The conditions in which Linebarger et al.'s original four aphasic subjects were consistently weakest were 5, 9,

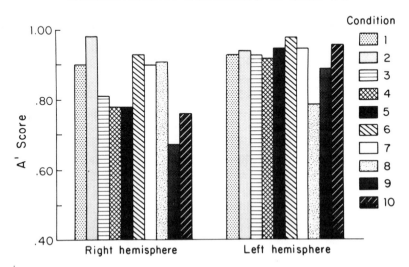

FIG. 1. A' scores of J.W.'s right and left hemispheres compiled judging grammaticality of binaurally presented sentences when the response choice is lateralized. In each condition, grammaticality tests were given for sentences constrained by a particular grammatical rule (see text).

GRAMMATICALITY JUDGMENTS OF CASE VP

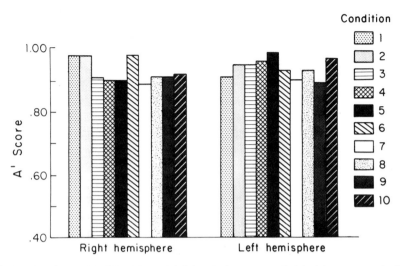

FIG. 2. A′ scores of V.P.'s right and left hemispheres compiled judging grammaticality of binaurally presented sentences when the response choice is lateralized. In each condition, grammaticality tests were given for sentences constrained by a particular grammatical rule (see text).

and 10. These conditions probed knowledge about three grammatical rules: (a) subject copying in the formation of a tag question ("Harry loved Mary, didn't it?"), (b) agreement between a reflexive pronoun and its antecedent ("Harry loves herself."), and (c) copying the auxiliary verb in the formation of a tag question ("Harry is waiting for Mary, doesn't he?").

As Fig. 1 illustrates, J.W.'s left hemisphere performs well. Although less accurate, his right hemisphere has the most difficulty with the same conditions as the agrammatic aphasics. Inspection of Fig. 1 also indicates that there is a much tighter relation between the pattern generated by J.W.'s right hemisphere and that generated by the aphasics. Moreover, the pattern of his left hemisphere appears to be distinct from that of his right hemisphere. The failure to find any interhemispheric similarity suggests that cross-cueing is not accounting for the good performance of the right hemisphere.

There is much less difference between the performances to the two hemispheres in V.P. than in J.W. (Fig. 2). V.P.'s and J.W.'s left hemispheres respond with similar accuracy (0.92 and 0.93, respectively), but V.P.'s right hemisphere is equally accurate (0.92), whereas J.W.'s mean accuracy falls to 0.84. The range of V.P.'s scores for her left hemisphere is from 0.89 to 0.99 and for her right hemisphere is 0.89 to 0.98. Moreover, the differences between the A′ scores of her two hemispheres in the comparable conditions range from only 0.01 to 0.09. In contrast, the between-hemisphere differences for J.W. range from 0.03 to 0.22, with the largest differences occurring in the crucial conditions of 5, 9, and 10.

What could account for J.W.'s accurate grammatical intuitions? Although he demonstrates accurate use of auditory information to decide whether a sentence is grammatically acceptable, he remains unable to use this information to derive meaning accurately from semantically reversible active and passive sentences.

J.W. is probably not using intonational cues when making grammaticality judgments. Berndt, Salasoo, Mitchum, and Blumstein (17) have demonstrated that normal and brain-damaged controls make accurate grammaticality judgments when the intonation contours are removed from sentences. Moreover, agrammatic aphasics are also able to make accurate grammaticality judgments without the information from the intonation contours and continue to demonstrate greater difficulty with sentences containing tag questions. The accuracy of grammaticality judgments by agrammatic aphasics, therefore, cannot be accounted for as the recognition of aberrant intonation cues in the ungrammatical sentences. As J.W.'s right hemisphere shows a similar pattern of performance it seems likely that it employs the same mechanism as that of the agrammatic aphasics.

V.P.'s results are more difficult to interpret because of the lack of a convincing difference between her left and right hemispheres. It is especially important to establish a difference in this subject because of the demonstration that some fibers of the splenium remain intact. Because V.P. has previously demonstrated greater right hemispheric syntactic competence than J.W. and because she appears to have some ability to generate speech from her right hemisphere, it would not be surprising that her right hemisphere would do well at this task. Without a greater dissociation of right and left hemisphere performance, little more can be said about V.P.'s performance at this time.

CONCLUSIONS

The most striking finding in these two commissurotomized patients with right hemisphere language is the dissociation between the ability to comprehend syntactically constrained sentences and the ability to judge their grammaticality. This dissociation can be found in two distinct populations, agrammatic aphasics and commissurotomy patients. Moreover, the presence of this dissociation in the intellectually impoverished right hemisphere suggests that grammaticality judgments may not depend on a developed intellectual capacity as much as the interpretation of sentences. The processing underlying grammaticality judgments may be automatic and data driven and, as a consequence, be independent of the adequate functioning of other cognitive systems, such as those involved in an inference task. Interpretation of syntactically constrained sentences may, however, require more interactive processing and depend crucially on inferential capacity.

We are not claiming that the processes responsible for grammaticality judgments are mediated solely by the right hemisphere [Berndt et al. (17) demonstrated that right hemisphere damaged patients are highly accurate in judging grammaticality]; nor are we claiming that the two hemispheres make grammatical judgments in the same way. There may be alternate processes for determining the well-formedness of sentences. We did not measure reaction time in J.W. and V.P., but V.P. was aware that she took longer to make a left than a right hemisphere decision. As she put it, when responding with her left hand to a right hemisphere presentation she felt the hand being "drawn to the screen like a magnet" before she had made up her mind about the answer. Rather we are arguing that the dissociation observed in J.W. suggests that grammaticality judgments and sentential interpretation involve different processes and that the preserved ability to judge the grammaticality of a sentence may rest in part on its relative independence from a more general intellectual capacity.

Other explanations of the findings are possible. Zurif and Grodzinsky (25), for instance, have argued that grammaticality judgments can be made on a degraded structural representation that does not contain sufficient information to process for comprehension. What this position seems to imply is that a full structural specification is necessary for normal comprehension [but see (2,6,7,13,20)]. A rough structural specification could be rapidly and automatically constructed as part of the normal comprehension process and our only conscious access to that process is our grammatical intuition. This rough specification may be all that the right hemisphere computes. Consequently, it may be able to make accurate grammaticality judgments, but still not have enough syntactic information to interpret the sentence accurately.

The present research cannot determine whether the processing underlying grammatical intuitions depends on a different system than the processing underlying comprehension—on which is data driven, automatic, and independent of higher order cognitive functioning—or whether the two processes involve the same system, but merely depend on different levels of syntactic representation. Clearly, further exploration of right hemisphere language must be undertaken, but the value of developing a model of right hemisphere language should be clear. As this model develops, the components and processes driving normal language function will be better understood.

ACKNOWLEDGMENTS

The research reported in this chapter was supported by NINCDS grant NS17778 and The Burke Foundation. We thank M.F. Schwartz, E.M. Saffran, O.S.M. Marin, and M. Linebarger for sharing their stimulus materials with us. Special thanks go to W. Hirst for his advice and support.

REFERENCES

1. Berndt, R.S., and Caramazza, A. (1980): A redefinition of Broca's aphasia: Implications for a neuropsychological model of language. *Applied Psycholinguistics*, 1:225–278.
2. Bever, T. (1970): The cognitive basis for linguistic structures. In: *Cognition and the Development of Language*, edited by J. Hayes, pp. 279–326. John Wiley, New York.

3. Caramazza, A. (1984): The logic of neuropsychological research and the problem of patient classification. *Brain Lang.*, 21:9–20.
4. Caramazza, A., Berndt, R.S., and Basili, A. (1983): The selective impairment of phonological processing: A case study. *Brain Lang.*, 18:128–174.
5. Caramazza, A., and Martin, R.C. (1983): Theoretical and methodological issues in the study of aphasia. In: *Cerebral Hemisphere Asymmetry: Method, Theory, and Application*, edited by J.B. Hellige, pp. 95–151. Praeger, New York.
6. Forster, K.I., and Obrei, I. (1973): Semantic heuristics and syntactic analysis. *Cognition*, 2:319–347.
7. Foss, D.J., and Hakes, D.T. (1978): *Psycholinguistics: An Introduction to the Psychology of Language*. Prentice Hall, Englewood Cliffs, NJ.
8. Gazzaniga, M.S. (1983): Right hemisphere language following brain bisection: A twenty year perspective. *Am. Psychol.*, 38:525–537.
9. Gazzaniga, M.S., and Hillyard, S. (1971): Language and speech capacity of the right hemisphere. *Neuropsychologia*, 9:273–280.
10. Gazzaniga, M.S., Holtzman, J.D., Deck, M.D.F., and Lee, B.C.P. (1985): MRI assessment of human callosal surgery with neuropsychological correlates. *Neurology*, 35:1763–1766.
11. Gazzaniga, M.S., and Smylie, C.S. (1984): Dissociation of language and cognition: A psychological profile of two disconnected right hemispheres. *Brain*, 107:145–153.
12. Gazzaniga, M.S., Smylie, C.S., Baynes, K., Hirst, W., and McCleary, C.A. (1984): Profiles of right hemisphere language and speech following brain bisection. *Brain Lang.*, 22:206–220.
13. Herriot, P. (1969): The comprehension of active and passive sentences as a function of pragmatic expectations. *J. Verb. Learn. Verb. Behav.*, 8:166–169.
14. Levy, J., and Trevarthen, C. (1977): Perceptual, semantic, and phonetic aspects of elementary language processes in split-brain patients. *Brain*, 100:108–118.
15. Linebarger, M., Schwartz, M.F., and Saffran, E.M. (1983): Sensitivity to grammatical structures in so-called agrammatic aphasics. *Cognition*, 8:1–71.
16. Newmeyer, F.J. (1986): *Linguistic Theory in America*, 2nd ed. Academic Press, Orlando, FL.
17. Berndt, R.S., Salasoo, A., Mitchum, C.C., and Blumstein, S.E. The role of intonation cues in aphasic patients' performance of the grammaticality judgment task. *Brain Lang. (in press).*
18. Schwartz, M.F., Saffran, E.M., and Marin, O.S.M. (1980): The word order problem in agrammatism: I. Comprehension. *Brain Lang.*, 10:249–262.
19. Sidtis, J.J., Volpe, B.T., Wilson, D.H., Rayport, M., and Gazzaniga, M.S. (1981): Variability in right hemisphere language after callosal section: Evidence for a continuum of generative capacity. *J. Neurosci.*, 3:323–331.
20. Slobin, D. (1966): Grammatical transformations and sentence comprehension in childhood and adulthood. *J. Verb. Learn. Verb. Behav.*, 5:219–227.
21. Zaidel, E. (1976): Auditory vocabulary of the right hemisphere following brain bisection of hemidecortication. *Cortex*, 12:191–211.
22. Zaidel, E. (1978): Auditory language comprehension in the right hemisphere following cerebral commissurotomy and hemispherectomy: A comparison with child language and aphasia. In: *Language Acquisition and Language Breakdown: Parallels and Divergencies*, edited by A. Caramazza and E.B. Zurif, pp. 229–275. The Johns Hopkins University Press, Baltimore.
23. Zaidel, E. (1983): Disconnection syndrome as a model for laterality effects in the normal brain. In: *Cerebral Hemisphere Asymmetry: Method, Theory, and Application*, edited by J.B. Hellige, pp. 95–151. Praeger, New York.
24. Zaidel, E. (1983): On multiple representations of the lexicon in the brain—The case of two hemispheres. In: *Psychobiology of Language*, edited by M. Studdert-Kennedy, pp. 105–122. MIT Press, Cambridge, MA.
25. Zurif, E.B., and Grodzinsky, Y. (1983): Grammatical sensitivity in agrammatism: A reply to Linebarger et al. *Cognition*, 15:207–213.

*Language, Communication, and
the Brain*, edited by F. Plum.
Raven Press, New York © 1988.

The Pathogenesis of Childhood Dyslexia

Albert M. Galaburda

*Department of Neurology, Harvard Medical School; and Neurological Unit,
Charles A. Dana Research Institute and Dyslexia Neuroanatomical Laboratory,
Beth Israel Hospital, Boston, Massachusetts 02215*

The notion that developmental dyslexia reflects a pathological brain and therefore requires a neuropathologic explanation is not without need of qualification. Abnormalities in cognitive and emotional behavior, and, within those categories, abnormalities in reading and writing acquisition, must be understood in the context of abnormal interactions between the brain and its environment because of abnormalities in the brain per se, abnormalities in the environment, abnormalities in the interaction itself, or all three. *A priori*, there is no strong argument that requires always the presence of an abnormal brain, since it is easy to conceive that a variety of exclusively environmental factors could interfere with the process of reading and writing acquisition. Thus, a seriously inadequate educational system, a difficult home situation, and other similar factors could interfere with the learning process. Moreover, other purely behavioral issues must be considered; thus, for instance, the exact nature of the linguistic demands of the task at hand might play a significant role, as is the case of the Japanese alphabetic script *Kana* and the ideographic *Kanji*, which appear to place different demands on the brain (23,32,38).

In the case that one *is* able to determine that the reading difficulties indeed arise from brain malfunction, there is again no *a priori* reason to predict that a single localization or a unique form of pathology must account for all the witnessed developmental reading disorders. An intuitively obvious distinction can be drawn between children with primary dyslexic symptoms in the face of a normal intellectual and emotional constitution and those who do not learn to read and write with ease in the context of a deeper emotional or intellectual deficiency, as is seen in childhood autism and in mental retardation. Even within the category of primary developmental dyslexia, a behavioral taxonomy might be developed in which different subtypes of dyslexia have separate and distinct neurological substrates.

The level of description of the anatomy may vary for different etiologies of the reading disorder. Thus, some types of dyslexia may be described at the neurochemical (molecular) level, whereas others may relate to gross anatomical changes. Take, for instance, *tachypnea* (rapid breathing), a symptom often encountered in clinical medicine. After subjecting the tachypneic patient to the appropriate behavioral scrutiny, e.g., noting the rate and pattern of breathing, as well as associated symptoms and signs, it is possible to describe the anatomical substrates at several levels, from the molecular to the social. Thus, the patient may be diabetic, and the tachypnea is the result of acute metabolic acidosis; conversely it may be a case of pneumonia, whereby abnormal inflammatory secretions can interfere with normal air exchange between alveoli and the blood and cause shunting of unoxygenated blood to the arterial circulation; one may be dealing with upper airway obstruction caused by aspiration of a foreign body, or it may even be caused by air pollution. The ability to describe the anatomy at the proper level is crucial to the design of appropriate therapies.

Assuming, furthermore, that the brain of a child with primary dyslexia is indeed different from that of a good reader at one or several levels of analysis, the question whether the difference can be accounted for by normal individual variability or by pathological oddity[1] must be raised. Does dyslexia arise from the interaction between the arbitrarily adopted environmental requirement of an inflexible educational system and normally diverse brain architectures, some of which do not do well under those particular requirements? Or does dyslexia arise outside of this normal variability, imposed on an individual because of a pathological brain architecture?

Anatomical approaches to the study of developmental dyslexia were made in our laboratory starting with the intuitive notion that odd brain architectures underlie the reading difficulty. The choice of level of analysis, at least at the early stages of the research, relied heavily on knowledge that the organization of the brain for language has been best demonstrated at the gross anatomical and histological levels and virtually not at all at the neurochemical or molecular level; furthermore, individual variability has been shown at these anatomical levels.

Specifically the research began with the hypothesis that dyslexics have primarily a linguistic deficiency, and, therefore, that known language substrates in the brain would be affected if odd anatomical architectures were to be demonstrated. Second, the behavioral literature suggested strongly that dyslexics exhibit disturbances in cerebral dominance, and, therefore, it would seem possible to demonstrate oddity in the manifestation of anatomical asymmetry. Finally, it was reasoned that, being a developmental problem, the allegedly odd brain architectures accompanying dyslexia might be uncovered and explained by tools and concepts derived from developmental neuroscience. In the following sections I describe the findings as they relate to these levels of inquiry, and in the last section I speculate on the possible mechanisms that could explain such findings.

ASYMMETRY IN THE BRAIN

It is now well accepted that some regions of the cerebral cortex are asymmetrical in size between the hemispheres. These asymmetries have been demonstrated at

---

[1]The term oddity, borrowed from Professor Mary-Louise Kean, implies an aberration that is not necessarily negative (see final section).

several levels, from the gross anatomical (including neuroradiologic procedures) (2,7,19,25,26,37), through histological (5–10), to neurochemical levels (1,29). One of the most striking of these asymmetries is visible in a gross anatomical landmark known as the *planum temporale*. This region, which is found on the supra-temporal plane just posterior to the transverse auditory gyrus of Heschl, is most often larger on the left side (2,19,37). We recently re-analyzed the brains reported by Geschwind and Levitsky (19), and found a bimodal distribution of these asymmetries with most brains asymmetrical toward the left or slightly toward the right, and a few brains strongly asymmetrical toward the right (13) (Fig. 1). The proportion of brains that are symmetrical in the planum temporale range from approximately 15% to 25% in published reports, and comprise approximately 15% in our study (arbitrarily defined by a coefficient of asymmetry, δ of -0.1 to $+0.1$). The odds of randomly finding a brain having symmetrical plana are approximately 1/6, and the odds of finding x consecutive brains with symmetrical plana approach $(0.15)^x$ (see below). Fewer than 5% of brains are strongly asymmetrical toward the right ($\delta > +1.0$), and the remainder ($\sim80\%$) are either asymmetrical toward the left ($\sim65\%$; δ ranging from -0.1 to -1.5) or slightly asymmetrical toward the right ($\sim15\%$; δ ranging from $+0.1$ to $+0.5$). Approximately 40% of brains are only moderately asymmetrical toward the left (δ ranging from -0.1 to -0.5, and about 10% are markedly asymmetrical toward the left (δ at least -1.0).

NATURE OF THE ANATOMICAL ASYMMETRY

The standard theory suggests that language is lateralized to the left, to the right, or shared between the two sides in varying proportions—implying that there is a somewhat uniform amount of language substrate to be distributed between the hemispheres according to the laterality of the individual. If, indeed, there is a

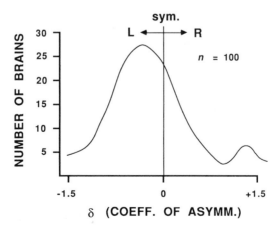

FIG. 1. Distribution of asymmetry coefficients [$\delta = (L - R)/0.5(L + R)$] for the *planum temporale* in a population of 100 normal adult human brains.

correlation between functional lateralization and anatomic asymmetry, the actual anatomical situation differs from that which would be predicted by the aforementioned theory. Thus, the theory predicts that some brains have large language areas on the left, others have large language areas on the right, and still others have medium-sized language areas, one in each hemisphere. Although the brains with marked asymmetry to the left and to the right appear to be mirror images of one another (Fig. 2), whereby the total amount of planum temporale (right + left) is similar in the two groups, the total amount of planum temporale in the rest of the brains, however, is not constant, varying instead with changes in the value of δ; consequently, the brains that are increasingly symmetrical have more total planum cortex than those that are mildly to moderately asymmetrical (Fig. 3). Moreover, leaving aside brains with extreme rightward asymmetry, the size of the left planum varies little in the population once corrections have been made for variations in total brain size. Instead, it is the size of the right planum that changes significantly in these brains (Fig. 4). We conclude, therefore, that there are two distinct populations of brains vis-à-vis the size of the planum temporale: one comprising the larger group in which the average asymmetry is moderately leftward; and one comprising a much smaller group with extreme rightward asymmetry. In the former group there is an inverse relationship between total amount of planum (left + right) and degree of asymmetry (defined by the δ value); the size of the left planum does not vary significantly in this population, and, instead, most of the variability takes place in the size of the right planum. There is an alternative interpretation of the functional implications of this arrangement; it appears as if the two hemispheres may not simply share language dominance in varying proportions, but rather that the relatively invariant left hemisphere dominance for language might be modulated to varying degrees and in different ways by homologous right hemisphere structures (13).

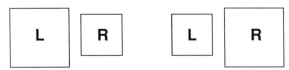

FIG. 2. Brains with extreme leftward asymmetry are mirror image to a small number of brains with extreme rightward asymmetry.

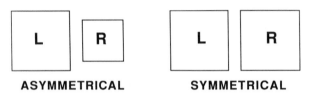

FIG. 3. Asymmetrical brains have a relatively smaller (rather than larger) region on one side, as compared with symmetrical brains.

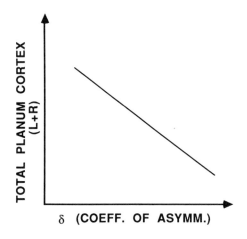

FIG. 4. There is an inverse relationship between degree of asymmetry (δ) and total amount of a particular region (R + L), e.g., symmetrical language areas are relatively larger than asymmetrical ones. (See Fig. 3).

We investigated the histological nature of cortical asymmetry and reasoned that asymmetry could be accounted for by side differences in the number of neurons, or in cell-packing density (which reflects the size of the dendritic arbor and local axons, as well as extraneuronal elements such as glia, myelin, vessels), or by a combination of both. The empirical evidence gathered from measurements of volumes of architectonic areas and neuronal counts in the cortical laminae in asymmetrical rat visual cortex showed that only side differences in total numbers of neurons correlated significantly with asymmetry (Fig. 5). Thus, the main reason for the differences in the volumes of homologous architectonic regions in asymmetrical brains is that they have different numbers of neurons rather than different local connectional architectures affecting cell-packing density.

Putting both sets of observations together, those regarding gross anatomical asymmetry and those of histological asymmetry, leads us to conclude that what best distinguishes two asymmetrical brain regions is that the former have a greater number of neurons in the usually nondominant side. Current research undertakes pinpointing the mechanisms by which asymmetrical brain regions achieve differences in numbers of neurons on the two sides. One working hypothesis, the arguments for which are beyond the scope of this summary, is that asymmetry in

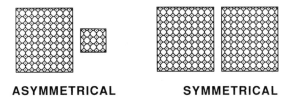

ASYMMETRICAL   **SYMMETRICAL**

FIG. 5. Asymmetrical areas exhibit side differences in the number of neurons. Brains with symmetrical cortical areas contain a relatively greater number of neurons in those areas than brains with asymmetrical cortical areas.

numbers of neurons is achieved through asymmetrical cell death during cortico-genesis. If asymmetrical cell death can account for the development of cerebral asymmetry, then developmental events capable of modulating cell death could lead to oddity in the manifestation of brain asymmetry and, consequently, of cerebral dominance.

SYMMETRY IN THE DYSLEXIC BRAIN

There have long been clinical observations suggesting anomalous cerebral dominance among dyslexics (30), and radiological studies have demonstrated deviations from the normal distribution of symmetry and asymmetry in that population (21,22), therefore we looked at brain asymmetry in the autopsy brains. The planum temporale was found to be of the symmetrical type in seven consecutively measured brains (Fig. 6); no brain from a dyslexic individual has thus far shown either the left- or right-asymmetrical type in our laboratory (11). Based on the chances of finding a single symmetrical brain at random (see above), it is distinctly unlikely [$\sim(0.15)^7$] that the consistent finding of symmetry in the dyslexic brains reflects a chance occurrence. Instead, we may safely surmise that the absence of standard asymmetry represents at least one of the anatomical accompaniments of the dyslexic syndrome, and, moreover, we may propose that dyslexic brains, at least in the region of the right planum temporale, contain excessive numbers of neurons.

MICRODYSGENESIS

Ectopias (small loci of abnormally placed neurons) or dysplasias (focally distorted cortical architecture) are found occasionally in routine autopsy studies (3,24,27,28,31,36). In reported studies the number of brains with anomalies and their distribution depends on the level of detail of the analysis, but it ranges between 3% and 15%, with lesions most commonly in the frontal lobe, right more often

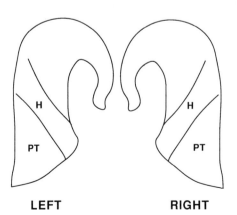

FIG. 6. Typically symmetrical appearance of the planum temporale in the brains of dyslexic individuals. Both plana are relatively large.

LEFT   **RIGHT**

than left. Five male dyslexic brains were sectioned whole at 35 μm and every 20th section was stained and examined. All brains showed microdysgenesis consisting of islands of subpial neurons (Fig. 7a) with occasional brainwart formation, underlying focal architectonic dysplasia (Fig. 7b) including one instance of micropolygyria, and many instances of microdysgenesis of small blood vessels including frank microangiomata (Fig. 7c) (11,12). The distribution of these anomalies was bilateral in all brains, but the number of disturbances was greater in the left hemisphere in all cases; within the hemisphere they affected the perisylvian cortices, particularly the frontal and temporal opercula. In our previous experience with at least 25 normative brains from the Yakovlev Collection at the Armed Forces Institute of Pathology and the Harvard Medical School (5–10), which were processed and examined in identical fashion, these types of cortical abnormalities were seen rarely and in single numbers.

EPIDEMIOLOGIC STUDIES AND PATHOGENETIC IMPLICATIONS

If the presence of microdysgenesis of the cortex characterizes the dyslexic brain, is there any evidence to help pinpoint possible mechanisms for such changes? There are data from the human and experimental developmental neuropathology literature to show that ectopias and dysplasias often result from focal cortical injury occurring during late corticogenesis when the last waves of neurons are migrating to the cortex

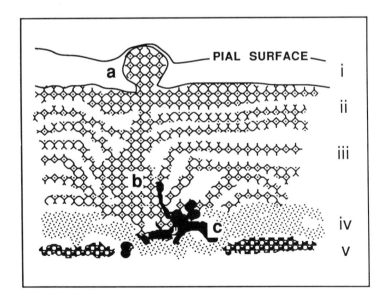

FIG. 7. Semistylized, composite diagram of the types of cerebrocortical dysgenesis seen in brains of dyslexics. An ectopic collection of neurons is seen in layer i (**a**); disorganization of cortical lamination (dysplasia) is seen predominantly in the upper layers (**b**); abnormal microarchitecture of cortical vessels often accompanies the dysplasia (**c**).

from the germinal zones (3,4): could injury be a cause of similar focal changes in the dyslexic brain? The answer may come from looking at the implications of clinical findings linking anomalous cerebral dominance (left-handedness and ambidexterity), learning disability, and certain diseases that implicate immune dysfunction (14–18). It is well known that fetal injury can be the consequence of autoimmune and allergic diseases (13). For example, it has been shown that pregnant mothers with systemic lupus erythematosus (SLE) carry antibodies that can lead to neonatal lupus. Moreover, there is evidence for the direct damage of the fetal heart tissue by toxic maternal antibodies crossing the placenta (33). There are several other examples of immune-based injury to fetal tissues, e.g., neonatal myasthenia gravis and erythroblastosis fetalis, and similar injury may take place against the fetal brain. Preliminary evidence from the laboratory of Dr. Peter Behan in Glasgow (*personal communication*) has shown that pregnant rabbits inoculated with autotoxic antibodies gave birth to offspring with marked cerebral dysmorphism, including holotelencephaly. Thus, although much more specific information is needed, there is now a possible pathogenetic link to the brain anomalies in the dyslexic brains. It remains possible, therefore, that individuals and families with increased risk for developing immune disorders may also have an increased risk for having focal brain injury during the late fetal period, which may lead to the brain changes seen in dyslexia. Part of the current efforts in our laboratory aims at disclosing evidence for immune injury to the developing brains of immune-defective mice with learning disorders and anomalies in cerebral dominance (34).

ANATOMICAL CONSEQUENCES OF EARLY BRAIN INJURY

Does the consistent co-occurrence of two unexpected events suggest that they are linked? Specifically, are the microdysgenesis and symmetry (both of which are unusual findings alone, and yet occur consistently in the dyslexic brains) linked? One way to explain this co-occurrence is to propose that the injury that causes the microdysgenesis leads to enhanced survival of neurons, and therefore increased symmetry. There is a considerable amount of evidence showing that injury to the brain during critical developmental stages (corresponding largely to late neuronal migration and neuronal maturation) leads to significant changes in neuronal architecture, among which it is possible, under some circumstances, to demonstrate enhanced survival of neurons and axons (20). We suggest that the focal dysplasias and ectopias reflect injury to the brain during analogous developmental epochs, which also leads to rearrangement of cortical architecture of neurons and connections and to changes in the patterns of asymmetry, symmetry, and cerebral dominance.

FUTURE RESEARCH AND GOALS

It appears essential to specify the exact interactions between anomalous brain architectures, possibly leading to increased risk for dyslexia, and immunological diseases. More epidemiological work is needed to uncover the immunological illnesses that increase this risk, and the developmental stages at which they do. Moreover, specific autoantibodies must be identified, which may serve, in part, as early markers for the risk for dyslexia. One of the possible general implications of the findings and hypotheses discussed in this chapter include the presence of a heretofore poorly understood group of disorders caused by abnormal immune interactions during fetal life, which may lead to a variety of intellectual deficits depending on the exact types and times of the interactions, as well as on the availability of compensatory mechanisms. Thus it is possible that developmental disorders of language, emotional behavior, and attention will eventually be explained by these mechanisms affecting different parts of the brain during different developmental epochs.

At the laboratory bench we need to specify the mechanisms of action of possible culprit immune reactions leading to brain injury, and the ways by which subtle focal injury leads to neural restructuring and its concomitant behavioral effects. There is the suggestion, even at this early stage, that anomalous cortical architectures may lead to increased risks not only for dyslexia, but also for some forms of epilepsy and other developmental cognitive disorders (35). It has, moreover, been suggested that pathological mechanisms such as those discussed in this summary could lead to brain reorganization that produces intellectual advantages. In some cases, therefore, it may be possible to characterize nonbehavioral, biological markers for giftedness. Finally, better understanding of the developmental processes that lead to brain oddity may help to explain later acquired disorders of the nervous system such as senile dementia.

ACKNOWLEDGMENTS

This work was supported in part by National Institutes of Health grants NICHD 14018 and 02711, and the General Dyslexia Grant and Orton Dyslexia Grant to the Beth Israel Hospital.

I thank Drs. Gordon F. Sherman and Glenn D. Rosen for their collaboration and comments.

REFERENCES

1. Amaducci, L., Sorbi, S., Albanese, A., and Gainotti, G. (1981): Choline-acetyltransferase (Ch AT) activity differs in right and left human temporal lobes. *Neurology*, 31:799–805.
2. Campain, R., and Minckler, J. (1976): A note on the gross configurations of the human auditory cortex. *Brain Lang.*, 3:318–323.
3. Caviness, V.S., Evrard, P., and Lyon, G. (1978): Radial neuronal assemblies, ectopia and necrosis of developing cortex: A case analysis. *Acta Neuropathol.*, 41:67–72.
4. Dvorak, K., Feit, J., and Jurankova, Z. (1978): Experimentally induced focal micropolygyria and status verrucosus deformans in rats: Pathogenesis and interrelations. *Acta Neuropathol.*, 44:121–129.
5. Eidelberg, D., and Galaburda, A.M. (1982): Symmetry and asymmetry in the human posterior thalamus. *Arch. Neurol.*, 39:325–332.

6. Eidelberg, D., and Galaburda, A.M. (1984): Inferior parietal lobule. Divergent architectonic asymmetries in the human brain. *Arch. Neurol.*, 41:843–852.
7. Galaburda, A.M., LeMay, M., Kemper, T.L., and Geschwind, N. (1978): Right-left asymmetries in the brain. *Science*, 199:852–856.
8. Galaburda, A.M., Sanides, F., and Geschwind, N. (1978): Human brain: Cytoarchitectonic left-right asymmetries in temporal speech region. *Arch. Neurol.*, 35:812–817.
9. Galaburda, A.M. (1980): La région de Broca: Observations anatomiques faites un siècle après la mort de son découvreur. *Rev. Neurol. (Paris)*, 36:609–616.
10. Galaburda, A.M., and Eidelberg, D. (1982): Symmetry ad asymmetry in the human posterior thalamus. II. Thalamic lesions in a case of developmental dyslexia. *Arch. Neurol.*, 39:333–336.
11. Galaburda, A.M., Sherman, G.F., Rosen, G.D., Aboitiz, F., and Geschwind, N. (1985): Developmental dyslexia: Four consecutive patients with cortical anomalies. *Ann. Neurol.*, 18:222–233.
12. Galaburda, A.M., Signoret, J.L., and Ronthal, M. (1985): Left posterior angiomatous anomaly and developmental dyslexia: Report of five cases. *Neurology*, 35(Suppl.):198.
13. Galaburda, A.M., Corsiglia, J., Rosen, G.D., and Sherman, G.F. (1987): Planum temporale asymmetry: Reappraisal since Geschwind and Levitsky. *Neuropsychologia (in press)*.
14. Geschwind, N., and Behan, P.O. (1982): Left-handedness: Association with immune disease, migraine, and developmental learning disorder. *Proc. Natl. Acad. Sci. USA*, 79:5097–5100.
15. Geschwind, N., and Behan, P.O. (1984): Laterality, hormones, and immunity. In: *Cerebral Dominance: The Biological Foundations*, edited by N. Geschwind and A.M. Galaburda, pp. 211–224. Harvard University Press, Cambridge, MA.
16. Geschwind, N., and Galaburda, A.M. (1985): Cerebral lateralization. Biological mechanisms, associations, and pathology: I. *Arch. Neurol.*, 42:428–459.
17. Geschwind, N., and Galaburda, A.M. (1985): Cerebral lateralization. Biological mechanisms, associations, and pathology: II. *Arch. Neurol.*, 42:521–552.
18. Geschwind, N., and Galaburda, A.M. (1985): Cerebral lateralization. Biological mechanisms, associations, and pathology: III. *Arch. Neurol.*, 42:634–654.
19. Geschwind, N., and Levitsky, W. (1968): Human brain: Left-right asymmetries in temporal speech region. *Science*, 161:186–187.
20. Goldman-Rakic, P.S., and Rakic, P. (1984): Experimental modification of gyral patterns. In: *Cerebral Dominance: The Biological Foundations*, edited by N. Geschwind and A.M. Galaburda, pp. 179–192. Harvard University Press, Cambridge, MA.
21. Haslam, R.H.A., Dalby, J.T., Johns, R.D., and Rademaker, A.W. (1981): Cerebral asymmetry in developmental dyslexia. *Arch. Neurol.*, 38:679–682.
22. Hier, D.B., LeMay, M., Rosenberger, P.B., and Perlo, V.P. (1978): Developmental dyslexia: Evidence for a subgroup with a reversal cerebral asymmetry. *Arch. Neurol.*, 35:90–92.
23. Iwata, M. (1986): Neural mechanisms of reading and writing in the Japanese language. *Functional Neurology*, 1:43–52.
24. Jacob, H. (1940): Die feinere Oberflächengestaltung der Hirnwindungen, die Hirnwarzenbildung und die Mikropolygyrie. *Z. Neurol. Psychiat.*, 178:64–84.
25. LeMay, M., and Culebras, A. (1972): Human brain: Morphological differences in the hemispheres demonstrable by carotid arteriography. *N. Engl. J. Med.*, 287:168–170.
26. LeMay, M., and Kido, D.K. (1978): Asymmetries of the cerebral hemispheres on computed tomogram. *J. Comput. Assist. Tomogr.*, 2:471–478.
27. McBride, M.C., and Kemper, T.L. (1982): Pathogenesis of four-layered microgyric cortex in man. *Acta Neuropathol.*, 57:93–98.
28. Morel, F., and Wildi, E. (1952): Dysgénésie nodulaire disséminée de l'écorce frontale. *Rev. Neurol.*, 87:251–270.
29. Oke, A., Keller, R., Mefford, I., and Adams, R.N. (1978): Lateralization of norepinephrine in the human thalamus. *Science*, 200:1411–1413.
30. Orton, S.T. (1925): "Word-blindness" in school children. *Arch. Neurol. Psychiat.*, 14:581–615.
31. Ranke, O. (1910): Beiträge zur Kenntnis der normalen und pathologischen Hirnrindenbildung. *Beitr. Path. Anat.*, 47:51–125.
32. Sasanuma, S., and Fujimura, O. (1971): Selective impairment of phonetic and non-phonetic transcription of words in Japanese aphasic patients: Kana vs. kanji in visual recognition and writing. *Cortex*, 7:1–18.
33. Scott, J.S., Maddison, P.J., Taylor, P.V., Esscher, E., Scott, O., and Skinner, R.P. (1983): Connective-tissue disease, antibodies to ribonucleoprotein, and congenital heart block. *N. Engl. J. Med.*, 309:209–212.

34. Sherman, G.F., Galaburda, A.M., and Geschwind, N. (1985): Cortical anomalies in the brains of New Zealand mice: A neuropathological model of dyslexia? *Proc. Natl. Acad. Sci. USA*, 82:8072–8074.
35. Taylor, D.C., Falconer, M.A., Burton, C.J., et. al. (1971): Focal dysplasias of the cerebral cortex in epilepsy. *J. Neurol. Neurosurg. Psychiatry*, 34:369–387.
36. Veith, G., and Schwindt, W. (1976): Pathologisch-anatomischer Beitrag zum Problem ''Nichtsesshaftigkeit.'' *Fortschr. Neurol. Psychiatr.*, 44:1–21.
37. Witelson, S.F., and Pallie, W. (1973): Left hemisphere specialization for language in the newborn. Neuroanatomical evidence of asymmetry. *Brain*, 96:641–646.
38. Yamadori, A. (1975): Ideogram reading in alexia. *Brain*, 98:231–238.

*Language, Communication, and
the Brain*, edited by F. Plum.
Raven Press, New York © 1988.

Dyslexia Subtypes: Genetics, Behavior, and Brain Imaging

*Herbert A. Lubs, †Shelley Smith, †William Kimberling,
‡Bruce Pennington, *Karen Gross-Glenn, and §Ranjan Duara

*Mailman Center for Child Development, Genetics Division,
University of Miami School of Medicine, Miami, Florida 33101;
†Boys Town National Institute, Omaha, Nebraska 68131;
‡University of Colorado Medical Center, Denver, Colorado 80262; and
§Departments of Radiology and Neurology,
University of Miami School of Medicine, Miami, Florida 33101, and Mount Sinai
Medical Center, Miami Beach, Florida 33140*

Advances in technology often provide new methods of approaching old problems. The work reported here is not only a new approach to the old problem of dyslexia but one that is also applicable to the study of the number of other possible genetic effects on brain development and behavior.

GENETIC STUDIES

Background and Methods

The project began over 10 years ago with Dr. Shelley Smith's Ph.D. thesis. At that time it was known from a study published by Hallgren (4) in 1950 that approximately 10% of families in Sweden appeared to have a dominantly inherited form of dyslexia. The world chose to ignore this report since the criteria for the diagnosis of dyslexia and selection of patients were not clearly defined. The genetic analysis was also not ideal but the data were highly suggestive for a genetic etiology of a significant portion of dyslexia. We decided to approach the problem through a linkage analysis. The value of the linkage study is clear: it is unlikely, because of the statistical criteria and the method of analysis of the data, that a significant positive linkage would be found unless there was a gene on a specific chromosome that led to the results. Thus, by carrying out family studies and a concomitant linkage study, it was possible to circumvent the problem of imprecise diagnostic criteria. After establishing a specific linkage, the phenotype, or description of the entity, can be redefined more precisely.

When chromosomes pair in meiosis, crossing over, or exchange of chromatin, occurs between the paired chromosomes with a frequency of about two crossovers per chromosome. Thus, chromosomes are not transmitted from generation to generation as a complete unit. The frequency with which any two genes will be concomitantly transmitted is directly related to their closeness on the chromosome. When two genes are transmitted together within a family 99% of the time, this is termed a recombination frequency of 0.01 or 1% and it is generally considered a close linkage. These results are expressed in terms of LOD scores or log of the odds of linkage. Since these scores are logarithms, a positive LOD score of 3 indicates 1,000-to-1 odds of linkage; a negative LOD score of 2 represents odds of 1 in 100 that there might be linkage. One of the advantages of using a logarithmic score is that the data from multiple matings within a family as well as between families can be directly added, and a cumulative LOD score can be developed.

The input of such a study includes two basic types of information: first, whether an individual within the family is affected, and second, a battery of genetic markers. Three types of markers can now be used in linkage studies: chromosomal variations, blood group and protein variations, and, in the last few years, normal variations in DNA constitution called restriction fragment length polymorphisms (RFLPs). The last, during the next few years, will probably be the only type of marker that is used. In the first part of this study, however, the first two were used, and they led to the identification of a positive linkage with chromosome 15 polymorphisms for a proportion of the families. The basis for this statement comes from the concomitant transmissions, not of a specific chromosomal variation, but from the collective set of variations present on chromosome 15. Normally, 5 to 10 variations are present on one or another chromosome. These do not represent abnormalities, but simply markers that can be transmitted or not transmitted concomitantly with the gene for dyslexia.

RESULTS

In the first part of this study, families were selected based on the following: a three-generation positive family history, normal intelligence, and performance on reading and spelling tests that was two or more years below an age-appropriate grade level. Anyone with other behavioral or central nervous system abnormalities by history or physical examination was excluded from the study. Thus, this method of selecting families results in a sample with relatively pure problems in reading and spelling.

The linkage studies in the first eight families from Denver and Miami were published in 1983 by Smith et al. (11). A maximum LOD score of 3.24 was found at a theta (or recombination frequency) of 0.13. These results indicated odds greater than 1,000 to 1 for linkage with chromosome 15 heteromorphisms. There was, however, a combination of positive and negative LOD scores with one family (432) being strongly positive and having no crossovers within that family. Another, however, was strongly negative, but not sufficiently negative to result in a significant test for genetic heterogeneity.

Since the available battery of genetic markers only covered 20% to 30% of the genome, the finding of a strongly suggestive result was, in a sense, a matter of luck. On the other hand, there are probably several different genes on different chromosomes that result in dyslexia, and in this sense, the positive result can be viewed as a likely finding. In the future we will be able to select DNA markers in such a way to increase and improve the distribution of these markers throughout the karyotype so that we will have a more complete screening battery.

Since the initial study, Dr. Pennington extended the studies of several of the original families and added additional families. This had the result of making the LOD scores either more positive or more negative, which has affected the testing for heterogeneity. Heterogeneity used in this sense means that more than one gene at one locus is involved in producing the clinical picture that we are now defining as developmental dyslexia. The most recent linkage analysis from the 16 families now available has shown a lower LOD score of 1.733 with a recombination fraction of 0.30 (13). More importantly, because of the greater size and number of families analyzed as well as the use of a more powerful analysis of heterogeneity (9), the testing for genetic heterogeneity was significantly positive and suggested that 30% of families showed a linkage to chromosome 15 polymorphisms. The chromosomal localizations of the other entities are unknown. Results of spelling and other testing in these families may be found in several publications by Smith et al. (11,13) and Pennington et al. (10).

Final acceptance of a linkage, however, depends on confirmation by an independent study. We are beginning such a study in Miami in collaboration with Drs. Gross-Glenn and Duara. In addition to the positron emission tomography (PET) and magnetic resonance imaging (MRI) studies, several visual and auditory psychophysical tests as well as a battery of neuropsychological tests (Table 1) will be included to determine the overall phenotype. We plan to analyze the remaining two-thirds of families not linked to chromosome 15 for other localizations and linkages. Ultimately, we hope to arrive at a final description of several subtypes of dyslexia, each attributable to a different gene, probably on different chromosomes, and to continue the linkage and related studies to the point of actually isolating and characterizing one or more genes for dyslexia. The entry criteria that we will be using are slightly different and are graded, as compared with the prior entry criteria of two grade levels below an age-appropriate norm (Table 2). We describe the preliminary brainscanning results in the next part of this chapter.

PET AND MRI STUDIES

Background

The diagnosis of developmental dyslexia is one of exclusion. It represents the failure of an individual of normal or superior intelligence, with no visual, auditory, social, or psychiatric handicaps, to learn to read normally. The heterogeneity of dyslexia has been investigated mainly from a behavioral standpoint. Although there

TABLE 1. *1986 Neuropsychological test
battery (three areas)*

Verbal subskills

  Peabody picture vocabulary
  Boston naming test
  "FAS" verbal fluency
  Token test
  Sentence repetition
  Rapid automatized naming
  Syntactic comprehension
  Gorham proverbs
  Rey auditory verbal learning
  Logical memory passages
  Paired association learning
  Digit span
  Consonant trigrams

Visuo-spatial/constructive skills

  Rey-Osterrieth complex figure
  Beery visual-motor integration
  Benton visual retention test
  Visual reproduction test
  Letter cancellation task
  Judgment of line orientation

Executive functions/set shifting

  Stroop test
  Rapid alternating stimuli
  Mazes

are likely to be specific neural bases for this group of disorders (1), it can be expressed as primarily an auditory-phonetic processing problem, a visuospatial processing problem, or as a mixture of the two (8).

There is a striking propensity for developmental dyslexia to afflict males, in whom the incidence is four to ten times that of females (1,7). Less striking, but still of interest, is the apparently lower prevalence of dyslexia in such countries as Italy and Spain (2) compared with northern Europe. Perhaps the most convincing evidence for a biological basis for developmental dyslexia is the accumulated evidence of a strong genetic factor in this disorder (1,4,6). Approximately 30% to 50% of developmental dyslexics have a positive family history of reading disability in first-degree relatives, and analyses of the hereditary pattern have generally suggested autosomal dominant transmission (14). (The current genetic and linkage studies are reviewed in the first section of this chapter.)

In contrast to the extensive behavioral studies on dyslexia and its subtypes, the reported anatomical and physiological studies are limited. In four dyslexics that came to autopsy, Galaburda et al. (3) discovered distinctive abnormalities such as

TABLE 2. *Entry criteria*

Age-appropriate grade level	Diagnostic criteria by grade (1986)
	Deviation (S.D.) from expected score on full-scale IQ in two of four reading/spelling criteria (word recognition, reading comprehension, phonics/decoding, spelling)
<Grade 3	−0.5
Grades 3–5	−1.0
Grades 6–8	−1.5
≥ Grade 9	−2.0

neuronal ectopias and architectonic dysplasias mainly in the left perisylvian regions. This group also described deviations in the size and shape of a specific part of the superior temporal convolution, i.e., the planum temporale, on autopsy.

MRI Scans—Methods and Results

We began a project to measure the length and describe the shape of the planum temporale from MRI scans obtained in the sagittal plane. Thus far, we have studied nine male controls and three male dyslexics, who are from a new sample of families that have not yet had genetic or linkage studies. Table 3 gives the length of the right and left planum temporale in these two groups of subjects. The linear measurement from the anterior-most point of Heschl's gyrus to the posterior-most point of the sylvian fissure was taken as the length of the planum temporale. This preliminary analysis showed a trend toward a smaller left planum temporale in dyslexia as compared with controls. These results should be viewed mainly as an attempt to quantify some aspects of brain anatomy in controls and dyslexics rather than a demonstration of a possible anatomical finding.

TABLE 3. *Length (mm) of planum temporale in dyslexia[a]*

	Controls (9 males)	Dyslexic group (3 males)
Age (years)	30.3 ± 5.0	31.0 ± 10.5
Right (mm)	17.4 ± 6.0	16.7 ± 9.2
Left (mm)	18.2 ± 2.0	12.9 ± 5.2

[a]Mean ± S.D.

PET Scans—Methods and Results

Methods

Brain physiological activity can best be studied in anatomical terms by recently developed PET techniques when used for quantifying cerebral glucose metabolism. Following the injection of a labeled analogue of glucose, [18F]fluorodeoxyglucose (FDG), the concentration in the brain of this tracer can be measured from the PET images. Glucose metabolic rate in various brain regions can be calculated, using the brain concentrations and the integrated plasma concentration of the tracer, with an operational equation (5).

Behavioral studies of dyslexics have suggested that they use strategies to read that are different from those of normal readers. Oral reading requires the use of visuo-spatial analysis of words to recognize graphemes, the conversion of graphemes into phonemes, the memory for the meaning of words, and finally the articulation of phonemes. Physiological dysfunction involving any one of these major steps may impede reading ability. Reading during the performance of a PET scan may indeed demonstrate the physiological analogue to the specific behavioral dysfunction producing a reading disability. Therefore, we studied eight normal subjects who read single words serially, five normal subjects who viewed pictures serially, and six dyslexics who read single words serially during the 30-min period between the intravenous bolus injection of FDG and the PET scan of the brain.

Criteria for subject selection for both groups were the following: age between 18 and 45 years, right-handedness (according to Edinburgh Questionnaire), normal or corrected-to-normal vision, no gross sensory, neurological, or psychiatric disorders, an educational level of at least high school, and good physical health.

Dyslexic subjects were those who reported a childhood history of reading and spelling problems severe enough to require treatment and/or disrupt their education, plus a similar history in at least one first-degree relative, and were of normal intelligence. Control subjects had a negative childhood history of reading and spelling problems, and reported no such history in their first-degree relatives.

We obtained psychometric data on dyslexic subjects. They showed normal intelligence (mean WAIS full-scale IQ, 107.4 ± 9.5); spelling deficits (Wide-Range Achievement Test, Level-II spelling, mean grade equivalent, 6.1 ± 3.0); and a considerable range of oral reading abilities (Gray Oral Reading Test, mean grade equivalent, 8.5 ± 4.5)

The activation tasks were as follows:

1. *Serial word reading.* We presented words sequentially at a rate of 1 every 5 sec, at a viewing distance of approximately 18 in. Lower-case letters were high contrast and subtended a visual angle of $0.6° \times 0.4°$. Words were high frequency nouns (A or AA, based on the Thorndike-Lorge count) of three to six letters in length. As instructed, subjects binocularly fixated on a small cross in the central field of view and pronounced each word as it appeared. Word reading began about 2 min prior to injection of FDG, and continued for 30 min, after which PET scanning

began, and lasted for 20 min. Ambient light level was low, and the room was quiet during the reading task.

2. *Serial picture viewing.* A slide projector presented a series of colored pictures of faces, animals, seascapes, landscapes, flowers, and inanimate objects, showing each slide for 10 sec. The test lasted 32 min (180 pictures per PET scan), beginning 2 min before the time of injection of the isotope. Subjects depressed a foot pedal with the right or left foot to indicate whether they did or did not like the picture. The responses were recorded.

Results of PET Scan Studies

Based on a total of 19 subjects (six dyslexics reading real words, eight age-matched control subjects reading real words, and five age-matched control subjects viewing pictures), preliminary data showed significant differences between the two groups. Average gray matter cerebral metabolic rate of glucose (CMRglc) was not significantly different between groups (Table 4).

However, when regional metabolic values were normalized, relative to overall gray matter metabolism (regional CMR/overall gray matter CMR), it was possible to assess the "landscape" of metabolic activation across the whole brain, and in this case, the groups appeared to differ (Table 4.)

Thus far there are two main findings. Normal readers showed relatively high levels of metabolic activity in bilateral peri-insular cortex during reading. Dyslexics

TABLE 4. *Glucose metabolism in dyslexia*

		Picture preference task (controls) ($N = 5$)	Oral word reading (controls) ($N = 8$)	Oral word reading (dyslexics) ($N = 6$)
Average gray matter		8.84 ± 0.84	7.07 ± 1.90	7.96 ± 2.26
Regional/overall gray matter CMRglc				
Occipital	R	1.15 ± 0.04	1.02 ± 0.17	1.15 ± 0.14
	L	1.13 ± 0.02	1.05 ± 0.17	1.14 ± 0.14
Superior temporal	R	0.98 ± 0.01	1.02 ± 0.03	0.97 ± 0.11
	L	0.96 ± 0.04	0.98 ± 0.05	0.96 ± 0.06
Inferior parietal	R	1.01 ± 0.06	1.05 ± 0.04	1.02 ± 0.08
	L	0.99 ± 0.03	1.01 ± 0.06	1.02 ± 0.08
Insula	R	1.04 ± 0.09[a]	1.15 ± 0.03	1.09 ± 0.06
	L	1.07 ± 0.03	1.13 ± 0.05	1.07 ± 0.05[a]
Premotor	R	1.09 ± 0.04	1.10 ± 0.07	1.06 ± 0.07
	L	1.09 ± 0.06	1.09 ± 0.05	1.06 ± 0.08
Prefrontal	R	0.97 ± 0.07	1.02 ± 0.08	1.00 ± 0.10
	L	0.96 ± 0.07	0.96 ± 0.10	0.99 ± 0.10

[a]Different from controls oral word reading ($p < 0.05$).

showed lower activation of this region bilaterally, although the comparison with control subjects reached statistical significance only for the left peri-insular cortex ($p < 0.05$). Controls who were activated by the picture viewing test had landscapes very similar to dyslexic readers. Furthermore, both dyslexics reading real words and controls viewing pictures tended to have greater relative occipital activation than did controls reading real words.

Second, when symmetry of activation was assessed by an unsigned laterality index, dyslexics showed more asymmetry than did controls in the region of the anterior superior temporal cortex ($p < 0.01$). Thus, the "normal" pattern during reading appeared to be a symmetrical one, with dyslexic subjects showing unequal activation of a homologous temporal lobe region. Direction of this asymmetry, however, varied across dyslexics, with some showing higher right-hemisphere activation; others, higher left-hemisphere activation.

As the major findings involve temporal cortex structures, they may suggest that dyslexics attend less to either the linguistic and/or phonetic aspects of words, as they are read aloud, than do normal readers, and tend to respond metabolically to the reading of words much like controls respond to the viewing of pictures. However, a clear-cut interpretation of these data awaits further PET scan studies with large samples of both normal and dyslexic readers.

SUMMARY AND CONCLUSIONS

This study was designed to identify inherited subtypes of specific dyslexia and to characterize these types by a variety of studies. A previous linkage study in large three-generation families resulted in a LOD score of 3.24 at a 13% recombination frequency between dyslexia and normal variations for the short arm of chromosome 15. The odds for linkage with chromosome 15 markers are better than 1,000 to 1. We estimate that 30% of an extended series of families show linkage to chromosome 15 polymorphisms. Other linkages remain to be identified.

PET scanning is being used to examine measures of regional cerebral glucose metabolism during two types of reading by (adult) dyslexics and normal readers. MRI is also being used to examine pertinent brain structures. Behavioral tests are also in progress.

The long-term goals of this study are to develop specific genetic and other diagnostic techniques that can be used to test children before beginning school and to develop sufficient understanding of the abnormal brain function of each subtype so that specific and effective remedial programs can be developed.

REFERENCES

1. Bettman, J.W., Jr., Stern, E.L., Whitsell, L.J., and Goffman, H.F. (1967): Cerebral dominance in developmental dyslexia. *Arch. Ophthalmol.*, 78:722–729.
2. Faglioni, P., Gatti, B., Pagnoni, A.M., and Robutti, A. (1969): A psychometric evaluation of developmental dyslexia in Italian children. *Cortex*, 5:15–26.

3. Galaburda, A.M., Sherman, G.F., Rosen, G.D., Aboitiz, F., and Geschswind, N. (1985): Developmental dyslexia: Four consecutive patients with cortical anomalies. *Ann. Neurol.*, 18:222–233.
4. Hallgren, B. (1950): Specific dyslexia ("congenital word blindness"): A clinical and genetic study. *Acta Psychiatry Neurol.* (Suppl. 65).
5. Huang, S.C., Phelps, M.E., Hoffman, E.J., et al. (1980): Non-invasive determination of local cerebral metabolic rate of glucose in man. *Am. J. Physiol.*, 238:E69–E82.
6. Ingram, T.T.S., Mason, A.W., and Blackburn, I. (1970): A retrospective study of 82 children with reading disability. *Dev. Med. Child. Neurol.*, 12:271–281.
7. Lovell, K., Shapton, D., and Warren, N.S. (1964): A study of some cognitive and other disabilities in backward readers of average intelligence as assessed by a non-verbal test. *Br. J. Educ. Psychol.*, 34:58–64.
8. Omenn, G.S., and Weber, B.A. (1978): Dyslexia: Search for phenotypic and genetic heterogeneity. *Am. J. Med. Genet.*, 1:333–342.
9. Ott, J. (1985): *Analysis of Human Genetic Linkage*. The Johns Hopkins University Press, Baltimore.
10. Pennington, B.F., Smith, S.D., McCabe, L.L., Kimberling, W.J., and Lubs, H.A. (1984): Developmental continuities and discontinuities in a form of familial dyslexia. In: *Continuities and Discontinuities in Development*, edited by R. Emde, and R. Harman, pp. 123–151. Plenum, New York.
11. Smith, S.D., Kimberling, W.J., Pennington, B.F., and Lubs, H.A. (1983): Specific reading disability: Identification of an inherited form through linkage analysis. *Science*, 291:1345–1347.
12. Smith, S.D., Pennington, B.F., Kimberling, W.J., Fain, P.R., Ing, P.S., and Lubs, H.A. (1986): Genetic heterogeneity in specific reading disability. *Am. J. Hum. Genet.* [*Prog. and Abst. for 1986 Annual Meeting*], 39 (Suppl.):A169.
13. Smith, S.D., Pennington, B.F., Kimberling, W.J., and Lubs, H.A. (1983): A genetic analysis of specific reading disability. In: *Genetic Aspects of Speech and Language Disorders*, edited by C. Ludlow and J. Cooper, pp. 169–178. Academic Press, New York.
14. Zahalkova, M., Urzal, V., and Kloboukova, E. (1972): Genetical investigations of dyslexia. *J. Med. Genet.*, 9:48–52.

Language, Communication, and
the Brain, edited by F. Plum.
Raven Press, New York © 1988.

Neurophysiological Studies in Dyslexia

*Frank H. Duffy, ‡Martha B. Denckla, *Gloria B. McAnulty, and
†Jane A. Holmes

Departments of *Neurology and †Psychiatry, Children's Hospital and
Harvard Medical School, Boston, Massachusetts 02115; and ‡Neurology Branch,
National Institutes of Neurological, Communicative Disorders, and Stroke,
Bethesda, Maryland 20205

BACKGROUND

In 1929 Berger's report of a rhythm recorded from the human scalp that appeared with eye closure and vanished with eye opening (5) astonished the neurological community and helped pave the way for the use of the electroencephalogram (EEG) as a tool to explore brain function. The observation by Gibbs et al. in 1935 (32) that clinical epilepsy was accompanied by a unique electrical rhythm known as the spike and wave advanced EEG into the forefront of neurodiagnostic technique. These early findings and the research that rapidly followed encouraged the belief that electroencephalography would form a major investigative tool and thereby enhance our understanding of both normal and abnormal brain function. It was commonly conceived that to decipher the workings of the brain would simply be a matter of gazing more intently at the erratic tracings from the brain on EEG recordings and eventually the "signature" of an underlying brain process would become readily apparent.

The passing years have made it clear, however, that EEG has failed to live up to the great hopes of the 1930s and 1940s. A major contribution of EEG has remained in the epilepsies, and only a few additional diagnostic signatures have been demonstrated. Regrettably, for many entities including the learning disabilities, the EEG abnormalities found were too nonspecific to form useful diagnostic constellations (38). For some time, we have believed that EEG data contain too much information to be easily assimilated by unaided visual inspection of polygraphic tracings. It is for this reason, rather than because of an inherent insensitivity to underlying brain function, that EEG has not completely realized our early optimistic expectations.

Some years ago, we recognized that a major limiting factor in the traditional extracting of information from EEG data was the inability of the human eye to discriminate the massive amounts of information contained within these complex multichannel renderings. Furthermore, interpretation of EEG's cousin, the long latency evoked potential (EP), suffered from the same information overload. For EEG the problem centered on the simultaneous needs to break down the signal visually into the classic EEG frequency bands, evaluate the distribution of these activities across the scalp, determine the "average" of these processes for the duration of the recording period, and detect deviations from a self-evolved concept of "normality." It was our opinion that the necessity to perform spectral, spatial, temporal, and statistical analyses by unaided inspection constituted a mental over-load, hindering the optimal extraction of information from EEG. From the EP perspective a similar limiting factor appeared to be the mental ability to assimilate the complex and rapidly changing spatio-temporal patterns. Indeed, it has been our observation that necessary clinical simplifications have primarily involved limiting the number of channels to be analyzed at the cost of losing spatial information.

The approach we have taken to enhance the value of both EEG and EP for the exploration of brain function is based primarily on topographic mapping (21). In a recent lecture entitled "From Graphein to Topos," Helmut Petsche (54) eloquently expressed our view that early EEG analyses had emphasized temporal relationships and waveshape morphology (Graphein) and that only with the advent of modern computing technology had EEG evolved sufficiently to place equal emphasis on spatial relationships (Topos). Therefore, in 1979, having developed our system for comprehensive electrocartographic analyses of brain signals, we undertook a re-investigation of the role of electrophysiological data in understanding learning disabilities, especially dyslexia.

BRAIN ELECTRICAL ACTIVITY MAPPING

Our approach to the extraction of further information from both EEG and evoked potential data has been termed brain electrical activity mapping (BEAM). As shown in Fig. 1, data are gathered from each of 20 active electrodes. For EEG data, spectral analysis is performed and the amount of delta, theta, alpha, and beta activity is numerically quantified for each electrode. By means of the topographic method shown in Fig. 1, displays are made of the spatial distribution of these different frequency ranges. Such maps are formed using 1- to 6-min segments of artifact-free EEG. For EP data, topographic images are made of the voltage distribution of EPs for every 4 msec over a range of 512 msec. Thus, a set of 128 serial images are viewed in rapid sequence (a form of cartooning) on a color video terminal. For both EEG and EP maps, the value of the variable being measured is displayed in "pseudo-color gray scale." These colored images of brain electrical activity are displayed and evaluated in much the same manner as are the colored topographic maps of temperature shown in certain popular newspapers. The result is a picture that is easily and rapidly interpretable by the clinician. These images have proved of great value in the assessment of EEG background activity. For EP they summarize complex spatio-temporal relationships. Essentially, the computer performs the spectral, temporal, and spatial analyses, thereby relieving the clinician of the burden of having to perform these complicated processes.

SIGNIFICANCE PROBABILITY MAPPING

From our initial topographic data it became clear that even within the normal population we could expect a certain degree of deviation from absolute symmetry.

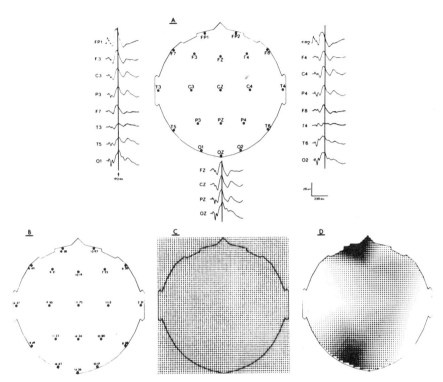

FIG. 1. Construction of beam images. Interpolation technique used in the formation of BEAM images (21). Although the technique is illustrated for EP data, the same process is used to map all other data, e.g., spectral functions of FFT, raw EEG activity, and statistical parameters. Data are gathered from a basic set of 20 scalp electrodes. These are shown (**A**) and labeled in the 10-20 format atop a schematic map of the head in vertex view with nose above, occiput below, left ear to the left, and right ear to the right. The set of 20 visual EPs derived from one subject is shown adjacent to the schematic head. The standard electrode from which each is derived is indicated. To illustrate the procedure a vertical line is drawn through all EPs at the 192 msec poststimulus latency point. The value of each EP is measured and placed next to the corresponding electrode in (**B**). Next the head outline is surrounded by a 64 × 64 matrix of 4,096 picture elements or pixels (**C**). The value at each pixel is obtained by interpolation based on the distance from the nearest three electrodes, a technique known as three-point linear interpolation. To the resulting matrix of numbers, a gray scale is attached with the result illustrated in (**D**). Note how visible the posterior and anterior asymmetries become when topographically mapped (D) as compared to when viewed in the raw EP tracings (A). To map another modality it becomes simply a matter of obtaining a suitable value for each electrode (e.g., EEG delta) and then creating a map (e.g., topographic distribution of delta). These maps are used to enhance visibility and to assist in the formation of summary variables or features from statistically derived templates (see text).

It was often not obvious when a focality or asymmetry constituted a clinical abnormality, or whether normal variation could account for the degree of asymmetry. To assist in this process of abnormality detection we developed a technique known as significance probability mapping (SPM) that forms maps of abnormality (20). In this process a single subject's topographic image can be compared with that of a control or reference data set. This results in a new image in which the delineation of individual deviation from comparable data collected on normal subjects replaces the original data. Essentially, the subject's data are replaced by their "Z-transform," thus displaying an image of standard deviation from the norm (Fig. 2). This fulfills the final and complicated step in the clinical evaluation of EEG and EP data, i.e., the delineation of regional abnormality. Clinically, the technique of SPM has proved singularly valuable in the diagnostic delineation of abnormalities in clinical subjects (16,21).

As further explained in Fig. 2, the SPM process can be applied not only to comparisons of one subject with a group (Z-transform) but also to comparisons

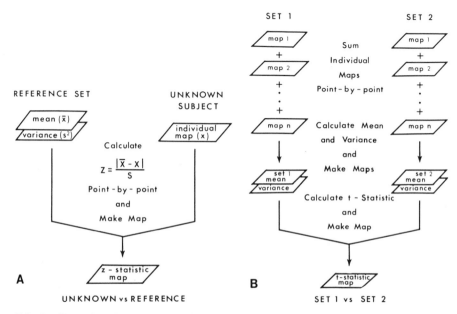

FIG. 2. Illustration of the process of SP M (20), a technique to form images of deviation from a standard to detect abnormality or difference. In general there are three SPM procedures: the first (**A**) facilitates detection of regions where an individual subject deviates from a control population by imaging the Z-transformation; the second (**B**) delineates regions where two groups differ by imaging Student's t-statistic; the third (not illustrated) delineates where three or more groups differ by imaging the ANOVA F-statistic. This approach is superior to simple difference maps formed by subtracting the 20 electrode values of a subject from the group normal mean values, i.e., A-Â. Since it would be unusual to expect a subject's values, A, to be exactly identical to the control group mean, Â, a difference map where A-Â is imaged will always show something. It does not help to illustrate when difference becomes abnormal. For the Z-transform SPM, this difference is normalized by the standard deviation (S), which is a reflection of the variability to be expected within a normal population. The Z-SPM images of [A-Â]/S reflect not just the difference of a subject from a group but the number of standard deviations the subject falls from the group mean. For all SPM conditions the appropriate statistic is formed independently for the data obtained from each electrode. The resulting Z, t, or F values are then formed into topographic images (Fig. 1). As an alternative the SPM process may also be performed on the elements of the pixel matrix after raw data is interpolated. In the first approach, statistics are performed and the results are interpolated. The second approach involves interpolation at the outset with statistical analysis of the larger interpolated matrix. Although not completely identical mathematically, both give comparable results. Accordingly, the first approach, computationally much less demanding, is most often used.

between two groups (t-statistic), and among three or more groups (F-statistic). Indeed virtually any statistical parameter can be similarly mapped, and these multigroup comparisons have proved useful in many research applications (17–19,22,23,51,52).

TOPOGRAPHIC MAPPING OF DYSLEXIA PURE

Background

In the late 1970s we became interested in the question of whether a specific reading disability was associated with a consistent, neurophysiologically detectable abnormality. Until recently (27–30), theories on the physiological cause of dyslexia had lacked neuropathological confirmation. Although many authors had employed clinical neurophysiological studies to analyze the problem (8,36,39,40,57,59,61), the EEG and EP findings in children with dyslexia were too nonspecific to form diagnostic constellations. With the exception of Hanley and Sklar (36), few had looked beyond the visual (occipital) or classic speech (temporoparietal) regions for abnormalities.

Another issue having an impact on results of neurophysiological studies of dyslexia centers on the *definition* of dyslexia and, thus, characteristics of this particular population and its comparability to other populations studied elsewhere. Reading disability, for example, can be caused by many factors and may be seen in children with associated neurological problems, as well as in children who are otherwise normal. Dyslexia, like epilepsy, has been interpreted as both symptom and disease. As the clinical neurologist reviews the learning disability (LD) literature relevant to dyslexia (2–4,6,7,11,24–30,37,38,41,46,47), a picture of apparent disorder appears, the clarification of which has been a consuming interest of countless dedicated individuals. Hughes (38,39) criticized many electrophysiological investigations for failure to adequately define the clinical population and for frequent omission of control groups. The World Federation of Neurology attempted to produce order through semantics by precisely defining developmental dyslexia as "a disorder manifested by difficulty in learning to read despite conventional instruction, adequate intelligence and sociocultural opportunity. It is dependent upon fundamental cognitive disabilities which are frequently of constitutional origin" (38). Many have soundly criticized this logic, especially Rutter (56), who pointed out that it begged a whole series of further questions such as the definitions of adequate intelligence, conventional instruction, and so forth.

In 1977 Denckla (15) brought the perspective of an adult neurologist to the study of dyslexia. She recognized the need to consider reading disability in concert with other evidence of brain dysfunction, such as low intelligence or attentional deficits, and separately from reading disability occurring as a relatively pure entity. These she labeled, "dyslexia-plus" and "dyslexia-pure," respectively. Following this lead, we restricted our first electrophysiological studies of dyslexia (22) to dyslexia-pure to the exclusion of plus. Operationally, we took the latter to include children with the common accompanying symptoms of hyperactivity, dyscalculia, and motor incoordination. Following the lead of Hughes, we defined "abnormality" in our dyslexic population as difference from a nondyslexic normative control population. This definition dovetailed with the SPM techniques developed to topographically delineate regions of between-group or among-groups difference.

Subjects

Our initial work was based on a small group of eight boys with dyslexia-pure (14,38) carefully selected from patients receiving a multidisciplinary workup for "reading difficulties" in the Learning Disabilities Clinic of Children's Hospital, Boston. None of these dyslexics had abnormalities on a traditional neurological examination by a neurologist; none demonstrated psychopathology by history or interview with a psychiatrist. All had oral reading scores at least 1.5 years below expectation as defined by Rutter (56), and none had a history of hyperactivity or received a score of 16 or above on the Connors rating scales for parents and teachers (9). To reduce variability, we chose to examine an all-male group 9.0 to 10.7 years of age with full-scale IQ scores ranging from 94 to 114. Two of the dyslexics were left-handed, two ambidextrous, and four right-handed.

Ten controls were recruited from a population of successful fifth grade suburban Boston students. This all-male group ranged in age from 9.0 to 10.7 years and came from a similar socioeconomic class to that of the dyslexics. All controls were administered the Raven Coloured Progressive Matrices test (55) and the Gray Oral Reading Test (33). To be included in the control group, each subject had to be above the 50th percentile on the former test and at fifth grade reading level on the latter. Two controls were left-handed, one ambidextrous, and seven right-handed.

Neurophysiological Test Procedures

All subjects were studied in the BEAM laboratory, Department of Neurology, Children's Hospital. Data were gathered from 20 EEG scalp electrodes placed in the standard 10-20 format, and four electrodes positioned to facilitate identification and elimination of eye movement and muscle artifact. Signals were amplified and monitored by a standard EEG polygraph (Grass Model 8-25 set to pass 1-300 Hz) and tape recorded (Honeywell 5600E) for subsequent computer analysis (Digital Equipment Corporation PDP-11/60). Trial markers were simultaneously recorded to mark onset of experimental states or stimulus presentations.

Spontaneous EEG was recorded for a period of 3 min during each of 10 different testing conditions or states. These were designed to permit recording during simple resting brain activity (with eyes open or closed) and during tests designed to activate the left hemisphere (speech and reading), the right hemisphere (music and geometric figures), and both hemispheres together (paired visual-verbal associations). The *10 EEG test states were*:

1. Speech (S): to listen carefully to a tape-recorded fairy tale ("The Elephant and the Butterfly," e.e. cummings) and answer simple questions about its content when completed.
2. Music (M): to listen to music (*Nutcracker Suite*, Tchaikovsky).
3. Kimura figures-instruction (KF-I) (43): to remember a set of six abstract figures on index cards presented by an examiner.
4. Kimura figures-test (KF-T): to select the six previously presented figures from a set of 38 figures, verbally indicating yes or no.
5. Paired associates-instruction (PA-I) (62): to associate each of four abstract figures on index cards with a particular artificial name (e.g., "mog") spoken by the examiner (i.e., the sound-symbol association test).
6. Paired associates-test (PA-T): to name each of the same four abstract figures when tested by the examiner.
7. Reading task-instruction (RT-I) (34): to read silently three previously unread paragraphs so as to answer questions subsequently.
8. Reading task-test (RT-T): to identify whether 34 typed sentences presented by the examiner were previously included in the three paragraphs (verbal yes or no response).
9. Eyes open (EO): to relax but remain still with the eyes open looking at a fixation target.
10. Eyes closed (EC): to relax but remain still with the eyes closed.

Data were gathered for the formation of *sensory EPs in three test states*:

1. Visual evoked potential (VEP): more than 500 flashes from a Grass PS-2 strobe stimulator were presented at random interstimulus intervals always exceeding 1.5 sec; the unit was set at intensity 8 and placed 30 cm from the subject's closed eyes.
2. Auditory evoked potential (AEP): more than 500 tone pips (40 msec, 1,000 Hz sine wave) were similarly presented via earphones at 92 db sound pressure level.
3. "Tight-tyke" auditory evoked potential (TTAEP): more than 250 presentations of the tape-recorded word "tight" were randomly presented, intermixed with a similar number of the word "tyke"; subjects were required to count the number of "tights" heard for half the presentation and "tykes" for the remainder of the presentation.

For both EEG and EP states, special care was taken to minimize the effects of eye blink, eye movements, and muscle artifact. In particular eye movements and eye blinks were monitored on line during the EEG recordings, and a number of maneuvers were used to reduce their frequency and extent. These included instructing the subjects to blink suppress, allowing frequent breaks for subjects to rest their eyes, making subjects aware of their blink frequency, and using longer recording sessions to obtain sufficient artifact-free tracing. Test materials were specially constructed to minimize eye movements and eye blinks. Similarly, time was spent during the recording session with each subject to obtain good relaxation and diminish muscle artifact.

Neurophysiological Analyses

In addition to the precautions noted above, great care was taken to minimize the effects of electrode artifact and 60 Hz mains interference on subsequent EEG spectral analysis. To minimize error induced by inadequate sampling rate (aliasing), data were bandpass filtered from 0.5 to 50 Hz at 24 db per octave during sampling.

Hanning, smoothing, and edge effects were handled in the conventional manner. This process was performed separately for all 10 EEG states. The 0–24-Hz segment was broken down into the following classic EEG frequency bands: delta (0–3.5 Hz), theta (4–7.5 Hz), alpha (8–11.5 Hz), beta 1 (12–15.5 Hz), beta 2 (16–19.5 Hz), and beta 3 (20–23.5 Hz). A single value representing the magnitude of EEG activity within each spectral range was obtained by integration across that 4-Hz range. Thus, for each frequency range, 20 values (one from each scalp electrode) were obtained for topographic mapping and four (one from each artifact electrode) for artifact analysis.

The off-line EP averaging program automatically rejected segments containing high voltage eye movement artifact. The background polygraphic record obtained during stimulation was inspected, and rejection level was individually optimized for each subject. No fewer than 100 stimuli were averaged for each subject, and most subjects had between 200 and 350 usable presentations. Two hundred fifty-six sampled data points were spaced over 1,024 msec. The stimulus occurred midway through the epoch. Thus, the first 512 msec formed a prestimulus baseline, and the next 512 msec represented the visual-evoked or auditory-evoked response. The prestimulus epoch provided the basis for establishing a 0-uV reference point for each channel's EP. Inspection of this pre-EP baseline epoch provided visual confirmation of the adequacy of signal averaging for all subjects. A single value representing the magnitude of evoked potential activity at each 4 msec poststimulus latency point was used for subsequent topographic mapping.

The sets of 20 spectra (one set from each of the 10 EEG states) and 20 EPs (visual, auditory, and tight-tyke) were processed into topographic maps as described in Fig. 1 (21). Between-group difference was delineated by the SPM process (20).

Results

Visual inspection of the *original EEG and EP topographic images revealed the following*:

1. Normals showed considerable between-state variability in their EEG and EP topographic distributions.

2. Dyslexics tended to show more state invariance in their plots.
3. Dyslexics seemed to show more EEG alpha overlying their left hemisphere.
4. Dyslexic EPs tended to be simpler, showing fewer transient asymmetries than normal.
5. Nonetheless, it was not possible to accurately classify subjects by simple visual inspection of their plot, because of an additional factor of considerable inter-subject (as well as intergroup) variability. However, subsequent inspection of the significance probability maps demonstrated large and coherent regions of between-group difference.

The *SPM derived from EP data demonstrated*:

1. little between-group difference in the VEP;
2. a large region of difference for AEP involving the middle posterior portions of the left temporal lobe, extending into adjacent parietal and occipital lobes;
3. large regions of difference of TTAEP involving not only the left posterior temporal regions as noted for AEP but also regions further posterior and also on the right, especially a prominent right posterior occipital-temporal region of group difference;
4. the activated TTAEP state showed the largest regions of difference, but the simple AEP state showed difference as well.

The *SPM derived from EEG data demonstrated*:

1. no between-group difference for the M, KF-I, and KF-T states (alpha);
2. large regions of between-group differences for the S-, RT-I-, PA-I-, and PA-T-activated states (alpha);
3. a large bilateral medial frontal difference with smaller, less consistent regional difference in the left temporal lobe the single most recurrent area (alpha);
4. lesser but distinct regional differences in the nonactivated EO and EC states, involving the frontal and left temporo-parietal lobes (alpha);
5. regions of between-group differences consistently associated with greater alpha for the dyslexics (alpha);
6. only the RT-I and KF-I states yielded between-group difference of significance, other states failed to reach a $p < 0.05$ (theta);
7. the RT-I difference again delineating the bilateral medial frontal region and the left mid-temporal region (theta);
8. the KF-I difference delineating the left anterolateral frontal region, an area not demarcated by alpha (theta).

Illustrations documenting the above findings may be found in the original publication (22). Results of the between-group comparison are shown in Fig. 3. This summary t-statistic SPM shows all regions of between-group difference reaching a $p < 0.02$ level or better in at least one of the experimental conditions. *Regions delineated are*:

1. bilateral medial frontal (supplementary motor area);

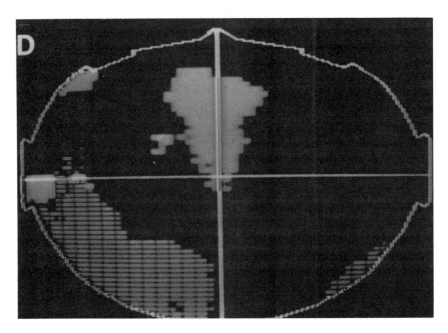

FIG. 3. Study 1 summary t-statistic SPM illustrating the regions where normal and dyslexic boys differ (22). It represents a summary of between group regions for all experimental states of the first study. Regions shown represent areas of dyslexic-nondyslexic difference reaching a t-statistic corresponding to the $p < 0.02$ level (two-tailed) at least once during all EEG and EP test states. Note that in addition to the expected left posterior and left anterior speech regions, the medial frontal region is also prominently involved.

2. left anterolateral frontal (Broca's area);
3. left midtemporal (auditory associative area);
4. left posterolateral quadrant (Wernicke's area, parietal associative areas and visual associative areas).

Discussion

The regions found to differ between normal and dyslexic boys (Fig. 3) are both reassuring and puzzling. Reassurance comes from the large left posterior regions characteristically involved in language disorders. The medial frontal regional involvement remains puzzling. The left midtemporal and left posterior quadrant regions represent the classical posterior speech area where differences between normals and dyslexics might be predicted by analogy to traditional aphasiology. Indeed, other neurophysiological studies have demonstrated differences in EEG and/or EP parameters overlying these regions (36,39,57,59,61). The frontal lobe regions of difference are more surprising and unpredicted. An explanation may stem from the work of Larsen and colleagues (44,45) who demonstrated, by xenon-labeled regional cerebral blood flow studies, a pattern of cortical activation during speech, oral reading, and silent reading in normal subjects that appears similar to all the regions demarcated in Fig. 3. These, in turn, correspond to brain regions which, when stimulated, interfere with patients' speech (53). The regions that we have shown to differentiate, electrophysiologically, between the brains of dyslexics and normal boys appear to be among the regions normally involved in speech and reading. Thus, the aberrant electrophysiological ''lesion'' of pure dyslexia does not appear confined to one locus, one lobe, or even one hemisphere. Rather, it appears to involve most of the extensive cortical system normally involved in speech and reading.

Regions of between-group differences demarcated by analysis of alpha activity have always been associated with greater mean alpha in the dyslexia group. Many investigators interpret relative increases in alpha as representing relative inactivity or ''idling'' of underlying cortex (31). Conversely, decreases in alpha are taken to represent cortical activation (12). Thus, the increased dyslexic alpha anteriorly may signify relative underactivation of frontal systems in dyslexics as compared with control boys.

Results of this study and those of Larsen et al. (44,45) are not the only ones to implicate the frontal lobe supplementary motor area in linguistic tasks. Penfield (53) reported both speech arrest and vocalization from stimulation of this region. Focal seizures emanating from lesions in this region have been reported to interfere with speech (35) or produce palilalia (1). Masdeu, Schoene, and Funkenstein (48) reported aphasia following infarction of the left supplementary motor region. Following a two- to three-week recovery period, the patient's residua consisted of a mild anomia with a ''marked impairment to both spontaneous writing and writing to dictation which persisted to . . . death.'' This was accompanied by ''a tendency to give up language tasks, particularly writing.'' Since isolated vascular accidents are less common in the anterior cerebral than middle cerebral territory, it may be that this region, prominently demarcated in our PI maps, plays a previously underemphasized role in aphasia and in concepts of dyslexia and dysgraphia.

Involvement of the frontal lobes in dyslexia may have additional implications. A slight enlargement of the aberrant frontal region might explain the clinical overlap and statistical association of dyslexia with the hyperactive syndrome and attentional deficits. Hughes and Denckla (38) referred to this association as dyslexia-plus.

The finding that differences of brain electrophysiological activity between normal and dyslexic boys do not necessarily require special or complex test conditions is of considerable interest. Whereas, the highly activated states requiring sound-symbol association (EEG alpha PA-I, PA-T) and a phonetic discrimination (TTAEP) produced the largest regions of difference between groups, sizable regional differences were demarcated during simpler conditions (e.g., alpha EO and EC, AER). Thus, the aberrant physiology of dyslexia is evident even when linguistic tasks are not being performed. Whether this differing physiology represents maturational lag or a fundamentally different brain organization is not known.

ELECTROPHYSIOLOGICAL DIFFERENCES AMONG SUBTYPES OF DYSLEXIA

Background

As we prepared to recruit new dyslexic subjects for the purpose of replicating our original findings, we became concerned that uncontrolled heterogeneity within dyslexia-pure might by chance render our second population incompatible with our first. Denckla (15), for example, argued that clearly recognizable differences in language function exist within the dyslexia-pure population. Moreover, by analogy with adult studies of aphasia, differences in language suggest differences in the loci of underlying microscopic neuropathology. If true, this would suggest that dyslexics with differing language function might show differing spatial patterns of aberrant electrophysiological activity.

Accordingly, the present study extends our previous neurophysiological investigations of dyslexia-pure to delineation of regional differences that characterize three of Denckla's language-based subgroupings, specifically anomic-repetition disorder, dysphonemic-sequencing disorder, and global-mixed language disorder (15).

Subjects

Forty-four boys fulfilling Denckla's criteria for dyslexia-pure were selected exactly as for our initial study. Following selection, the dyslexic subjects were interviewed and given a neuropsychological test battery designed to permit classification into Denckla's subcategories of dyslexia-pure. We chose to select three relatively common dyslexic subgroups based on patterns of linguistic deficit as shown below.

Dyslexia-Pure: Clinical Characteristics

Global-mixed language disorder:

1. All tests of language fell below age expectations (comprehension, repetition, and naming tests).
2. Verbal IQ was below 90 and performance IQ was at least 95.

Dysphonemic-sequencing disorder:

1. Sentence memory and digit span "failed" by virtue of omissions, substitutions, and errors of sequence.
2. Naming errors (not excessive in number) were also characteristically phonemic and/or sequential details.
3. Complex syntactical constructions were misunderstood.
4. Articulation and verbal IQ were at least average.

Anomic-repetition disorder:

1. Circumlocutory and paraphasic errors accounted for most excessive errors on confrontation naming.
2. Sentence and digit span was shorter than, as well as qualitatively worse than, expected for age group (not true after 10 years).
3. Articulation and comprehension were normal.
4. There was "scatter" among subjects on verbal IQ.

Language assessment included evaluation of comprehension, naming (confronation and repeated), and repetition (for both meaningful and nonmeaningful material). The tests used included the Token Test (58), the Peabody Picture Vocabulary Test (24), Menyuk Syntactic Comprehension Test (50), the Boston Naming Test (42), Rapid Automatized Naming (15), Sentence Memory (Stanford-Binet Intelligence Scale) (60), and Digit-Span (Wechsler Intelligence Scale for Children-Revised) (63).

Each subject was tentatively assigned to one dyslexic category or was designated unclassifiable independently by two neuropsychologists and one neurologist on the basis of test scores and written summaries from the Children's Hospital Learning Disabilities Clinic. From the 44 dyslexics, these three LD specialists identified 26 that they agreed represented the most characteristic examples of the three dyslexic subgroups. These 26 exemplars were represented for statistical purposes by the six neuropsychological variables used in their definition:

1. BOSNTS: Boston Naming Test
2. PPVTST: Peabody Picture Vocabulary Test
3. TOKTST: Token Test
4. MENYUK: Menyuk Syntactic Comprehension Test
5. SENMEN: Sentence Memory subtest of the Stanford-Binet Intelligence Scale
6. DIGSPN: Digit Span subtest from the WISC-R

Each variable was expressed as years above or below age expectancy in half-year increments. To improve the security and objectivity of subject classification, this data set was submitted to a multigroup statistical classification algorithm (program CLASIF) using Geisser's equal dispersions, small samples procedure as described by Cooley and Lohnes (10). This program develops rules and thereby assigns subjects to one of several categories based on probabilistic measures derived from considerations of the data-set structure (i.e., variance and covariance matrices). CLASIF was used to develop categorization rules based on the 26-member "training set" of subjects who were securely assigned to a subgroup by all three examiners. Next, these CLASIF-derived rules were applied to all 44 subjects. Subjects were assigned to a particular subgroup by CLASIF when the probability level reached 75% or more. Thirty subjects were statistically assigned at this high probability level: nine global, eight dysphonemic, and 13 anomic. The subsequent neurophysiological investigations were based on this carefully defined 30-member subset of dyslexics. The territorial map resulting from discriminant function analysis among the three groups is shown in Fig. 4.

Neurophysiological Test Procedures

Test procedures were the same as for the previous study described.

Neurophysiological Analyses

For the neurophysiological data, regions of between-group difference were delineated on the basis of two strategies. First, t-SPM were formed by comparing each dyslexic subgroup with all other dyslexics treated as a group. This "within-dyslexia" group comparison analysis (GRP) directly delineated regions where an individual subgroup differs from other dyslexics as a group. Ninety GRP regions were identified by SPM. Second, SPMs were formed between each dyslexic subgroup

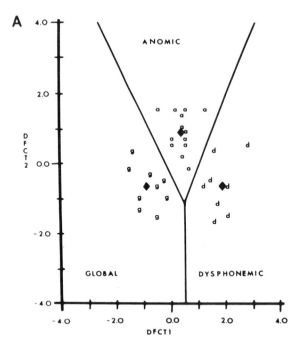

FIG. 4. Territorial map produced by stepwise discriminant analysis of the three dyslexic subgroups. Each subject was represented by his six neuropsychological measures. Subjects in the anomic-repetition subgroup are represented by "a." Those in the dysphonemic-sequencing subgroup are represented by "d." Those in the global processing disorder are represented by "g." Subgroup definitions are given in the text. The complete separation among these three subgroups by the two resulting discriminant functions (vertical and horizontal axes) is illustrated. This population served as the basis for the neurophysiological studies of subgrouping.

and the control group. This control group comparison analysis (CON) delineated regions where each dyslexic subgroup differed from controls, but not necessarily from other dyslexic subgroups. Fifty-nine CON regions were identified by SPM. The next step was to identify which of the 149 SPM delineated regions were unique to each subgroup. To facilitate this search, single numerical variables were generated from each subject corresponding to each t-SPM. In other words, t-SPMs were used to derive single numerical measurements or features descriptive of group separation. This involved the creation of a "template" from each t-SPM encompassing a region delineated by t-values above an *a priori* criterion corresponding to the 5% probability level, usually a t-value of 2.00. Such templates were then applied to each individual subject's raw topographic data to form numerical features by summation of all values bounded by the state-appropriate template.

A t-SPM region was considered uniquely different for a particular subgroup when its corresponding template-derived feature separated that group significantly from the other two dyslexic subgroups combined into one larger group. The Mann-Whitney U-test was used for this criterion.

Results

Six anomic, 16 dysphonemic, and 12 global features reached or exceeded the $p < 0.02$ level on the two-tailed U-test. Of these 34 features, 25 were developed from within dyslexia group comparisons (GRP features) and nine from control group comparisons (CON features). Thirty of the 34 were developed from EP states and only four from EEG states. EP latencies ranged from 36 to 476 msec. Eighteen of the 30 EP features were derived from the TTA, seven from the AER, and five from the VER. EEG frequency bands were restricted to delta (0–4 Hz) and slow beta (12–20 Hz). There were two RTT-, one PAT-, and one SPE-derived EEG features. The SPMs that generated the features were evenly divided between the hemispheres. Overall, eight were equally bihemispheric, 12 were preponderantly left sided and 14 right sided. There was no clear hemispheric bias to any subgroup.

To clarify this complex analysis, a single topographic map was formed for each subgroup to demonstrate those regions where the particular subgroup differed from the other dyslexic subgroups (Fig. 5). This was done by forming a summary t-SPM. In Fig. 5, the complexity of regional between-subgroup difference is summarized for each subgroup in single maps. These maps characterize regions where, for each subgroup, between-group differences were found within the set of all SPMs for that subgroup. Where regions were identified by more than one SPM, the highest t-value was assigned to the summary map.

To address the question of the "meaning" of the individual features and their corresponding templates, these features were individually correlated with the six neuropsychological variables (used to define the subgroups) and the two neuropsychological discriminant function scores (derived from the analysis shown in Fig. 3). Next, the templates were passed over all the control subjects to determine the relative feature values for controls, index subgroup, and nonindex subgroup.

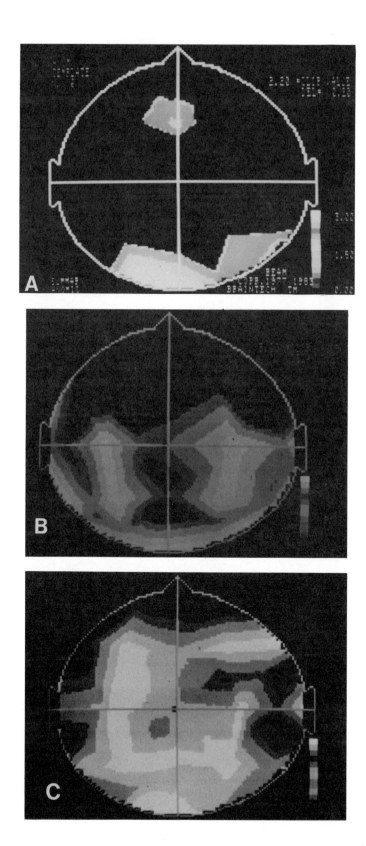

Then all neuropsychological variables were ordered so that larger values were better. To determine whether larger or smaller neurophysiological feature values are "better," the value of each feature for the control group was taken as the "best" value to have. Knowing the sign of the correlation coefficient and the "better" direction of both the features and variables, it became possible to determine whether a neurophysiological feature correlated with better or worse neuropsychological performance.

Two hundred seventy-two correlations were formed, the product of 34 neurophysiological features and eight neuropsychological variables. Fifty-three of the correlations reached statistical significance at the 0.02 level, 36 at the 0.01 level, and 10 at the 0.001 level. This exceeds the number expected by chance alone (49). Four of the six anomic, 10 of the 16 dysphonemic, and 11 of the 12 global features correlated with one or more variables.

For all 12 significant global features, the sign of the correlation coefficient indicated that the more electrically aberrant (compared with control) the feature value for the global population, the worse the neuropsychological score. In contrast, all six anomic and 10 dysphonemic variables showed the opposite effect, i.e., the more aberrant the neurophysiological feature, the better the neuropsychological performance.

Discussion

Results of this study may best be visualized by the summary templates shown in Fig. 5. First, it can be seen that electrophysiological difference can be found for each subgroup. Second, the spatial patterns of the differences are unique. The anomic subgroup differs from the nonanomic population in the frontal and occipital regions (Fig. 5A). On the other hand, the dysphonemic and nondysphonemic groups

---

FIG. 5. Three composite t-SPM images summarizing the results of the dyslexic subgrouping study. The maps delineate regions where, for each subgroup, significant between group differences were found across all EEG and EP states for comparison of that particular dyslexic subgroup with all other dyslexics grouped together. (**A**) depicts the comparison of the anomic and nonanomic population. Note the prominent distinctions contributed by the bilateral medial frontal and occipital regions. (**B**) compares the dysphonemic with the nondysphonemic population. Note the prominent distinguishing feature in the bilateral central-parietal regions and the somewhat complementary regional involvement in (A) and (B). More aberrant electrical activity in the regions shown in (A) and (B) were associated with better neuropsychological test performance. These regions may signal widespread compensatory brain activity. (**C**) compares the global with the nonglobal population. Note the much greater overall spatial involvement for this comparison. Greater electrical aberrance in the regions shown in (C) were associated with poorer performance on neuropsychological testing.

differ in a spatially different pattern involving the bilateral parietal-central regions (Fig. 5B). The globals differ from the nonglobals (Fig. 5C) over most regions, more or less a combining of the maps above. Third, there is an obvious absence of among-group difference in the classic left temporal speech areas. The relative lack of differentiating regions involving left temporoparietal areas is consistent with the language-deficit substrate of the reading-disabled subgroups (27,28,30). Whereas there are prominent left temporal differences between controls and all dyslexics, subtypes do not differ substantially among each other in this region. Regional subgroup differences appear to lie primarily outside this classic region. Fourth, the degree of regional involvement as shown in Fig. 5 roughly parallels the overall degree of clinical impairment, i.e., global > dysphonemic > anomic.

The degree to which the discriminating regions involve both hemispheres is quite surprising. Recent studies of cerebral metabolism as evidenced from blood flow measurements have emphasized the unexpectedly widespread, bihemispheric involvement of cortex during tasks once believed to be quite focal or restricted in nature. Larsen et al. (44), using the intracarotid xenon technique, found that the acts of reading silently, reading aloud, and speaking activated surprisingly wide areas of cortex outside of the classic left temporal language areas. The other areas include prominent and consistent involvement of both left and right medial frontal lobes. Presumably this widespread involvement of brain during cognition and communication speaks for the complexity of the processes and the need to call on many brain systems to execute the desired task. The simple act of reading, for example, calls upon complicated interaction between the visual and oculomotor systems, in addition to activation of the visual-verbal association of memory areas. Moreover, reading is seldom a neutral activity. In addition to changing levels of arousal and attention, the content of the material read may call up unknown sensory and/or emotional associations. It is not surprising, therefore, that such cognitive tasks which appear to be behaviorally discrete may activate widespread cortical areas. Accordingly, in the face of pathology, widespread physiological alterations might be expected. Our findings within dyslexia suggest that subtypes differ among themselves not as much in the primary language areas as in the more widespread bihemispheric cortical regions.

Whereas all regions shown in Fig. 5 manifest themselves on the basis of aberrant brain electrical activity, it should not be presumed that the regions are necessarily delineated on the basis of greater underlying pathology. Indeed, for the anomic and dysphonemic groups, the greater the electrical aberrance from control values, the better the performance on the neuropsychological tasks. This raises the possibility that the aberrant electrical activity (Fig. 5A, B) may represent compensatory overactivity rather than simple pathological overactivity. We may be visualizing compensatory activity from regions not ordinarily called on to function during a neuropsychological challenge. Although it is notoriously difficult to make reliable inferences from correlational data, we speculate that the widespread neurophysiological involvement need not necessarily signal correspondingly widespread pathology but may demonstrate regions of relatively more normal function. If this is true, the data may suggest that the anomic and dysphonemic subgroups show evidence compatible with bihemispheric compensatory activity whereas the global subgroup shows bihemispheric evidence of pathological hypofunction.

The fact that nine of the 34 neurophysiological features failed to correlate with neuropsychological variables may simply indicate that our test battery was language oriented and that the dyslexic subgroups may also differ by behavioral variables (e.g., spatial ability, attention) not measured. Indeed, it could be that the widespread neurophysiological involvement mirrors associated pathology outside of language/communication cortex, despite the lack of obvious clinical differences.

The neural circuitry involved in comprehension of the written word is complex and widespread. By limiting our study to the language-deficit-based subgroup of dyslexia-pure, we had anticipated differences in left hemisphere brain systems. The finding of prevalent bihemispheric among-group differences was unforeseen and may reflect pathology in bihemispheric language cortex, associated pathology in nonlanguage related areas, and/or widespread compensatory activity. These data speak to problems inherent in the establishment of a physiologically meaningful taxonomy of dyslexia and the future need for careful investigations in this area.

From the methodological perspective our findings of electrophysiological differences among subgroups serve as a warning that future studies must adequately characterize their study populations. Failure to do so may result in excessive variance and loss of power as well as nonreproducible results.

SUMMARY AND CONCLUSIONS

Using sophisticated computer graphics technologies and sensitive methods, our original dyslexia study of dyslexic boys delineated specific areas of the brain which in combination could constitute a "physiological signature" of dyslexia. In addition to identifying aberrant brain function in the traditional language-associated left posterior region, we also observed medial frontal lobe differences from normals, a finding confirmed by others in recent research.

Our subsequent study sought to refine further current definitional subgroupings within the broad entity known as dyslexia-pure. Indeed language-based subgroups appear to have identifiable and differing topographic signatures. Furthermore, based on correlations between neuropsychological test scores and neurophysiological measurements, we suggest that subgroup electrophysiological differences may reflect compensatory as well as pathological brain activity.

We believe that the currently expanding understanding of the neurophysiology of dyslexia will lead eventually to improved diagnosis and remediation of this learning disability. The detailed mapping of brain electrical activity shows promise of providing the neuropsychologist and learning disability specialist with another "perspective" on reading disability. This technique *may* prove valuable in the diagnosis of dyslexia at an early age and in the tailoring of the learning experience to a child's specific deficits and capabilities.

ACKNOWLEDGMENTS

I acknowledge my associates in our original dyslexia study, Drs. Giulio Sandini and Peter H. Bartels. I also acknowledge the meticulous work and long hours of our many EEG technologists who have contributed to our research data. Special thanks go to our subjects, their parents, and educators for their sacrifice and generosity in contributing to our studies.

REFERENCES

1. Alajouanine, T., Castaigne, P., and Sabouraud, O. (1959): Palilalie paroxystique et vocalisations itératives au cours de crises épileptiques par lésion intéressant de l'aire motrice supplémentaire. *Rev. Neurol.*, 101:685–697.
2. Bannatyne, A. (1971): *Language, Reading and Learning Disabilities.* Charles C. Thomas, Springfield, IL.
3. Bender, L.A. (1975): A fifty-year review of experience with dyslexia. *Bull. Orton Soc.*, 25:5–23.
4. Benton, A.L., and Pearl, D. (eds.) (1978): *Dyslexia—An Appraisal of Current Knowledge.* Oxford University Press, Oxford, England.
5. Berger, H. (1929): Ueber das Elektrenkephalogram des Menschen: I. Mitteilung. *Arch. Psychiatr. Nervenkr.*, 87:527–528.
6. Boder, E. (1971): Developmental dyslexia: Prevailing diagnostic concepts and a new diagnostic approach. In: *Progress in Learning Disabilities,* edited by H. Myklebust, pp. 293–321.
7. Boder, E. (1973): Developmental dyslexia: A diagnostic approach based on three atypical reading patterns. *Dev. Med. Child Neurol.*, 15:663–687.
8. Connors, C.K. (1970): Cortical visual evoked response in children with learning disorders. *Psychophysiology*, 7:418–428.
9. Connors, C.K. (1973): Rating scales for use in drug studies with children. *Psychopharmacol. Bull.*, (special issue): 24–29.
10. Cooley, W.W., and Lohnes, P.R. (1971): *Multivariate Data Analysis.* John Wiley, New York.
11. Critchley, M. (1970): *The Dyslexic Child.* Charles C. Thomas, Springfield, IL.
12. Davidson, R.J., and Schwarz, G.E. (1977): The influence of musical training on patterns of EEG symmetry during musical and non-musical self-generation tasks. *Psychophysiology*, 14:58–63.
13. Davidson, R.J., and Schwarz, G.E. (1977): Minimal brain dysfunction and dyslexia: Beyond diagnosis by exclusion. In: *Child Neurology*, edited by M.E. Blau. Spectrum, New York.
14. Davidson, R.J., and Schwarz, G.E. (1977): The neurological basis of reading disability. In: *Reading Disability: A Human Approach to Learning*, edited by F.G. Roswell and G. Natchez. Basic Books, New York.
15. Denckla, M.B. (1979): Childhood learning disabilities. In: *Clinical Neuropsychology*, edited by K. Heilman and E. Valenstein, pp. 535–573.
16. Duffy, F.H. (1982): Topographic display of evoked potentials: Clinical applications of brain electrical activity mapping (BEAM). *Ann. NY Acad. Sci.*, 388:183–196.
17. Duffy, F.H., Albert, M.S., and McAnulty, G. (1984): Brain electrical activity in patients with presenile and senile dementia of the Alzheimer's type. *Ann. Neurol.*, 16:439–448.
18. Duffy, F.H., Albert, M.S., and McAnulty, G. (1984): Age-related differences in brain electrical activity mapping of healthy subjects. *Ann. Neurol.*, 16:430–438.
19. Duffy, F.H., and Als, H. (1983): Neurophysiological assessment of the neonate: An approach combining brain electrical activity mapping (BEAM) with behavioral assessment (APIB). In: *New Approaches to Developmental Screening of Infants*, edited by T.B. Brazelton, pp. 175–196. Elsevier, New York.
20. Duffy, F.H., Bartels, P.H., and Burchfiel, J.L. (1981): Significance probability mapping: An aid in the topographic analysis of brain electrical activity. *Electroencephalogr. Clin. Neurophysiol.*, 51:455–462.

21. Duffy, F.H., Burchfiel, J.L., and Lombroso, C.T. (1979): Brain electrical activity mapping (BEAM): A method for extending the clinical utility of EEG and evoked potential data. *Ann. Neurol.*, 5:309–321.
22. Duffy, F.H., Denckla, M.B., and Sandini, G. (1980): Dyslexia: Regional differences in brain electrical activity by topographic mapping. *Ann. Neurol.*, 7:412–420.
23. Duffy, F.H., Jensen, F., Erba, G., Burchfiel, J..L., and Lombroso, C.T. (1984): Extraction of clinical information from electroencephalographic background activity—The combined use of brain electrical activity mapping and intravenous sodium thiopental. *Ann. Neurol.*, 15:22–30.
24. Dunn, L.M. (1965): *Peabody Picture Vocabulary Test.* American Guidance Service Inc., Circle Pines, MN.
25. Fletcher, J.M. (1984): Book review of classification of learning disabled children. *J. Clin. Neuropsychol.*, 6:229–234.
26. Gaddes, W.H. (1976): Prevalence estimates and the need for definition of learning disabilities. In: *The Neuropsychology of Learning Disorders: Theoretical Approaches*, edited by R.M. Knights and D.J. Bakker, pp.3–24. University Park Press, Baltimore.
27. Galaburda, A.M., and Eidelberg, D. (1982): Symmetry and asymmetry in the human posterior thalamus. II. Thalamic lesions in a case of developmental dyslexia. *Arch. Neurol.*, 39:333–336.
28. Galaburda, A.M., and Kemper, T.L. (1979): Cytoarchitectonic abnormalities in developmental dyslexia: A case study. *Ann. Neurol.*, 6(2):94–100.
29. Galaburda, A.M., Sherman, G.F., Rosen, G.D., Aboitiz, F., and Geschwind, N. (1985): Developmental dyslexia: Four consecutive patients with cortical anomalies. *Ann. Neurol.*, 18:222–233.
30. Galaburda, A.M., Sherman, G.F., Rosen, G.D., Aboitiz, F., and Geschwind, N. (1985): Left posterior angiomatous anomaly and developmental dyslexia: Report of five cases. *Neurology*, 35(Suppl. 1):198.
31. Gevins, A.S., Zeitlin, G.M., Doyle, J.C., et al. (1979): Electroencephalogram correlates of higher cortical functions. *Science*, 203:665–668.
32. Gibbs, F.A., Davis, H., and Lennox, W.G. (1935): The electroencephalogram in epilepsy and in conditions of impaired consciousness. *Arch. Neurol. Psychiatry*, 34:1133–1135.
33. Gray, W.S. (1963): *Gray Oral Reading Test.* Bobbs-Merrill, Indianapolis.
34. Gray, W.S. (1973): *Gray Oral Reading Tests.* Western Psychological Services, Los Angeles.
35. Guidetti, B. (1957): Désordres de la parole associés à des lésions de la surface interhémisphérique frontale postérieure. *Rev. Neurol.*, 97:121–131.
36. Hanley, J., and Sklar, B. (1976): Electroencephalographic correlates of developmental reading dyslexias: Computer analyses of recordings from normal and dyslexic children. In: *Basic Visual Processes and Learning Disability*, edited by G. Leisman, pp. 217–243. Charles C. Thomas, Springfield, IL.
37. Hanley, J., and Sklar, B. (1976): Biochemical and electroencephalographic correlates of learning disabilities. In: *Neuropsychology of Learning Disorders: Theoretical Approaches*, edited by R.M. Knights, University Park Press, Baltimore.
38. Hughes, J.R., and Denckla, M.B. (1978): Outline of a pilot study of electroencephalographic correlates of dyslexia. In: *Dyslexia—An Appraisal of Current Knowledge*, edited by A.L. Benton and D. Pearl. Oxford University Press, Oxford, England.
39. Hughes, J.R., and Park, G.G. (1969): Electro-clinical correlation in dyslexic children. *Electroencephalogr. Clin. Neurophysiol.*, 26:117–121.
40. John, E.R., Karmel, B.Z., Corning, W.C., et al. (1977): Neurometrics. *Science*, 196:1393–1410.
41. Johnson, P.J., and Myklebust, H.R. (1967): *Learning Disabilities.* Grune and Stratton, New York.
42. Kaplan, E., Goodglass, H., and Weintraub, S. (1976): *Boston Naming Test.* Experimental Edition, Veterans Administration Hospital, Boston.
43. Kimura, D. (1963): Right temporal lobe damage. *Arch. Neurol.*, 8:264–271.
44. Larsen, B., Skinhoj, E., and Lassen, N.A. (1978): Variations in regional cortical blood flow in the right and left hemispheres during automatic speech. *Brain*, 101:193–210.
45. Larsen, B., Skinhoj, E., and Lassen, N.A. (1978): Brain function and blood flow. *Sci. Am.*, 239:62–71.
46. Levin, H.S., Hamsher, K.DeS., and Benton, A.L. (1975): A short form of the Test of Facial Recognition for clinical use. *J. Psychol.*, 91:223–228.
47. Lewitter, F.I., DeFries, J.C., and Elston, R.C. (1980): Genetic models of reading disability. *Behav. Gen.*, 10:9–30.
48. Masdeu, J.C., Schoene, W.C., and Funkenstein, H. (1978): Aphasia following infarction of the left supplementary motor area: A clinicopathologic study. *Neurology*, 28:1220–1233.

49. Maus, A., and Endresen, J. (1979): Misuse of computer-generated results. *Med. Biol. Eng. Comput.*, 17:126–129.
50. Menyuk, P. (1963): Syntactic structures in the language of children. *Child Dev.*, 34:407–422.
51. Morihisa, J.M., Duffy, F.H., and Wyatt, R.J. (1983): Brain electrical activity mapping (BEAM) in schizophrenia patients. *Arch. Gen. Psychiatry*, 40:719–728.
52. Morihisa, J.M., Duffy, F.H., and Wyatt, R.J. (1983): Altered P300 topography in schizophrenia. *Arch. Gen. Psychiatry*, 40:729–734.
53. Penfield, W., and Roberts, L. (1959): *Speech and Brain Mechanisms.* Princeton University Press, Princeton, NJ.
54. Petsche, H. (1987): From graphein to topos. In: *Proceedings of the Wuerzburg Conference on Topographic Mapping*, edited by K. Maurer. Springer-Verlag, Frankfurt *(in press)*.
55. Raven, J.C. (1962): *Coloured Progressive Matrices.* Silver End Press, London.
56. Rutter, M. (1978): Prevalence and types of dyslexia. In: *Dyslexia—An Appraisal of Current Knowledge*, edited by A.L. Benton and D. Pearl, p. 3. Oxford University Press, Oxford, England.
57. Sobotka, K.R., and May, J.G. (1977): Visual evoked potentials and reaction time in normal and dyslexic children. *Psychophysiology*, 14:18–24.
58. Spreen, O., and Benton, A.L. (1969): *Neurosensory Center Comprehensive Examination for Aphasia.* Neuropsychology Laboratory, Victoria, BC.
59. Symann-Louett, N., Gascon, G.G., Matsumiya, Y., and Lombroso, C.T. (1977): Wave form difference in visual evoked responses between normal and reading disabled children. *Neurology*, 27:156–159.
60. Terman, L.M., and Merrill, M.A. (1973): *Stanford Binet Intelligence Scale, Manual for the 3rd Edition, Form L-M.* Houghton Mifflin, Boston.
61. Torres, R., and Ayers, F.W. (1968): Evaluation of the electroencephalogram of dyslexic children. *Electroencephalogr. Clin. Neurophysiol.*, 24:281–294.
62. Vellutino, F.R., Steger, J.A., Harding, C.J., and Phillips, F. (1975): Verbal versus non verbal paired associates learning in poor and normal readers. *Neuropsychologia*, 13:75–82.
63. Wechsler, D. (1963): *Wechsler Intelligence Scale for Children-Revised.* Psychol Corp, New York.

*Language, Communication, and
the Brain*, edited by F. Plum.
Raven Press, New York © 1988.

Language Sequelae of Unilateral Brain Lesions in Children

Dorothy M. Aram

*Department of Pediatrics, Case Western Reserve University and Rainbow Babies and
Children's Hospital, Cleveland, Ohio 44106*

Central to the study of unilateral brain lesions in children and the effect on language have been two related issues. First, the degree of early brain specialization for higher cognitive functions—here language (32); and second, the degree of plasticity or reorganization of higher cognitive functions following lesions incurred early in life. (30). Although evidence from multiple perspectives suggests considerable brain specialization early in life for language (35,42), most observations also evidence that young children sustaining unilateral brain lesions recover cognitive functions much more rapidly and completely than do adults with similar lesions. What is not well understood is how recovery relates to the aspect of language examined, the age of lesion onset, or the site and extensiveness of lesions within a hemisphere.

This chapter reviews the literature pertaining to early unilateral brain lesions and language in children and summarizes the work undertaken in our laboratory with particular attention to the factors of age of lesion onset and site of lesion within a hemisphere.

HISTORICAL PERSPECTIVE

Surprisingly little objective investigation has occurred in this area, and work that has been reported typically includes serious methodological problems that limit interpretation of results. The older literature [and by this I generally mean pre-computerized tomography (CT) scan era] has come from three overlapping sources: (a) the *acquired lesion* or *acquired aphasia* (2,22,24,25,37,47–49) literature involving reports of cognitive functioning following lesions acquired after a period of presumably normal development; (b) studies of *hemiplegic infants or children* (1,3,11,12,21,23,26,28,38); and (c) studies of *hemidecorticate individuals* who function with one remaining hemisphere (13,14,16–18,31). Although the hemidecorticate studies have been exemplary in specifying anatomical involvement and instructive in detailing cognitive abilities among the subjects studied, generalization

171

from those data to children with other forms of unilateral brain lesions is not appropriate owing to the important difference between functioning with one hemisphere (which by necessity assumes all functioning and in many instances probably represents a different brain organization from very early in development), and functioning with two hemispheres (in which the early normal organization of brain functioning was disrupted at the time of lesion onset). The hemidecorticate data, therefore, are not reviewed here. The early work addressing childhood hemiplegia or acquired lesions rarely specified lesion unilaterality or reported objective measures of behavior beyond IQ scores, thus much of this work is of limited contribution. During the past eight years, several case studies (15,19,20,33,39) and group reports (29,36,40,41,43,44,48) of children with unilateral lesions have appeared in which attempts to specify unilaterality have been included and objective measures of behavioral parameters other than IQ scores have been reported. Yet even in these more recent studies, serious methodological problems appear to underlie often contradictory findings. Among these methodological problems, which in large part I believe account for the inconclusive data reported, are the following. Important subject variables not adequately accounted for in previous work include:

1. *Specification of lesion unilaterality*, involving the related issues of how lesion location was determined and the etiology of the lesion. Crucial to inferences made about the relationship between site of lesion and any behavior measured is careful specification of lateralization of lesion location. Early studies typically based lateralization on clinical findings; in more recent studies in which CT scans have been reported, children have been included with negative CT findings but positive physical findings. In addition, virtually all investigators have included children with lesions suggesting bilateral or more diffuse involvement, e.g., head trauma, tumors, asphyxia, and systemic infections. Aram and colleagues (4–10) appear to present the only studies confined to children with vascular lesions and the only group study attempting to relate intrahemispheric localization and behavioral findings.

2. *Inclusion of patients with seizure disorders* confounds the unilateral effect of a lesion for at least three reasons: (a) the effect of the epileptiform discharge on behavior, particularly if it spreads bilaterally; (b) the effect of anticonvulsants on higher cognitive functions; and (c) the long-term effect of the epileptiform discharges on brain cells.

3. *Premorbid physical or cognitive status of subjects* typically is not stated or that which is known often implicates more diffuse involvement, e.g., neonatal asphyxia or prematurity.

4. *Use of control subjects* often has been absent or questionable. What variables to control for or what constitutes an appropriate comparison group may be debatable, yet it is doubtful that "standardized" normative data suffice given the multitude of factors known to influence higher cognitive functions.

The primary limitation in measurement has been the reliance on clinical impression that introduces the issues of the reliability and criteria by which judgments are made, but, until the past eight years, formed the dominant data other than IQ scores.

Fortunately, during the past several years, investigators began to include objective language measures in their assessment batteries. Limited longitudinal study has also been undertaken, thus presenting two important limitations: the recovery and developmental process cannot be charted, and unless testing is undertaken well beyond what is considered the period of normal development, any differences may represent a delay, presumably necessitated by hemispheric reorganization rather than a permanent deficit.

AUTHOR'S DATA BASE

The nature of the data base from our laboratory will be described briefly, as most of the summary that follows is based on that work. During the past six years, we have been involved in an ongoing study of the effects of unilateral left or right brain lesions on children's cognitive development, most importantly language (4–10). All lesioned children entered into our study have met the following strict criteria for inclusion, with many more children being excluded than included.

1. Presence of a static, unilateral left or right hemisphere lesion as evidenced by clinical neurological examination and a technically acceptable CT scan or magnetic resonance imaging (MRI). Children have been excluded with: (a) identified or suspected bilateral involvement, including those in whom lesions were sustained secondary to trauma, tumor, or systemic infections; (b) ongoing seizure disorders, requiring anticonvulsant therapy; and (c) lack of an observable lesion on CT or MRI, i.e., clinical findings alone are insufficient criteria for inclusion.

2. Evidence of normal neurological and behavioral development prior to lesion onset for all patients sustaining lesions after the perinatal period, and no evidence of genetic or other neurological problems. Children have been excluded with: (a) neonatal complications beyond congenital heart disorders, including prematurity, respiratory distress syndrome, asphyxia, and Rh-incompatibility; (b) identified or suspected genetic syndromes, such as trisomy 21; or (c) abnormal motor, mental, or social development prior to lesion onset per parent report or chart review.

3. Written parental consent to participate in the study.

Currently, 24 left-lesioned and 14 right-lesioned children are being followed, as summarized in Table 1. In the studies undertaken thus far, however, not all children have participated because of the age requirements of the measures used, and the number and age of children enrolled when a study was reported. Thus, depending on the study, our N ranges from case studies of two children to the entire complement of all lesioned children. Of the left-lesioned children, current age range is five years to 18 years, with a mean of almost 11 years. Six sustained pre- or perinatal lesions (usually porencephalic cysts) with the latest lesion onset occurring at 15.96 years of age, with a mean age of lesion onset at 4.41 years. Among the rights, the youngest is now 2½ years of age, the oldest is 19 years, with a mean age of 8.44 years. Three right-lesioned subjects sustained perinatal lesions, and the oldest sus-

TABLE 1. *Left- and right-lesioned children: subject characteristics*

No.	Date of birth	Age at lesion	Sex	Race	SES	Etiology	Lesion location
Lefts							
1	4/15/81	PN	M	W	3	PN	Subcortical
2	2/9/81	PN	F	W	3	PN	Pre & retro +BG
3	2/1/81	PN	M	W	3	PN	Pre & retro −BG
4	1/7/81	0.41	M	W	1	CVA	Pre & retro +BG
5	7/23/79	0.49	M	W	2	CVA	Pre & retro −BG
6	6/3/79	0.16	M	W	2	CVA	Pre & retro −BG
7	5/7/79	0.42	M	W	3	AVM	Pre +BG
8	12/8/78	4.33	M	W	2	CVA	Subcortical
9	9/25/78	PN	M	W	1	PN	Retro −BG
10	4/23/78	0.10	M	W	2	CVA	Retro −BG
11	3/22/78	7.72	M	W	1	CVA	Pre & retro +BG
12	3/28/77	0.27	M	W	2	CVA	Pre & retro −BG
13	9/14/76	1.96	M	B	3	CVA	Retro −BG
14	7/31/75	8.00	M	W	2	CVA	Retro −BG
15	5/21/74	6.19	M	W	3	CVA	Pre & retro +BG
16	5/7/74	7.42	F	W	2	CVA	Subcortical
17	9/19/73	PN	M	W	1	PN	Pre +BG
18	9/12/72	PN	M	W	3	PN	Retro +BG
19	9/7/72	4.50	M	W	3	CVA	Retro −BG
20	5/31/71	11.58	M	W	4	CVA	Pre −BG
21	7/31/70	11.25	F	W	1	AVM	Pre −BG
22	9/17/69	14.25	M	W	2	AVM	Pre & retro +BG
23	10/26/68	10.83	F	W	1	Complex migraine	Subcortical
24	7/29/68	15.96	F	W	2	AVM	Pre & retro +BG
Rights							
1	3/13/84	PN	M	W	2	PN	Pre & retro −BG
2	5/30/80	1.37	M	W	3	CVA	Pre −BG
3	3/12/80	4.17	M	W	2	CVA	Subcortical
4	8/21/79	0.72	F	W	2	CVA	Pre −BG
5	8/17/79	PN	F	W	1	PN	Subcortical
6	7/15/79	5.27	M	W	3	CVA	Subcortical
7	7/1/79	4.92	F	W	2	CVA	Subcortical
8	4/24/78	0.33	M	B	5	CVA	Retro −BG
9	3/21/78	3.11	M	B	5	CVA	Pre −BG
10	3/13/78	3.67	M	W	5	CVA	Pre & retro +BG
11	2/28/78	PN	F	W	3	PN	Subcortical
12	7/17/77	2.72	F	W	3	CVA	Subcortical
13	3/15/77	0.56	F	W	3	CVA	Pre −BG
14	11/16/67	1.09	F	W	3	CVA	Retro +BG

PN, pre- or perinatal; CVA, cerebrovascular accident; AVM, arteriovenous malformation; pre & retro, prerolandic/retrorolandic; BG, basal ganglia.

tained lesion onset at 5.27 years of age, with a mean lesion onset of 2.00 years. The older mean age of onset for the left-lesioned children is predominantly the result of five left-lesioned children all sustaining lesions after 10 years of age. When these five older subjects are removed, mean age of lesion onset for the left group is 2.20, thus closely approximating the mean age of onset for right subjects. In our more recent studies, we have reanalyzed our data both with and without these older five left-lesioned subjects, with negligible difference in results. As can be seen in Table 1, five of the left-lesioned children are girls and 19 boys; whereas for the right, seven are girls and seven boys. Social class for the lefts, with a mean Hollingshead score of 2.17 (SD = 0.75), is somewhat higher than for the rights (mean Hollingshead score, 3; SD = 1.54). All children sustained single vascular lesions, usually secondary to congenital heart disorders. The vast majority had experienced cerebrovascular accidents (CVA) with other etiologies listed on Table 1. Most involved the middle cerebral artery, with half of the left lesions and two of the right lesions involving both pre- and retrorolandic areas with or without basal ganglia involvement. With our increasing number of subjects, we now have a greater number with more discrete lesion sites.

Given the significant discrepancy in age, sex, and social class, we have not been able to compare left- and right-lesioned children directly. Therefore, each lesioned child has been matched individually to a neurologically normal child with a congenital heart disorder. Children with congenital heart disorders were selected as a comparison group since the majority of lesioned children also presented congenital heart disorders and this condition represents a chronic disease state necessitating hospitalization, special medical consideration, and parental care and concern similar to children with CNS involvement, but in the absence of neurological complications affecting CNS functioning and cognitive development. Control subjects were matched individually based on the following: (a) age; (b) sex; (c) race; (d) socioeconomic status using the Hollingshead 4-factor index; and (e) arterial blood oxygen saturation level, with lesioned children who do not have congenital heart disorders matched only to acyanotic (defined at 92% oxygen saturation level) control children and lesioned children with congenital heart disorders matched as closely as possible by arterial oxygen saturation levels. When both lesioned and control subjects have congenital heart disorders, attempts have also been made to match as closely as possible for severity of heart disorders and for number of hospitalizations. All controls are right-handed.

Turning to what we now know about early brain lesions and language abilities in children, the following discussion reviews first the findings related to overall level of cognitive functioning in children with unilateral lesions, and then addresses in turn these children's comprehension of connected language, spoken syntax, and the lexical/semantic aspects of language. Included will be consideration of the effect of age of lesion onset and a somewhat speculative discussion of the relationship between the site of lesion within a hemisphere and the behavioral sequelae observed.

COGNITIVE LEVEL AND PROFILES

Although IQ scores have been the most extensively reported measure of cognitive ability of children with lateralized brain lesions, this area has yielded probably the most contradictory results—in large measure owing to the inclusion in virtually all previous studies of children with probable bilateral involvement and seizure disorders. Most of the earlier studies reported intelligence test findings for large groups of left-hemiplegic and right-hemiplegic children heterogeneous in terms of etiologies included age of lesion onset, severity of motoric disorders, and degree of bilateral involvement (3,23,28,38). Although there is considerable variability in findings, generally these earlier studies reported reduced IQs for both left- and right-hemiplegic children and failed to demonstrate the adult pattern of lower verbal IQ following left-hemisphere lesions and lower performance IQ following right-hemisphere lesions. Variables suggested to explain this lack of relationship between lateralized brain damage and verbal and performance IQ discrepancies have focused on the early age of lesion onset and the presumed plasticity of young children's brains. Yet four recent studies, all of which reported CT scan confirmation of lesion location for the majority of subjects and specifically addressed Verbal and Performance IQ, lesion laterality, and age of lesion onset, present conflicting results (Table 2) (36,41,43,47).

Woods's data (47) suggested that early right-hemisphere, and both early and late left-hemisphere lesions impaired both verbal IQ (VIQ) and performance IQ (PIQ), whereas late right-hemisphere lesions lowered PIQ alone. Riva and Cazzaniga's (41) replication of Woods's study, however, failed to support Woods's findings. In their study, both early and late onset right-lesioned patients presented significant VIQ-PIQ discrepancies, with PIQ but not VIQ significantly lower than for siblings. Among children with early onset left lesions, both performance IQs were significantly lower than those for siblings, although significant verbal-performance differences were not present. Children with late onset left lesions tended to have lower scores than siblings, but neither the difference between lesioned children and siblings nor the difference between verbal and performance scores was significant. Vargha-Khadem, O'Gorman, and Watters (43) reported IQ scores for children with prenatal, early (2 months to 5 years), or late (5 years to 13 years) lesion onset, contradicting

TABLE 2. Lesion laterality and IQ results of recent studies

Investigators	Lesion onset	Subjects' hemisphere involved	
		Left	Right
Woods (47)	<1 year	↓ VIQ ↓ PIQ	↓ VIQ ↓ PIQ
	>1 year	↓ VIQ ↓ PIQ	↓ PIQ
Riva and Cazzaniga (41)	<1 year	↓ VIQ ↓ PIQ	VIQ > ↓ PIQ
	>1 year		VIQ > ↓ PIQ
Vargha-Khadem, O'Gorman, and Watters (43)	Prenatal		
	Early postnatal	VIQ ↓ [a] <PIQ	
	Late postnatal	VIQ ↓ NS <PIQ	
Nass, Koch, Janowsky, and Stiles-Davis (36)	All pre- and perinatal	VIQ ↑ PIQ[a]	>VIQ[a] = PIQ

VIQ, Verbal IQ; PIQ, Performance IQ; NS, not significant.
[a] Authors reported significant findings.

both the Woods and the Riva and Cazzaniga studies. Although there was a tendency for children with early and late postnatal left lesions to have lower VIQs than PIQs, and for all groups of right-lesioned children to have lower PIQs than VIQs, the only lesioned group to present a significant VIQ-PIQ discrepancy was the early onset left-lesioned group. Finally, in a recent study of children who sustained prenatal or perinatal damage, Nass, Koch, Janowsky, and Stiles-Davis (36) suggested yet another relationship between VIQ and PIQ and lateralized brain lesions in childhood. The children with prenatally or perinatally incurred left lesions presented significantly higher VIQs than the right-lesioned children, with no differences between PIQs.

Many factors undoubtedly contribute to these variable findings, chief of which I believe to be the limited sensitivity of VIQ and PIQ measures to reflect linguistic, visuo-perceptual and/or performance deficits, and the inclusion of children with variable degrees of bilateral involvement. Annett (3), in a review of many of the earlier studies, has addressed a number of variables related to IQ among hemiplegic children including motor performance in the dominant and nondominant hand (thereby assessing bilaterality of involvement), familial sinistrality, and the presence or absence of seizure disorders.

We have reported the level and pattern of the *Wechsler Preschool and Primary Scale of Intelligence* (WPPSI) (45) and *Wechsler Intelligence Scale for Children-Revised* (WISC-R) (46) performance for 18 left- and 13 right-lesioned children in comparison with their controls (4). VIQ, PIQ, and Full Scale Intelligence (FIQ) were well within normal limits for all groups, although right-lesioned children had scores significantly lower than those of right controls (Table 3). The high level of performance among the lesioned children studied here was striking and contrasts with earlier reports of lower IQs and lateralized brain damage in children. The exclusion of children with diffuse brain involvement and seizures were factors felt to contribute to the high overall performance of the lesioned children studied here.

No significant differences between VIQ, PIQ, and FIQ were found within the left- or right-lesioned or control groups; thus VIQ and PIQ discrepancy was not found to relate to lesion laterality, contrary to findings of adults with acute lesions. However, when WISC-R subtests were recategorized according to Kaufman's factors (27) (verbal comprehension, perceptual organization, freedom from distractibility), the freedom from distractibility factor was impaired in both left- and right-lesioned children and right-lesioned children were also deficient in perceptual organization.

Left lesion onset prior to one year of age was associated with homogeneous VIQ, PIQ, and FIQ scores, whereas after one year of age, left-lesioned children's VIQ tended to be lower than PIQ (Table 4). PIQ was significantly lower for left-lesioned children with lesion onset prior to one year than after one year, suggesting either verbal sparing at the expense of performance abilities prior to one year or alternatively, greater impairment of VIQ following lesions sustained after one year of age. Similarly, for the right-lesioned children, a nonsignificant tendency was present for those sustaining lesions prior to one year to have more homogeneous IQ scores, whereas for lesions sustained after one year, PIQ was lower than VIQ.

TABLE 3. WPPSI and WISC-R IQs: descriptive and two-factor repeated Anovas

IQ scores

IQ		Left children (N = 18)		Right children (N = 13)	
		Subject	Control	Subject	Control
Verbal	$\bar{X}$	109.56	116.89	107.08 [a]	114.54
	SD	18.15	14.40	14.59	12.98
Performance	$\bar{X}$	113.78	115.00	102.08 [a]	116.46
	SD	12.27	13.21	12.24	9.03
Full Scale	$\bar{X}$	112.56	117.61	104.92 [a]	117.00
	SD	15.16	14.53	13.06	12.00

Source	df	SS	MS	F	p	df	SS	MS	F	p
Group	1,17	555.79	555.79	1.73	0.206	1,12	2493.35	2493.35	22.50	<0.001
IQ	2,34	63.69	31.84	0.51	0.606	2,24	45.54	22.77	0.62	0.545
Interaction	2,34	171.69	85.84	2.27	0.118	2,24	161.54	80.77	2.91	0.074

Kaufman factors

		Left children (N = 18)		Right children (N = 10)	
		Subject	Control	Subject	Control
IQ					
Verbal comprehension	$\bar{X}$	11.69	12.78	11.35	12.15
	SD	2.99	2.12	2.36	2.04
Perceptual organization	$\bar{X}$	12.46	12.22	10.35	12.15
	SD	1.71 [b]	2.13	1.16 [c]	1.23
Freedom from distractibility	$\bar{X}$	10.17 [b]	11.96	9.83 [c]	12.47
	SD	2.18	2.30	1.64	2.15

	Left children (N = 18)					Right children (N = 10)				
Source	df	SS	MS	F	p	df	SS	MS	F	p
Group	1,17	20.96	20.96	4.18	0.057	1,9	45.65	45.65	23.95	0.001
IQ	2,34	36.12	18.06	5.81	0.007	2,18	4.13	2.07	1.00	0.389
Interaction	2,34	19.14	9.57	4.52	0.018	2,18	8.43	4.21	3.41	0.005

[a] Tukey 6.68.
[b] Tukey 1.48.
[c] Tukey 1.57.
From Aram and Ekelman (4).

TABLE 4. IQ scores: age of lesion onset and site of lesion

IQ and lesion onset before or after one year of age (mean performance and Mann Whitney U Results)

	Left-lesioned subjects				Right-lesioned subjects			
	Onset <1 year (N = 7)	Onset >1year (N = 11)	U	p	Onset <1 year (N = 5)	Onset >1 year (N = 8[a])	U	p
IQ score								
Verbal IQ								
Mean	108.14	110.45	36.5	0.8561	105.40	106.83	17.5	0.7140
Mean rank	9.79	9.32			6.50	7.31		
Performance IQ								
Mean	107.86	117.55	15.0	0.0321	107.20	97.83	11.5	0.2121
Mean rank	6.14	11.64			8.70	5.97		
Full scale IQ								
Mean	108.57	115.09	35.0	0.7513	106.40	102.67	15.5	0.5071
Mean rank	9.00	9.82			7.90	6.44		
Kaufman factors in standard scores								
Verbal comprehension								
Mean	11.54	11.80	36.5	0.8562	11.05	11.29	17.0	0.6588
Mean rank	9.79	9.32			6.40	7.38		
Perceptual organization								
Mean	11.79	12.89	22.5	0.1456	10.55	10.25	19.0	0.8833
Mean rank	7.21	10.95			7.20	6.88		
Freedom from distractibility								
Mean	9.71	10.45	31.5	0.5248	10.67	8.94	4.0	0.0427
Mean rank	8.50	10.14			8.20	4.17		

Site of lesion, mean IQ and mean scaled scores for Kaufman factors

	N	WISC-R (Mean IQ)			Kaufman factors[b] (Mean scaled scores)		
		VIQ	PIQ	FIQ	VC	PO	FD
Lefts							
Prerolandic only	4	115.00	119.75	119.00	12.81	12.94	11.17
Retrorolandic only	6	107.50	104.00	106.33	11.42	11.21	9.78
Cortical only	9	107.89	109.33	109.22	11.33	11.72	10.63
Subcortical only	3	108.00	125.67	118.00	11.17	13.75	11.00
Rights							
Prerolandic only	3	97.00	107.33	101.33	9.83	10.08	9.89
Retrorolandic only	2	103.50	98.00	101.00	10.50	10.25	9.50
Cortical only	5	98.20	102.00	99.40	9.90	10.05	9.20
Subcortical only	5	115.80	102.40	110.20	12.80	10.65	10.47

[a]Two children received the WPPSI and are therefore not included in the Kaufman factors.
[b]Kaufman factors: VC, verbal comprehension; PO, perceptual organization; FD, freedom from distractibility.
From Aram and Ekelman (4).

Any relationship between site of lesion and IQ is speculative given the small number of children presenting discrete lesion sites (Table 4). Trends, however, can be noted. With the exception of the right-lesioned children with prerolandic-only involvement, all groups classified by lesion site demonstrated the lowest scores on the freedom from distractibility factor, suggesting that distractibility may be associated with brain damage in children irrespective of specific lesion site. Further, it appears that left-lesioned children with retrorolandic involvement may have relatively lower IQ scores than those with prerolandic involvement, where IQ scores are comparable to controls. The suggestion of a lateralized relationship between VIQ and PIQ and subcortical lesions, with notably lower VIQ and PIQ scores for left-lesioned children and the converse observed for right-lesioned children, is particularly interesting. In summary, the findings demonstrate that IQ scores of children with unilateral brain lesions and no ongoing seizure activity may be expected to be well within normal limits, but may not be sensitive indicators of differences in these children's language or learning abilities.

SYNTACTIC COMPREHENSION

Earlier reports based on clinical observation suggested that, except acutely, comprehension is rarely impaired among children with acquired brain lesions (2,24,25). The few data-based studies, however, generally have demonstrated the presence of at least subtle deficits among left brain lesioned children (Table 5). Woods and Carey (48) appear to have been the first investigators to report objective measures of comprehension, including three measures (Token Test, identification of syntactically anomalous that-clause sentences; demonstration of ask-tell distinctions through puppets) in their assessment battery of left-lesioned children. These investigators were particularly interested in age of lesion onset, reporting that the 16 children with lesion onset after one year of age were significantly impaired on all three measures, whereas the 11 children with lesions prior to one year of age (and the onset of language) differed from comparison subjects only on the Token Test. Dennis (15), who documented the acute recovery of a nine-year-old girl with a left temporoparietal infarct, administered an array of syntactic comprehension tasks including the Token Test and a task of metalinguistic judgment of word relatedness. Across all syntactic comprehension tasks, this child demonstrated marked impairment, although unlike the other studies summarized in Table 5, testing was conducted acutely following lesion onset. Kiessling, Denckla, and Carlton (29) administered a syntactic awareness task to eight right- and eight left-hemiplegic children documenting right hemiplegics' inferior performance in comparison to left-hemiplegic or comparison children. Finally, two additional studies, Rankin, Aram, and Horwitz (40) and Vargha-Khadem, O'Gorman, and Watters (43) found children with left hemisphere lesions to perform more poorly than right-lesioned or control children on the Token Test, irrespective of age of lesion onset.

Although at least four previous studies had administered the Token Test to children with lateralized brain lesions, except for Rankin et al. (40), none had

TABLE 5. *Review of syntactic comprehension and lateralized brain lesions in children*

Investigators	Subjects				Measures	Findings
Woods and Carey (48)	Left-brain lesioned: Onset: 11, <1 year 16, >1 year				Token Test, That-clause sentences, Ask-tell distinctions	Lesion onset: <1 year: ↓ Token Test; >1 year: ↓ all 3 measures
Kiessling, Denckla, and Carlton (29)	8 right, 8 left hemiplegics (<1 year)				Syntactic awareness task	Right-hemiplegics < lefts or controls
Rankin, Aram, and Horwitz (40)	3 right, 3 left, hemiplegics (≤birth)				Token Test	Right-hemiplegics < lefts
Vargha-Khadem, O'Gorman, and Watters (43)		Pre-natal	Postnatal		Token Test	Lefts in all age groups <controls; Rights = controls
			Early	Late		
	Left:	18	6	4		
	Right:	16	5	5		

analyzed performance by subtest, thus not evaluating the relative contribution of memory load versus syntactic comprehension to the results obtained. Therefore, we administered the Revised Token Test (RTT) (34) to 17 children with left hemisphere lesions and 11 with right hemisphere lesions. Left-lesioned children's lower performance on several subtests than that of controls appeared to be related predominantly to the memory demands of these subtests rather than the limited syntactic elements assessed by the RTT (Fig. 1). Although right-lesioned children's performance tended to be lower than their matched controls, these differences were not significant nor readily related to either the memory or specific linguistic structures assessed (Fig. 2). A trend for left-lesioned children with retrorolandic lesions to perform more poorly than those with left prerolandic lesions was suggested. No systematic difference in performance was apparent for children with left cortical versus left subcortical lesions or among discrete sites of lesion within the right hemisphere. Children with left-hemisphere lesions prior to one year of age performed no better and, in several instances, significantly more poorly than left-lesioned patients sustaining lesions after one year of age. Among right-lesioned subjects, a trend was noted for those sustaining lesions after one year of age to have greater difficulty than those with lesion onset before one year of age, especially in linguistic elements that were dependent on visuospatial properties.

Overall, all studies to date demonstrate at least subtle deficits in syntactic comprehension following left but not right hemisphere lesions. Further studies, however, need to more fully evaluate comprehension of more complex linguistic stimuli than assessed by the Token Test and the role of more primary cognitive abilities such as memory and attention in contributing to the comprehension deficits observed.

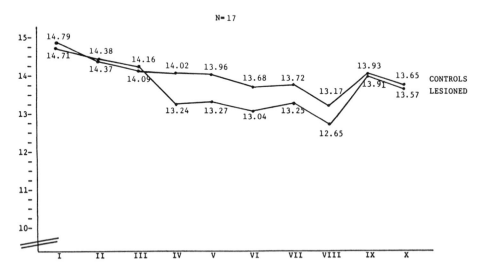

FIG. 1. Mean performance on Revised Token Test subtests by left-lesioned subjects and controls.

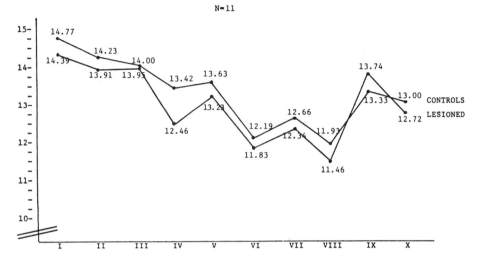

FIG. 2. Mean performance on Revised Token Test subtests by right-lesioned subjects and controls.

SYNTACTIC PRODUCTION

Most observations of children sustaining acquired left (2,22,24,25,29) and occasionally right brain lesions (19,32) report mutism acutely and telegraphic expressive language during recovery. An occasional report of fluent aphasia following left lesions in children has appeared (44), yet the anticipated result of acquired lesions in young children irrespective of age of onset or site of lesion within the left hemisphere is reduced output.

Besides clinical observations or a few well-described case studies, few investigators have documented expressive language abilities after acute recovery. Exceptions include Woods and Carey (48) who administered a sentence completion task to their 27 subjects sustaining left lesions many years prior to testing. These investigators found left-lesioned subjects sustaining insult after but not before one year of age to be impaired on this task in comparison to normally developing peers. Kiessling et al. (29) administered the Binet Sentences, a repetition task, to eight right and eight left hemiplegics. In contrast to the findings of Woods and Carey, Kiessling et al. found the right hemiplegics, all of whom sustained injury prior to one year of age, performed more poorly than left hemiplegics or sibling controls (Table 6).

Except for Dennis's (15) case study of the acute recovery of a nine-year-old with a temporoparietal infarct, we know of no work other than our own that has described the syntax of spontaneous spoken language of children with unilateral lesions. As one of the earlier studies (8) we undertook, we analyzed the spontaneous spoken language of eight left-lesioned children who at that time were between two and

TABLE 6. *Syntactic production and lateralized brain lesions in children*

Investigators	Subjects	Measures	Findings
Woods and Carey (48)	Left-lesioned: Onset: 11, <1 year 16, >1 year	Sentence completion task	↓ lesion onset >1 year; not <1 year
Kiessling, Denckla, and Carlton (29)	8 right, 8 left hemiplegics	Binet sentence repetition	Right hemiplegics < Lefts and Controls

eight years of age, and eight right-lesioned children aged 1½ to six years of age. Based on analyses of spontaneous language samples (Table 7), left-lesioned subjects were found to perform more poorly than controls on most measures of simple and complex sentence structures. In contrast, right-lesioned subjects performed similarly to controls on these measures except for a tendency to make more errors in simple sentence structures. Given the small number of children studied and the limited variability in age of onset and lesion location, no attempt was made to relate spoken syntax to these factors.

TABLE 7. *Spoken syntax in children with left or right lesions*

	Left subjects/ left controls	Right subjects/ right controls
Overall sentences		
Mean length of utterance	*[a]	*
DSS: complexity score	*	NS
% Total sentences correct	*	*
Simple sentences		
% Attempted	*	NS
% Correct	*	*
Complex sentences		
% Attempted	*	NS
% Correct	*	NS
Embeddings		
Number	*	NS
% Correct		
Conjunctions		
Number	NS[b]	NS
% Correct	NS	NS
DSS		
Pronouns		
Mean	NS	NS
Total	NS	NS
Main verb		
Mean	*	NS
Total	*	*
Interrogative reversals		
Mean	*	NS
Total	*	NS
Wh-questions		
Mean	*	NS
Total	*	NS
Negatives		
Mean	*	*
Total	NS	NS
GMN	*	NS
GME	*	*

[a] Significant at <0.05.
[b] Not significant; randomization test for matched pairs.
From Aram, Ekelman, and Whitaker (8).

At the present time, follow-up analyses of spoken syntax among the larger and now generally older groups of lesioned and control children are under way. Experimental syntactic measures are being administered as well, and we anticipate findings with this older and expanded group of children will further evidence long-standing deficits in expressive syntax following left brain lesions in children.

LEXICAL/SEMANTIC ASPECTS OF LANGUAGE

As with spoken syntax, the lexical or semantic aspects of either language comprehension or production have rarely been described among children sustaining unilateral brain injury, except during acute recovery stages (28,29,39,44). Beyond case studies, I am aware of only four studies of children with long-standing left or right brain lesions that have included naming or other semantic measures, and the results from these studies are contradictory (Table 8).

Once again, Woods and Carey (48) appear to be the first to administer a systematic measure of naming to subjects sustaining left hemisphere lesions in childhood. Using the Oldfield and Wingfield Naming Test, these investigators found left-lesioned subjects sustaining lesions after but not before one year of age were significantly less accurate in naming than control subjects. Three studies reported results on naming tasks for both left- and right-lesioned children. Kiessling et al. (29) reported that mean z-scores on the Boston Naming Test were lower for both the left (mean z-score, -1.47) and the right (mean z-score, -1.42) groups of brain lesioned children than for sibling comparison children, although these differences were not statistically significant, and differences between the left- and right-lesioned groups were negligible. Vargha-Khadem et al. (43) administered the Oldfield and Wingfield Naming Test to 28 left- and 25 right-lesioned subjects, grouped according to age at lesion onset. All groups of left-lesioned subjects (prenatal, early postnatal, and late postnatal) and the early postnatal right group were impaired in accuracy of naming in comparison to control subjects. A significant negative relationship between age of lesion onset and naming accuracy was reported. Finally, we (7) administered the Expressive One-Word Picture Vocabulary Test (EOWPVT), a confrontation naming task, and the Peabody Picture Vocabulary Test (PPVT), a vocabulary comprehension task, to eight left- and eight right-lesioned children and their controls, demonstrating poorer performance of both the left- and right-lesioned children in comparison with control subjects on both the naming and vocabulary comprehension tasks. Overall, these few studies evidence that both left- and right-lesioned children may have persistent naming and possibly lexical comprehension deficits.

In light of these preliminary findings, we then went on to assess further the nature of these naming or lexical retrieval difficulties. In order to evaluate the effect of retrieval cues and semantic category on rate of lexical retrieval, we administered two additional naming tasks to 19 left- and 13 right-brain-lesioned children and their controls (8) (Table 9). On the Word Finding Test, left-lesioned subjects were

TABLE 8. *Lexical abilities and lateralized brain lesions in children*

Investigators	Subjects				Measures	Findings
Woods and Carey (48)	Left-lesioned: Onset: 11, <1 year 16, >1 year				Oldfield and Wingfield Naming Test	Lesion onset <1 year: no differences; >1 year: significance ↓
Kiessling, Denckla, and Carlton (29)	8 right, 8 left hemiplegics				Boston Naming Test	Both left and right hemiplegics nonsignificantly lower than controls
Vargha-Khadem, O'Gorman, and Watters (43)		Pre-natal	Postnatal Early	Late	Oldfield and Wingfield Naming Test	All left groups and early postnatal right group < controls
	Left:	18	6	4		
	Right:	16	5	5		
Aram, Ekelman, Rose and Whitaker (7)	8 right-, 8 left-lesioned				Expressive One-Word, Picture Vocabulary Test, Peabody Picture, Vocabulary Test	Left- and right-lesioned < controls on both measures

TABLE 9. *Lexical retrieval and left or right brain lesions in children*

Word-Finding Test
Latencies in seconds for semantic, rhyming, and visual cues

	Overall		Semantic		Rhyming		Visual	
	M̄	SD	M̄	SD	M̄	SD	M̄	SD
Lefts								
L	1.82	0.49	1.70	0.88	2.74	0.97	1.30	0.58
C	1.54	0.32	1.26	0.47	2.58	0.87	1.02	0.33
t[a]	3.12[b]		3.01[b]		0.77		2.64[c]	
Rights								
L	1.68	0.32	1.81	0.50	1.85	0.57	1.44	0.43
C	1.95	0.41	2.12	0.80	2.62	0.83	1.49	0.36
t	−1.63		−1.09		−2.40[c]		−0.33	

Rapid Automatized Naming Test
Latencies in seconds for colors, numbers, objects, and letters

	Overall		Color		Number		Object		Letter	
	M̄	SD	M̄	SD	M̄	SD	M̄	SD	M̄	SD
Lefts										
L	52.57	29.09	64.42	39.87	41.46	24.49	86.83	50.16	45.04	36.10
C	34.87	17.81	43.07	19.97	26.18	14.65	56.71	28.06	25.39	15.44
t	3.19[b]		2.74[c]		3.68[b]		3.43[b]		3.01[b]	
Rights										
L	60.61	17.54	80.95	41.31	56.75	18.96	87.80	28.82	49.92	20.34
C	62.20	33.02	66.12	18.87	53.15	36.04	80.75	27.98	55.38	40.49
t	0.16		1.48		0.31		0.79		−0.44	

[a] Matched t.
[b] $p < 0.01$.
[c] $p < 0.05$.
From Aram, Ekelman, and Whitaker (9).

significantly slower in response time than left controls when given semantic and visual cues and made more errors when given rhyming cues. On the Rapid Automatized Naming Test, left-lesioned subjects were significantly slower than left controls in naming all semantic categories, including colors, numbers, objects, and letters. In contrast, right-lesioned subjects responded as or more quickly than did right controls in all access conditions and in naming semantic categories, yet tended to produce more errors than their controls, suggesting a speed-accuracy trade-off. Children sustaining left brain lesions before one year of age appeared to be as impaired as those whose lesions occurred after one year of age. Diverse lesion sites within the left hemisphere were associated with increased lexical retrieval latencies.

SUMMARY OF FINDINGS

Language Abilities

In summary of language sequelae described thus far (Table 10), left-lesioned children have shown deficits in language comprehension, spoken syntax, latency

TABLE 10. *Summary of cognitive and language findings*

Area assessed	Findings to date	
	Left-lesioned (LL)	Right-lesioned (RL)
Cognitive level and pattern	WPPSI and WISC-R IQs and Kaufman factors	
	IQs normal; no difference between LLs and LCs on VIQ, PIQ, and FIQ; lesion laterality not reflected in VIQ-PIQ discrepancy. LL < LC on freedom from distractibility.	IQs normal; RL < RC on VIQ, PIQ, and FIQ; lesion laterality not reflected in VIQ-PIQ discrepancy. RL < RC on freedom from distractibility and perceptual organization.
Syntactic comprehension	Revised Token Test	
	LL significance < LC on several subtests of RTT; deficit appears secondary to memory rather than syntactic features.	Nonsignificant tendency for RL performance to be lower than RC across tasks; question role of attention; suggestion of deficit on linguistic elements based on visuospatial properties.
Spoken syntax	Spontaneous language	
	LL < LC on most measures of simple and complex sentence structures.	RL = RC on most measures except greater tendency for error on simple sentence structures.
Semantics	Lexical retrieval	
	LL latencies and errors > LC	RL ≤ RC in latencies. RL > RC in errors on lexical retrieval tasks.

From Aram and colleagues.

of word retrieval and percentage of errors in word retrieval, whereas children with right hemisphere lesions have not shown similar deficits. These findings may suggest considerable early left hemisphere specialization for these aspects of language. Studies are under way to determine whether deficits in spoken syntax persist over time and whether the phonological characteristics of speech are impaired by lateralized brain lesions. Children with right hemisphere lesions have been found to be essentially comparable to controls on syntactic comprehension and production, but to be impulsive in naming, producing reduced latencies on naming tasks and an increased percentage of errors. Future studies are needed to assess more fully: the role of complex sentence structure, attention, and memory in contributing to the left-lesioned children's difficulty with comprehension of connected language; lateralized lesions and the ability to understand more conceptually based aspects of semantics; and the relationship between phonological deficits observed in speech, reading, and spelling.

Age of Lesion Onset

Summarizing our findings in respect to the age of lesion onset (Table 11), among left-lesioned subjects, lesion onset prior to or after one year of age does not appear to be related to observed performance in most areas examined thus far, with the exception of VIQ and PIQ, which appear to be more comparable among children with left lesions before one year of age and to reflect lesion laterality after one year of age. To date, therefore, age of lesion onset is not emerging as a factor related to outcome for left subjects. Among right-lesioned subjects, some tendency was suggested for lesion onset after one year to be associated with poorer performance on aspects of the RTT related to visuospatial properties and more errors on the lexical retrieval tasks. Again mirroring left-lesioned findings, right lesion onset prior to one year of age was associated with comparable verbal and performance IQs, whereas after one year, PIQ tended to be notably lower than VIQ. Whether these findings are idiosyncratic to the small group of right-lesioned children studied here, or evidence age of onset as a variable important to outcome will require study of additional children with a fuller range of tasks considered to be sensitive to right hemisphere lesions.

Site of Lesion

Our attempts to relate site of lesion within hemisphere to behavioral sequelae (Table 11) have been limited by two factors: (a) the low number of children presenting discrete lesion sites—the majority evidencing both pre- and retrorolandic and often both cortical and subcortical involvement; and (b) the use of CT scans, obtained for clinical purposes over a considerable span of years and on differing scanners, on which to base determination of anatomic involvement. Therefore, any

TABLE 11. Summary of relationships suggested between behavioral area assessed, age of lesion onset, and site of lesion within a hemisphere

| Behavioral area | Age of lesion onset (< or > 1 year) | | Site of lesion | | | |
| | Lefts | Rights | Lefts | | Rights | |
			Pre-/retrorolandic	Cortical/subcortical	Pre-/retrorolandic	Cortical/subcortical
Cognitive abilities			Low scores on Freedom from Distractibility factor associated with diverse sites.			
Wechsler profiles/Kaufman factors	<1 year, VIQ = PIQ >1 year, VIQ < PIQ	<1 year, VIQ = PIQ >1 year, VIQ > PIQ	Trend for retro-IQs to be lower than prerolandic.	Trend for lateralized subcortical effect; VIQ < PIQ.		Trend for lateralized subcortical effect; PIQ < VIQ.
Language abilities Syntactic comprehension	<1 year of age performance equal to or poorer than >1 year of age.	>1 year performance poorer than <1 year especially on tasks related to visuospatial properties.	Retrorolandic < prerolandic.	No apparent differences.	No apparent differences.	No apparent differences.

(continued)

TABLE 11. (continued)

| Behavioral area | Age of lesion onset (< or > 1 year) | | Site of lesion | | | |
| | Lefts | Rights | Lefts | | Rights | |
			Pre-/retrorolandic	Cortical/subcortical	Pre-/retrorolandic	Cortical/subcortical
Lexical retrieval	Comparably increased latency and percentage of error at > and <1 year of age.	>1 year variable, but tendency to have more errors than those before 1 year.	Diverse lesion site associated with lexical retrieval problems. Tendency for retrorolandic to have greater difficulty than prerolandic.	Diverse lesion site associated with lexical retrieval problems.	Not analyzed.	Not analyzed.

conclusions relating site of lesion to behavior are offered tentatively and somewhat speculatively.

Among left-lesioned children a trend was observed for children with only retro-rolandic involvement to have greater difficulty with tasks of syntactic comprehension, lexical retrieval, and overall IQ than children with only prerolandic lesions. Although no differences were observed between left cortical and left subcortical lesions on syntactic comprehension and lexical retrieval tasks, children with sub-cortical-only lesions tended to have lower VIQs than PIQs. (Data not reported here demonstrate that subcortical left lesions also are associated with slower diado-chokinetic repetition rates and lower performance on perceptual speed, reasoning, math, and reading clusters.) Among the right-lesioned children, few differences were observed to relate to site of lesion within the right hemisphere, owing in part to the limited number of children presenting discrete lesions as well as perhaps to the nature of the tasks measured. Mirroring the left subcortical lesioned children, right subcortical lesioned children tended to present more discrepant IQs with PIQ being notably poorer than VIQ.

CONCLUSION

Finally, I would like to comment that, although we are identifying significantly poorer performance in left-lesioned children than controls across a range of syntactic and lexical language tasks, by and large these deficits are mild, and often subtle, with few children remaining clinically aphasic. These children, however, are typically having academic problems (data are not reported here). Although the right-lesioned children appear to be functioning well based on the findings presented here, it must be kept in mind that the tasks discussed were confined predominantly to language tasks generally thought to be left-hemisphere dependent. Right-lesioned children appear to have their own set of difficulties, exemplified here by naming errors, also in areas of attention, impulse inhibition, memory, and other areas that we are only beginning to explore. Overall, I am not convinced that age of lesion onset bears much relationship to the sequelae we are observing for left-lesioned children, at least for the age group we have been studying. I am, however, intrigued by the tentative findings relative to site of lesion within a hemisphere, particularly involvement of cortical versus subcortical structures, an aspect we plan to study in a more detailed and systematic manner through the aid of MRI.

ACKNOWLEDGEMENTS

The work on which this chapter is based was supported by NINCDS Grant NS17366 awarded to the author.

REFERENCES

1. Aicardi, J., Amsili, J., and Chevrie, J.J. (1969): Acute hemiplegia in infancy and childhood. *Dev. Med. Child Neurol.*, 11:162–173.
2. Alajouanine, T.H., and Lhermitte, F. (1965): Acquired aphasia in children. *Brain*, 88:653–662.
3. Annett, M. (1973): Laterality of childhood hemiplegia and the growth of speech and intelligence. *Cortex*, 9:4–33.
4. Aram, D.M., and Ekelman, B.L. (1986): Cognitive profiles of children with early onset unilateral lesions. *Dev. Neuropsychol.*, 2:155–172.
5. Aram, D.M., and Ekelman, B.L. Scholastic aptitude and achievement among children with unilateral brain lesions (*submitted*).
6. Aram, D.M., and Ekelman, B.L. Unilateral brain lesions in childhood: Performance on the *Revised Token Test. Brain Lang. (in press).*
7. Aram, D.M., Ekelman, B.L., Rose, D.F., and Whitaker H.A. (1985): Verbal and cognitive sequelae following unilateral lesions acquired in early childhood. *J. Clin. Exp. Neuropsychol.*, 7:55–78.
8. Aram, D.M., Ekelman, B.L., and Whitaker, H.A. (1986): Spoken syntax in children with acquired unilateral hemisphere lesions. *Brain Lang.*, 27:75–100.
9. Aram, D.M., Ekelman, B.L., and Whitaker H.A. (1987): Lexical retrieval in left and right brain lesioned children. *Brain Lang.*, 61–87.
10. Aram, D.M., Rose, D.F., Rekate, H.L., and Whitaker, H.A. (1983): Acquired capsular/striatal aphasia in childhood. *Arch. Neurol.*, 40:614–617.
11. Basser, L.S. (1962): Hemiplegia of early onset and the faculty of speech with special reference to the effect of hemispherectomy. *Brain,* 85:427–460.
12. Byers, R.K., and McLean, W.T. (1962): Etiology and course of certain hemiplegias with aphasia in childhood. *Pediatrics*, 29:376–383.
13. Day, P.S., and Ulatowska, H.K. (1979): Perceptual, cognitive, and linguistic development after early hemispherectomy: Two case studies. *Brain Lang.*, 7:17–33.
14. Dennis, M. (1980): Capacity and strategy for syntactic comprehension after left or right hemidecortication. *Brain Lang.*, 10:187–307.
15. Dennis, M. (1980): Strokes in childhood: Communicative intent, expression and comprehension after left hemisphere arteriopathy in a right-handed nine-year-old. In: *Language Development and Aphasia in Children*, edited by R.W. Rieber, pp. 45–67. Academic Press, New York.
16. Dennis, M., and Kohn, B. (1975): Comprehension of syntax in infantile hemiplegics after cerebral hemidecortication: Left hemisphere superiority. *Brain Lang.*, 2:472–482.
17. Dennis, M., and Whitaker, H.A. (1976): Language acquisition following hemidecortication: Linguistic superiority of the left over the right hemisphere. *Brain Lang.*, 3:404–433.
18. Dennis, M., and Whitaker, H.A. (1977): Hemispheric equipotentiality and language acquisition. In: *Language Development and Neurological Theory*, edited by S. J. Segalowitz and F. A. Gruber, pp. 93–106. Academic Press, New York.
19. Ferro, J.M., Martins, I.P., Pinto, F., and Castro-Caldas, A. (1982): Aphasia following right striato-insular infarction in a left-handed child: A clinico-radiological study. *Dev. Med. Child Neurol.*, 24:173–182.
20. Ferro, J.M., Martins, I.P., and Tavora, L. (1984): Neglect in children. *Ann. Neurol.*, 15:281–284.
21. Gold, A.P., and Carter, S. (1976): Acute hemiplegia of infancy and childhood. *Pediatr. Clin. North Am.*, 23:413–433.
22. Guttmann, E. (1942): Aphasia in children. *Brain*, 65:205–219.
23. Hammil, D., and Irwin O.C. (1966): IQ differences of right and left spastic hemiplegic children. *Percept. Mot. Skills*, 22:193–194.
24. Hecaen, H. (1976): Acquired aphasia in children and the ontogenesis of hemispheric functional specialization. *Brain Lang.*, 3:114–134.
25. Hecaen, H. (1983): Acquired aphasia in children: Revisited. *Neuropsychologia*, 21:581–587.
26. Hood, P.N., and Perlstein, M.A. (1955): Infantile spastic hemiplegia: II. Laterality of involvement. *Am. J. Phys. Med.*, 34:457–466.
27. Kaufman, A.S. (1975): Factor analysis of the WISC-R at 11 age levels between 6 and 16½ years. *J. Consult. Clin. Psychol.*, 43:135–147.

28. Kershner, J.R., and King, A.J. (1974): Laterality of cognitive functions in achieving hemiplegic children. *Percept. Mot. Skills,* 39:1283–1289.
29. Kiessling, L.S., Denckla, M.B., and Carlton, M. (1983): Evidence for differential hemispheric function in children with hemiplegic cerebral palsy. *Dev. Med. Child Neurol.,* 25:727–734.
30. Kinsbourne, M., and Hiscock, M. (1977): Does cerebral dominance develop? In: *Language Development and Neurological Theory,* edited by S.J. Segalowitz and F.A. Gruber, pp. 171–191. Academic Press, New York.
31. Kohn, B., and Dennis, M. (1974): Selective impairments of visuo-spatial abilities in infantile hemiplegics after right cerebral hemidecortication. *Neuropsychologia,* 12:505–512.
32. Lenneberg, E. (1967): *Biological Foundations of Language.* Wiley, New York.
33. Martins, I.P., Ferro, J.M., and Trindade, A. (1984): Acquired crossed aphasia in a child. Paper presented at the meeting of the International Neuropsychology Society, Aachem, Germany, June.
34. McNeil, M.R., and Prescott, T.E. (1978): *Revised Token Test,* Pro-Ed, Inc., Austin, TX.
35. Molfese, D.L., and Segalowitz, S.J. (eds.) *The Developmental Implications of Brain Lateralization,* Guilford Press, New York *(in press).*
36. Nass, R., Koch, D.A., Janowsky, J., and Stiles-Davis, J. (1985): Differential effects on intelligence of early left versus right brain injury. *Ann. Neurol.,* 18:393.
37. Oelschlaeger, M.L., and Scarborough, J. (1976): Traumatic aphasia in children: A case study. *J. Commun. Disord.,* 9:281–288.
38. Perlstein, M.A., and Hood, P.N. (1957): Infantile spastic hemiplegia: Intelligence and age of walking and talking. *Am. J. Ment. Defic.,* 61:534–542.
39. Pohl, P. (1979): Dichotic listening in a child recovering from acquired aphasia. *Brain Lang.,* 8:372–379.
40. Rankin, J.M., Aram, D.M., and Horwitz, S.J. (1981): Language ability in right and left hemiplegic children. *Brain Lang.,* 12:292–306.
41. Riva, D., and Cazzaniga, L. (1986): Late effects of unilateral brain lesions before and after the first year of age. *Neuropsychologia,* 24:423–428.
42. Segalowitz, S.J. (ed.) (1983): *Language Functions and Brain Organization.* Academic Press, New York.
43. Vargha-Khadem, F., O'Gorman, A.M., and Watters, G.V. (1985): Aphasia and handedness in relation to hemispheric side, age at injury and severity of cerebral lesion during childhood. *Brain,* 108:677–696.
44. Visch-Brink, E.G., and Van De Sandt-Koenderman, M. (1984): The occurrence of paraphasias in the spontaneous speech of children with an acquired aphasia. *Brain Lang.,* 23:258–271.
45. Wechsler, D. (1967): *Wechsler Preschool and Primary Scale of Intelligence.* Psychological Corporation, New York.
46. Wechsler, D. (1974): *Wechsler Intelligence Scale for Children-Revised.* Psychological Corporation, New York.
47. Woods, B.T. (1980): The restricted effects of right-hemisphere lesions after age one: Wechsler test data. *Neuropsychologia,* 18:65–70.
48. Woods, B.T., and Carey, S. (1979): Language deficits after apparent clinical recovery from childhood aphasia. *Ann. Neurol.,* 6:405–409.
49. Woods, B.T., and Teuber, H.L. (1978): Changing patterns of childhood aphasia. *Ann. Neurol.,* 3:272–280.

Language, Communication, and the Brain, edited by F. Plum.
Raven Press, New York © 1988.

Linguistic Deficits in Aphasia

Sheila E. Blumstein

*Department of Cognitive and Linguistic Sciences, Brown University,
Providence, Rhode Island 02912*

In theory, language comprises a number of structural components or levels of representation, each with its own vocabulary and principles of operation. These components include the sound structure of language (its phonetics and phonology), the vocabulary or words of the language (its lexicon), the sentence structure of the language (its syntax), and the representation of meaning (its semantics). Research on the underlying bases of the language deficits in aphasia has placed a great deal of emphasis on the selectivity of aphasic deficits with respect to these components of the linguistic grammar. In this chapter, we review the nature of linguistic deficits in aphasia focusing on phonetic, syntactic, and lexical-semantic impairments. We consider in detail the view that Broca's aphasics have selective phonetic and syntactic deficits, in contrast to Wernicke's aphasics who have selective lexical-semantic deficits.

PHONETIC DEFICITS IN BROCA'S APHASICS

Linguistic theory makes a clear-cut distinction between phonetics, i.e., the realization of the physical properties of the speech signal in both articulation and perception, and phonology, i.e., the organization and structure of the sound system of a language. The facts of aphasia support such a distinction, particularly in the investigation of speech production deficits. Phonological errors in aphasia reflect patterns consistent with the view that the underlying phonological system of the patient is still governed by structural principles intrinsic to the phonology of language as well as to the particular language affected (3,8,18,23,26,30,35,37).

There is another source of errors that indicates that the articulatory implementation of these phonological patterns may be impaired in some patients. The evidence for selective phonetic deficits in Broca's aphasics comes from acoustic analyses of the speech production of both Broca's and Wernicke's aphasics. For example, the contrast between voiced and voiceless stop consonants in English, [b d g] versus [p t k], turns on, in part, a phonetic dimension called voice-onset time (VOT). VOT is an acoustic parameter that reflects the timing relation between the release of the stop closure and the onset of glottal pulsing or voicing. Figure 1 shows the

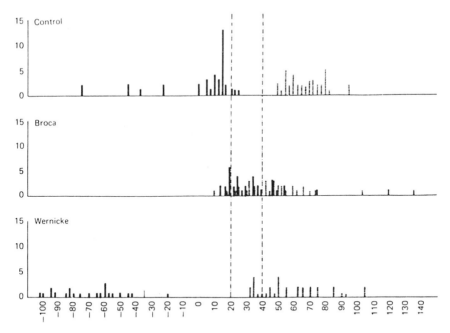

FIG. 1. The distribution of VOT productions for the alveolar stop consonants for a normal control (top panel), a Broca's aphasic (middle panel), and Wernicke's aphasic (bottom panel). The abscissa represents VOT in milliseconds, and the ordinate represents the total number of utterances produced by the subject. Target voiced tokens, [d], are indicated by the *solid lines*, and target voiceless tokens, [t], by the *striped lines*. The *stippled lines* at 20 and 40 ms represent the defined boundary ranges for normal voiced and voiceless productions. From Blumstein et. al. (4).

VOT distribution for a normal subject, a Wernicke's aphasic, and a Broca's aphasic. As the figure shows, for normal subjects producing a set of words beginning with voiced and voiceless alveolar stops such as "dot" versus "tot," voiceless stops have a longer VOT or longer delay in the onset of voicing relative to the release of the stop compared to voiced stops. Voiced stops have a shorter VOT than voiceless stops or they show prevoicing. In the case of prevoiced stops, vocal cord vibration begins prior to the release of the stop. As the top panel shows, there are two distinct categories of voiced and voiceless productions (as a function of VOT). There is no overlap between the two categories, and there are some 10s of ms where no utterances fall. Wernicke's aphasics also maintain the distinction between voiced and voiceless stops. In contrast, the Broca's aphasics show a tremendous inconsistency in their voicing productions with a failure to maintain a systematic distinction between the two categories, and a large number of productions falling in the boundary region between the two categories. These results suggest a clear-cut dichotomy between Broca's and Wernicke's aphasics, with Broca's showing a selective impairment in articulatory implementation and, in particular, in articulatory timing.

These patterns of results emerge not only in English and Japanese for which VOT serves to distinguish voiced and voiceless phonetic categories (5,6,13,22,39) but also in Thai for which VOT serves as a three-category distinction among prevoiced, [b], short-lag VOT, [p], and voiceless aspirated VOT, [p^h], stops (14).

THE NATURE OF AGRAMMATISM

Broca's aphasics also show syntactic impairments. Clinically, many of these patients show productive agrammatism. In productive agrammatism, grammatical markers of the language seem to be selectivity affected, particularly grammatical markers such as inflectional and plural endings, and grammatical words such as articles, e.g., "the," and verb modals, e.g., "have," "be." Investigations of agrammatism in English-speaking subjects suggest that grammatical markers such as inflections and plurals, and grammatical words such as articles, verb modals, and prepositions are lost or are used inconsistently. However, analyses of agrammatic patients in languages other than English indicate that grammatical markers are dropped *only* if the subsequent string constitutes an allowable word in the language (19). Thus, in infixing languages like Hebrew, the patient does not produce the phonologically ungrammatical skeletal root in the absence of grammatical inflections, e.g., */ktb/ "write" for /katab/, "he wrote," nor does s/he produce a phonologically permissible jargon string maintaining the root with a series of vowels infixed in the string. Instead, s/he produces a fully inflected form that may in effect be inappropriate to the context and seems to reflect a reduction in the markedness of the particular inflectional ending, e.g., for past tense producing present tense (25). Similarly, in an inflected language like German, the patient does not produce a phonologically unallowable verb form consisting solely of a verb stem, e.g., /singe/ "he sings"→ */sing/. Rather s/he produces an inflected form that again seems to be generally less marked grammatically. As a result, inflected verbs are often produced as infinitives by these patients, e.g., /singen/.

One of the most interesting findings in the study of agrammatism across languages is the similarity of the agrammatic patterns. In particular, whether a language is agglutinative as in Japanese or inflected as in German or Russian, it is the grammatical markers that seem to be selectively affected (30,36,37). Thus, the grammatical structures of human language seem to be subserved by similar neural substrates despite different surface instantiations of such structure. Interestingly, even aphasic deaf signers display agrammatism with damage to similar neural structures as those implicated in agrammatic hearing subjects (1a).

Productive agrammatism is usually accompanied by a severe restriction on the syntactic structures of sentences. The occurrence of embedded sentences, complementizers, and relative clauses or complex phrases in which several adjectives precede a noun is rare. Further, in severe cases of agrammatism, even the domain of a simple sentence is limited to either a noun phrase (NP) or verb phrase (VP) with the juxtaposition of an NP VP occurring only on occasion (15,16).

Of great importance is that the agrammatic deficits of Broca's aphasics is not restricted to speech production. Broca's aphasics show comprehension impairments as well, and these impairments seem to be grammatical in nature. Zurif, Caramazza, and Myerson (43) investigated the linguistic intuitions of agrammatic patients by asking them to judge how words in a written sentence "go best together." Results from normals as shown in Fig. 2 indicate that they cluster words very much like a linguist, i.e., as a phrase structure tree representing the hierarchical syntactic relations of the words in the sentence. In contrast, as the figure shows, Broca's aphasics do not show normal grammatical intuitions. They cluster content words together, and group articles and function words on a random basis.

Further studies have shown that the comprehension deficit in these patients goes well beyond processing function words and grammatical markers; the processing of syntactic structures is also affected. Such impairments emerge particularly when the semantic interpretation of the sentence is determined by the syntactic structure alone. In contrast to a sentence like "the boy eats a hamburger," in which the lexical items basically dictate the semantic interpretation of the sentence, in a sentence like "the boy kisses the girl," it is necessary to know the syntactic structure in order to unequivocally determine who did what to whom. Broca's aphasics show impairments in comprehension in these latter types of sentences when meaning is determined solely on the basis of the syntactic structure. Particularly vulnerable are embedded subject and object relatives (particularly object relatives), object cleft

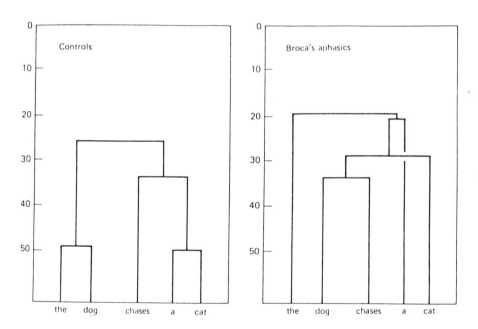

FIG. 2. Hierarchical clustering schema for four normal controls and three Broca's aphasics for the sentence "the dog chases a cat." From Blumstein (4).

sentences, and reversible passives (9,12,42). Even simple reversible active declaritive sentences may be poorly understood, e.g., "the boy chases the girl" (38).

On the basis of such evidence, it has been suggested that Broca's aphasics have a central syntactic disorder, i.e., a disorder affecting the *representation* of the syntactic structures of language (2,11,38). Different claims have been made concerning the structural basis of this syntactic disorder. However, they all implicate an impairment in the use of grammatical formatives as syntactic placeholders to mark phrasal constituents as they enter into grammatical relations. One of the most detailed accounts is that of Grodzinsky (19–21) who suggests that agrammatism turns on a structural impairment in the assignment of thematic roles because of the failure to co-index empty categories or traces with their antecedents. In contrast, Caplan and colleagues (9,10) argue that syntactic structures are "simplified" for agrammatic patients, and these structures are analyzed for meaning in terms of a linear rather than hierarchical grouping of major lexical categories.

LEXICAL-SEMANTIC DEFICITS IN APHASIA

Studies with Wernicke's aphasics have emphasized their lexical-semantic impairment. Clinically, the speech output of Wernicke's aphasics seems syntactically full, but semantically empty. They have naming impairments and often produce semantic paraphasias. The auditory comprehension of these patients is also very poor, and they often fail to correctly point to an auditorily presented word. More systematic studies support the view that these impairments reflect a deficit at the level of lexical representation, and in particular, a deficit in the structural representation of words in the lexicon. For example, Zurif, Caramazza, Myerson, and Galvin (44) explored Wernicke's aphasics subjective judgments about how words go together. Subjects were asked to group the two words of a set of three that went best together. The words used (mother, wife, cook, partner, knight, husband, shark, trout, dog, tiger, turtle, crocodile) varied along several semantic dimensions. Results showed that normals grouped the words along these dimensions, e.g., human, nonhuman, and gender. Wernicke's aphasics produced random clusters, i.e., they were as likely to group "husband" with "turtle" as with "wife." The authors concluded that at least part of the word-finding problem in Wernicke's aphasics is rooted in the disruption of stored semantic representations.

The results reviewed in this chapter thus far are in themselves very exciting for they suggest an instantiation of linguistic levels of representation or components of the grammar in the neurology of language. They also imply a direct relation between particular neural structures and language functions. Nevertheless, although this evidence suggests selectivity with respect to particular components of the grammar, the nature of language deficits in aphasia is in reality a good deal more complicated. First, it is the case that clinically and in experimental investigations nearly all aphasics display impairments at all linguistic levels (27). Broca's aphasics show phonological, lexical, and semantic impairments as well as phonetic and syntactic deficits, and Wernicke's aphasics show phonological and syntactic impairments as well as lexical and semantic deficits (4). What is not clear is whether such deficits necessarily reflect impairments to the same underlying mechanisms in all of these aphasic patients. Moreover, as we will review, there are a series of more recent studies that show interesting dichotomies for Wernicke's aphasics in lexical-semantic tasks, and Broca's aphasics in syntactic tasks. These dichotomies challenge the view that these patients have deficits in the structural components of the grammar per se. Instead, they suggest the need to make a distinction between deficits related to the integrity of stored lexical or grammatical representations, i.e., the linguistic knowledge base itself, and deficits related to the processes needed to access or search through these stored representations for normal language use.

STRUCTURAL VERSUS PROCESSING DEFICITS
IN LEXICAL ACCESS

Let us consider evidence concerning lexical-semantic deficits in Wernicke's aphasics. Using an adaptation of a procedure developed by Meyer and Schvaneveldt (31), aphasic patients were asked to make lexical decisions about words and nonwords (7,32). In each case, the target word to be judged (dog) was preceded by a prime that was semantically related (cat-dog), unrelated (table-dog), or neutral (glub-dog) with respect to the prime. Normal subjects showed semantic facilitation in such a lexical decision task; that is, they showed a faster lexical decision reaction-time to a word that is preceded by a semantically related prime word compared with a semantically unrelated or neutral prime.

If Wernicke's aphasics have an impairment in the representation of words in the lexicon, we would expect to find no semantic facilitation or a reduction in semantic facilitation in a lexical decision task compared with normals. However, these results were not obtained (Fig. 3). Although slower in making lexical decisions than either normals or Broca's aphasics, Wernicke's aphasics showed semantic facilitation in a lexical decision task. These results were obtained whether the stimulus pairs were presented visually (32) or auditorily (7).

Interestingly, these semantic facilitation effects were observed even in those patients who are unable to perform reliably a metalinguistic task requiring them to judge whether two words are related. For example, patients were given the same real word pairs as in the lexical decision task and asked whether "cat-dog" are related. Wernicke's aphasics performed very poorly and even randomly on such tasks; Broca's aphasics did very well. Thus despite severe auditory comprehension deficits and an inability to judge overtly the semantic values of words, Wernicke's aphasics displayed sensitivity to semantically associated words.

Before considering the implications of such results, let us consider one other experiment. It is possible that the semantic facilitation effects were obtained in the previous experiment because the stimuli were closely related associates, i.e., the

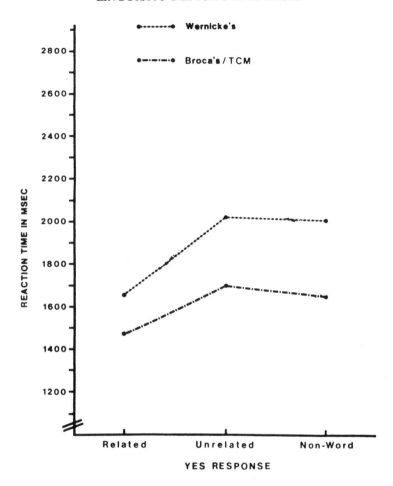

FIG. 3. Mean reaction-time latencies of correct responses for seven nonfluent patients (three Broca's and four transcortical motor) and seven Wernicke's aphasics for yes responses as a function of condition, related, unrelated, and nonword.

particular stimulus pairs may have been overlearned, and thus, might not reflect the underlying organization of the lexicon itself. In other words, less highly related word pairs may not show such normal performance in Wernicke's aphasics. To explore this question, the semantic relations of ambiguous words were examined (34). Word triplets were presented auditorily. The middle word was ambiguous, and the semantic relations of the first and third words varied systematically. In one condition, the meaning of the first and third word was *concordant*—coin-bank-money. In a second, they were *discordant*; the first word was related to one meaning of the ambiguous word and the third word was related to another meaning—river-bank-money. In the third, *neutral*, condition, only the third word was related to the ambiguous word—nose-bank-money, and in the fourth, *unrelated*, condition, none of the words was related—nose-watch-money. Figure 4 shows the results for normal subjects. Reaction times varied as a function of the semantic relations to the ambiguous words. Subjects were faster, i.e., showed semantic facilitation, in the concordant and neutral conditions relative to the unrelated condition. In contrast, they showed no semantic facilitation in the discordant condition.

Figure 5 shows the results for the Broca's and Wernicke's aphasics. Note that the results for Wernicke's aphasics are similar to normals. In contrast, and surprisingly, the Broca's aphasics did *not* show sensitivity to the semantic relations of the ambiguous words.

The pattern of results are fairly clear-cut for Wernicke's aphasics, and the following conclusions can be drawn. The fact that semantic facilitation occurs in the auditory as well as the visual modality is evidence that the performance of the Wernicke's patients reflects the characteristics of the lexical access system independent of the modality of word presentation. Perhaps more important, this system of organization seems to be relatively spared, and semantic information appears to be available to the aphasic patient as long as no overt semantic manipulation or

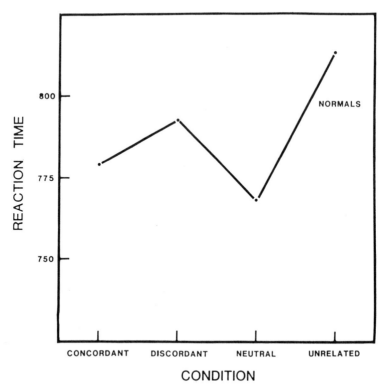

FIG. 4. Mean reaction-time latencies as a function of priming condition for 20 normal subjects. From Milberg et al. (34).

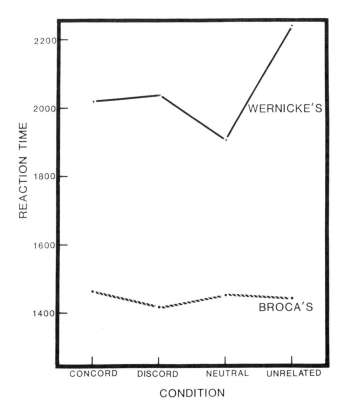

FIG. 5. Mean reaction-time latencies as a function of priming condition for seven Broca's and six Wernicke's aphasic subjects. From Milberg et al. (34).

judgment is required. Thus, semantic organization, at least at the level of semantic relatedness, seems to be relatively spared in Wernicke's aphasia. Although these findings do not unequivocally demonstrate normal semantic structure in Wernicke's aphasics, they decrease the likelihood that auditory comprehension deficits are due to semantic organization per se and increase the likelihood that the deficits lie in one of the many processes involved in access to that information.

What might be the nature of this processing impairment? Recent claims have emerged in the study of lexical processing in normals that there are two distinct types of processing contributing to lexical access. Both processes are based, in part, on the assumption that semantic memory or the mental lexicon is represented as a network of lexical entries organized in terms of shared semantic features or attributes. In this view, accessing a lexical item with a particular meaning automatically reduces the threshold for all of those words sharing semantic properties with the lexical item. The more closely related the words, the more likely they will be "excited" and the lower their threshold of activity will be. Although this process occurs in real time, it is assumed to be very rapid, of short duration, and to be virtually unlimited in capacity. Further, the initiation and termination of this process are assumed not to be under the voluntary control of the subject. On the basis of these characteristics, this process has been called *automatic* (24,40).

The second process involved in lexical access is less consistently labeled in the literature, but it is defined by the fact that it is under the subject's voluntary control (either consciously or unconsciously), is slow, is of relatively long duration, and is limited in capacity (40). The second process is called *strategic* or *controlled* processing. Controlled processing is also involved in lexical access, but it is influenced by the subject's expectancies and attentional demands.

The results of the lexical decision experiments with aphasics may be characterized in terms of these two processes. Wernicke's aphasics showed consistent evidence of semantic facilitation in the lexical decision tasks, but did not appear to be able to analyze word meaning in a simple semantic judgment task. Therefore, they seemed to be able to access the lexicon using processing routines that are "automatic" in the sense that they are rapid, of short duration, and not under voluntary control. In contrast, these patients were unable to use this knowledge of the rules about semantic features or semantic relations to consciously make a semantic judgment about how words go together.

For Broca's aphasics, the results are less clear-cut. The lack of consistent priming effects suggests that they may have impairments in processing routines for accessing the lexicon in an automatic, on-line manner. Nevertheless, they may still be able to access the lexicon through strategic, direct search processes, and thus can make judgments about the semantic relations among words.

STRUCTURAL VERSUS PROCESSING DEFICITS FOR SYNTAX

The different processing impairments suggested here may help to account for recent dissociations in performance found for Broca's aphasics in syntactic tasks. It will be recalled that earlier research suggested that Broca's aphasics displayed a selective syntactic deficit affecting both the comprehension and production of language. Nevertheless, a recent study by Linebarger, Schwartz, and Saffran (28) showed that patients who were agrammatic in language comprehension and production were nonetheless able to make correct grammatical judgments often of sentences that were only subtly ungrammatical. For example, they recognized correctly that the following sentences were ungrammatical: "he shut the window that the door was open," "the girls laughed the clown," "my father knew they would give the job to." These results challenge the view that Broca's aphasics have impaired syntactic representations. If the representations themselves were impaired, then the patients should be unable to recognize the ungrammaticality of the above sentences.

Linebarger et. al. (28) suggested that the underlying syntactic representations of agrammatic aphasics are spared. Instead, they have a processing impairment affecting the "mapping" of syntactic structures onto their appropriate semantic interpretations. Recent results from several lexical decision experiments are consistent with this view. Instead of focusing on semantic/associate relations between words as reviewed above, these studies focused on the syntactic-grammatical relations among words.

One current study focuses on the relation between the auxiliary and verb (33). Twenty real word targets consisting of a verb form marked for tense and aspect were preceded by four different priming conditions. Normals showed faster reaction-times to the word "going" in a lexical decision task (Fig. 6), if it was preceded by the correct aux—"is going" than if preceded by an incorrect aux (poor)— "could-going," an incorrect part of speech (wrong) "very-going," or a nonword "plib-going" [see (17,29,41) for similar results with normals]. Of the patients tested thus far, Broca's aphasics did not show such sensitivities to grammatical relations (Fig. 7). Only three Wernicke's aphasics have been tested thus far, and the graph represents the results for only one patient. The results for this patient as well as the other two tested showed similar patterns to normals. As to the patients' ability to make syntactic judgments, i.e., to determine whether the word pairs such as "is-going" can go together, normals made 5% errors, Broca's made 23% errors, and Wernicke's aphasics made 47% errors. Thus, again, we see a dissociation between the performance of Broca's and Wernicke's aphasics. Broca's aphasics did

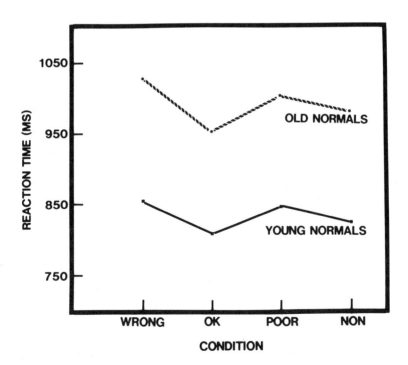

FIG. 6. Mean reaction-time latencies of old and young normal subjects as a function of syntactic priming condition.

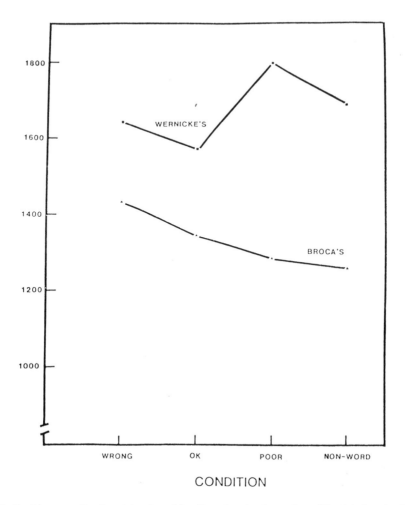

FIG. 7. Mean reaction-time latencies of five Broca's aphasics and one Wernicke's aphasic as a function of syntactic priming condition.

not show syntactic facilitation in a lexical decision task, although they could make syntactic judgments. In contrast, Wernicke's aphasics did show such facilitation, and yet were unable to judge reliably syntactic relations.

In a recent study, Baum (1) compared directly agrammatic patients' performance on grammaticality judgment tasks with a lexical decision task using the same stimuli. In one condition, subjects were required to make a grammatical judgment on a sentence, and in another condition, they were required to make a lexical decision on the last word of that sentence, e.g., "at 6 o'clock, he came to *dinner*" versus "at 6 o'clock he came *dinner*." Overall, results were consistent with those reported earlier. In particular, unlike normal controls, agrammatic patients did not show faster reaction-times in a lexical decision task when the sentence was grammatical compared with when it was ungrammatical. Nevertheless, the same patients generally were able to make grammatical judgments, although not as well as those reported by Linebarger et. al. (28).

The implications of these results are that both Broca's and Wernicke's aphasics show lexical and syntactic deficits. However, their deficits are of a different kind. The nature of the processing limitations affects the language behavior and language abilities of Broca's and Wernicke's aphasics in qualitatively different ways. Although the character of the disorder for Broca's aphasics seems primarily syntactic and the Wernicke's primarily semantic, it is suggested that the underlying basis of their deficits is a processing one—simultaneously cutting across different components of the grammar. For both groups, the components of the grammar themselves seem to be relatively spared, whereas access to them is impaired in different ways. Broca's aphasics show impairments in accessing rule-bound relations or linguistic associations in a rapid, on-line fashion. Nevertheless, the data structures are available through direct search and thus can be used for metalinguistic judgments. In contrast, Wernicke's aphasics show relatively spared lexical and syntactic representations, and they can access rule-bound relations of both a semantic and syntactic nature. However, they fail to be able to "use" such knowledge via direct strategic search, and thus to make appropriate linguistic judgments. Consequently, the nature of the processing deficits in Broca's and Wernicke's aphasics cuts across what have been generally considered to be dissociable linguistic levels—in this case, lexical-semantic and morphological-grammatical.

CONCLUSION

Studies of linguistic deficits in aphasia suggest that language is organized into subsystems similar to components of the grammar proposed in linguistic theory, and although these subsystems have their own vocabulary, structure, and operating characteristics, they probably do not have a direct instantiation in localized areas of the brain. More recent research has challenged the view that the structure of the linguistic components themselves is affected in aphasia, but rather suggests that the processing operations affecting access to and communication between these components are impaired.

ACKNOWLEDGMENTS

This research was supported in part by NIH grant NS 15123.

REFERENCES

1. Baum, S. (1986): Syntactic processing in aphasia. Unpublished doctoral dissertation, Brown University.
1a. Bellugi, U., Poizner, H., and Klima, E. S. (1987): *What the Hands Reveal about the Brain.* Bradford Books, Cambridge, MA. (*in press*).

2. Berndt, R.S., and Caramazza, A. (1981): Syntactic aspects of aphasia. In: *Acquired Aphasia*, edited by M.T. Sarno, pp. 129–156. Academic Press, New York.
3. Blumstein S.E. (1973): *A Phonological Investigation of Aphasic Speech*. Mouton, The Hague.
4. Blumstein, S.E. (1981): Neurolinguistic disorders: Language-brain relationships. In: *Handbook of Clinical Neuropsychology*, edited by S.B. Filskov and T.J. Boll, pp. 227–256. Wiley, New York.
5. Blumstein, S.E., Cooper, W.E., Goodglass, H., Statlender, S., and Gottlieb, J. (1980): Production deficits in aphasia: A voice-onset time analysis. *Brain Lang.*, 9:153–170.
6. Blumstein, S.E., Cooper, W.E., Zurif, E., and Caramazza, A. (1977): The perception and production of voice-onset time in aphasia. *Neuropsychologia*, 15:371–383.
7. Blumstein, S., Milberg, W., and Shrier, R. (1982): Semantic processing in aphasia: Evidence from an auditory lexical decision task. *Brain Lang.*, 17:301–315.
8. Bouman, L., and Grunbaum, A. (1925): Experimentell-psychologische Untersuchungen sur Aphasie und Paraphasie. *Zeitschrift fur die gesamte Neurologie und Psychiatrie*, 96:481–538.
9. Caplan, D., Baker, C., and Dehaut, F. (1985): Syntactic determinants of sentence comprehension in aphasia. *Cognition*, 21:117–175.
10. Caplan, D., and Futter, C. (1986): Assignment of thematic roles to nouns in sentence comprehension by an agrammatic patient. *Brain Lang.*, 27:117–134.
11. Caramazza, A., Berndt, R.S., Basili, A., and Koller, J. (1981): Syntactic processing deficits in aphasia. *Cortex*, 17:333–348.
12. Caramazza, A., and Zurif, E.B. (1976): Dissociation of algorithmic and heuristic processes in language comprehension: Evidence from aphasia. *Brain Lang.*, 3:572–582.
13. Freeman, F.J., Sands, E.S., and Harris, K.S. (1978): Temporal coordination of phonation and articulation in a case of verbal apraxia: A voice-onset time study. *Brain Lang.*, 6:106–111.
14. Gandour, J., and Dardarananda, R. (1984): Voice onset time in aphasia: Thai II. Production. *Brain Lang.*, 23:177–205.
15. Gleason, J.B., Goodglass, H., Green, E., Ackerman, N., and Hyde, M. (1975): The retrieval of syntax in Broca's aphasia. *Brain Lang.*, 2:451–471.
16. Goodglass, H., Gleason, J., Bernholtz, N.A., and Hyde, M.R. (1972): Some linguistic structures in the speech of a Broca's aphasic. *Cortex*, 8:191–212.
17. Goodman, G.O., McClelland, J.L., and Gibbs, R.W. (1981): The role of syntactic context in word recognition. *Memory and Cognition*, 9:580–586.
18. Green, E. (1969): Phonological and grammatical aspects of jargon in an aphasic patient: A case study. *Lang. Speech*, 12:103–118.
19. Grodzinsky, Y. (1984): The syntactic characterization of agrammatism. *Cognition*, 16:99–120.
20. Grodzinsky, Y. (1986): Language deficits and the theory of syntax. *Brain Lang.*, 27:135–159.
21. Grodzinsky, Y., Swinney, D., and Zurif, E. (1985): Agrammatism: Structural deficits and antecedent processing disruptions. In: *Agrammatism*, edited by M.L. Kean, pp. 65–82. Academic Press, New York.
22. Itoh, M., Sasanuma, S., Tatsumi, I.F., Murakami, S., Fukusako, Y., and Suzuki, T. (1982): Voice onset time characteristics in apraxia of speech. *Brain Lang.*, 17:193–210.
23. Jakobson, R. (1968): *Child Language, Aphasia, and Phonological Universals*. Translated by A.R. Keiler. Mouton, The Hague.
24. LaBerge, D., and Samuels, S.J. (1974): Towards a theory of automatic information processing in reading. *Cognitive Psychology*, 6:293–323.
25. LaPointe, S. (1985): A theory of verb form use in the speech of agrammatic aphasics. *Brain Lang.*, 24:100–155.
26. Lecours, A.R., and Lhermitte, F. (1969): Phonemic paraphasias: Linguistic structures and tentative hypotheses. *Cortex*, 5:193–228.
27. Lesser, R. (1978): *Linguistic Investigations of Aphasia*. Arnold, London.
28. Linebarger, M., Schwartz, M., and Saffran, E. (1983): Sensitivity to grammatical structure in so-called agrammatic aphasics. *Cognition*, 13:361–392.
29. Lukatela, G., Kostic, A., Feldman, L.B., and Turvey, M.T. (1983): Grammatical priming of inflected nouns. *Memory and Cognition*, 11:59–63.
30. Luria, A.R. (1966): *Higher Cortical Functions in Man*. Basic Books, New York.
31. Meyer, D.E. and Schvaneveldt, R.W. (1971): Facilitation in recognizing pairs of words: Evidence of a dependence between retrieval operations. *J. Exp. Psychol.*, 90:227–234.
32. Milberg, W., and Blumstein, S.E. (1981): Lexical decision and aphasia: Evidence for semantic processing. *Brain Lang.*, 14:371–385.

33. Milberg, W. Blumstein, S.E., and Dworetzky, B. (1985): Sensitivity to morphological constraints in Broca's and Wernicke's aphasics: A double dissociation of syntactic judgements and syntactic facilitation in a lexical decision task. Paper presented at the Academy of Aphasia, Pittsburgh.
34. Milberg, W., Blumstein, S.E., and Dworetzky, B. (1986): Processing of lexical ambiguities in aphasia. *Brain Lang.*, 31:138–150.
35. Niemi, J., Koivuselka-Sallinen, P., and Hanninen, R. (1985): Phoneme errors in Broca's aphasia: Three Finnish cases. *Brain Lang.*, 26:28–48.
36. Panse, F., and Shimoyama, T. (1973): On the effects of aphasic disturbance in Japanese: Agrammatism and paragrammatism. In: *Psycholinguistics and Aphasia*, edited by H. Goodglass and S. Blumstein, pp. 171–182. Johns Hopkins University Press, Baltimore.
37. Peuser, G., and Fittschen, M. (1977): On the universality of language dissolution: The case of a Turkish aphasic. *Brain Lang.*, 4:196–207.
38. Schwartz, M.F., Saffran, E.M., and Marin, O.S.M. (1980): The word order problem in agrammatism. I. Comprehension. *Brain Lang.*, 10:249–263.
39. Shewan, C.M., Leeper, H.A., and Booth, J.C. (1984): An analysis of voice onset time (VOT) in aphasic and normal subjects. In: *Apraxia of Speech: Physiology, Acoustics, Linguistics, Management*, edited by J. Rosenbek, M. McNeil, and A. Aronson, pp. 197–220. College-Hill Press, San Diego.
40. Shiffrin, R.M., and Schneider, W. (1977): Controlled and automatic human information processing. II. Perceptual learning, automatic attending and a general theory. *Psychol. Rev.*, 84:127–190.
41. Wright, B., and Garrett, M. (1984): Lexical decision in sentences: Effects of syntactic structure. *Memory and Cognition*, 12:31–45.
42. Zurif, E.B., and Caramazza, A. (1976): Psycholinguistic structures in aphasia: Studies in syntax and semantics. In: *Studies in Neurolinguistics*, edited by H. Whitaker and H. Whitaker, pp. 261–292. Academic Press, New York.
43. Zurif, E., Caramazza, A., and Myerson, R. (1972): Grammatical judgements of agrammatic aphasics. *Neuropsychologia*, 10:405–417.
44. Zurif, E., Caramazza, A., Myerson, R., and Galvin, J. (1974): Semantic feature representations for normal and aphasic language. *Brain Lang.*, 1:167–187.

*Language, Communication, and
the Brain*, edited by F. Plum.
Raven Press, New York © 1988.

Cortical-Subcortical Differences in Aphasia

*Michael P. Alexander and †Margaret A. Naeser

*Aphasia Program, Braintree Rehabilitation Hospital,
Braintree, Massachusetts 02184, and
†CT Laboratory of the Aphasia Research Center, Psychology Service,
Boston Veterans Administration Medical Center, Boston, Massachusetts 02130 and
Department of Neurology, Boston University School of Medicine,
Boston, Massachusetts 02215*

In this chapter we relate the clinical phenomenology of adult aphasia to the pathologic anatomy as determined by computerized tomography (CT) scan. We place particular, but not sole, emphasis, on the role of damage to subcortical structures in the generation of clinical signs.

In the history of aphasia research, the investigation of subcortical structures has had a fitful place. There have been two traditional motivations for the study of subcortical (SC) damage and aphasia that we feel are not germane. First, it is not a method by which the classical cortical aphasic syndromes can be invalidated. The classical syndromes are clusters of neurological signs that, when occurring together, carry a high correlation with damage to specific cortical regions. The collection of individual signs needs not have any more basic biologic coherence than do facial paresis and contralateral hemiparesis (Millard-Gubler syndrome). They represent evidence of damage to individually coherent, perhaps even overlapping, neural systems that are seen together because of anatomic propinquity. Lesions occurring in different regions (e.g., purely subcortical) could not necessarily be expected to proffer any direct evidence for or against the diagnostic accuracy or anatomical coherence of the syndromes of cortical lesions. This does not mean that the two lesion types must be irrelevant to each other.

Second, the study of SC lesions is not simply a search for the "smallest" lesions that cause some sign or syndrome. There is no absolute *a priori* reason to anticipate that SC lesions will be smaller (convergence of critical pathways?) or larger (divergence of critical pathways?) than cortical lesions. There are, it is true, parallels from sensory-motor systems that suggest that convergence of pathways will play a role in subcortical lesion effects; small lesions may, then, be common.

We believe that the study of SC lesions is a valuable approach to aphasia for other reasons. First, many clinical phenomena (of whatever syndromes they may be part) have been classically attributed to cortical lesions but are seen after purely subcortical lesions as well. When these subcortical lesions lie within the known or suspected afferent or efferent pathways of the "classical" cortical area, the SC lesion may be producing a dysconnection of the cortical area. Norman Geschwind often taught that dysconnection phenomena would be very common if we knew how to look for them. SC lesions may provide an arena in which to investigate that assertion. Second, the constellations of signs that define classical cortical syndromes often disassociate in cases of purely subcortical lesions; not that evidence was really needed, but the ready dissociation of key elements of syndromes may serve as additional proof that the classical syndromes did not describe the biologic units of language breakdown. Third, cortical lesions often disrupt multiple functional systems; the separate pathophysiologies of the various individual systems can be identified only with great difficulty. SC lesions may disrupt functional systems along different anatomic or physiologic dimensions, permitting another window to open on the anatomy and physiology of the individual signs in aphasia.

During recent years there has been a growing interest in defining the anatomy of cognitive functions as neural networks. A network is a number of discrete cortical and subcortical areas and their interconnections that operate together to perform some cognitive or behavioral function. Mesulam (18) provided the most coherent example of such a network with his analysis of the complex function of attention. A network may be interrupted in many areas, but the involved cognitive domain will be impaired wherever the structural lesion is located. What might differ with different lesion locations would be the severity and the clinical profile that accompanies the damage. Analysis of subcortical lesions points to the existence of neural networks and their interconnections for the complex functions of language.

For this review we emphasize the anterior aphasias and their anatomy because the greatest amount of research has focused there. (The alexias are another domain in which similar investigations have been performed and in which a neural network can be defined.) We define the effects of small lesions in various subcortical territories and then the effects of larger combinations of lesions. We try to relate the clinical phenomena and the responsible anatomy to the classical syndromes when appropriate.

CASE MATERIAL

We restrict our analysis of subcortical-aphasia relationships to cases of stroke and intracerebral hemorrhage. As much as possible we restrict our investigations and assertions to an interval 2 to 12 weeks after injury. There are several justifications for this approach. Interpretation of clinical-anatomic relationships in other etiologies is more difficult. Many mass lesions have deep and remote pressure effects or are infiltrative and not actually destructive. Some disorders are inherently bilateral. Slowly progressive disorders (mass lesions or degenerative diseases) may allow compensatory avenues of function to develop over the course of the illness. The more robust brain-behavior relationships eventually emerge in most diseases (a left occipital tumor is still more likely to result in alexia than a nonfluent aphasia), but these disorders are less appropriate for establishing the primary functional relationships. It is likely that at least the degenerative disorders have their own rules for the study of brain-behavior relationships that are just as interesting as acute focal lesions (14), simply more difficult to define.

Intracerebral hemorrhages have some limitations for study. In the acute phase, mass effects may be dramatic and remote functional disturbances will be present. Deep hemorrhages may compromise attention or alertness. Hemorrhages often dissect through the planes of brain tissue, producing an initial area of visible blood much larger than the actual destroyed brain. We believe that hemorrhages are properly studied once alertness is regained and when CT demonstrates disappearance of mass effect and perhaps even of blood; otherwise the anatomical correlations are feeble. Because hemorrhages are *unilateral* and *sudden* lesions, and because they open to analysis territories not routinely isolated by ischemic stroke, we believe that it is both appropriate and important to include cases of hemorrhage with the caveats above.

Several excellent longitudinal studies have shown that aphasias spontaneously change over time (15–17, 25). It is likely that the proper study of aphasia requires inclusion of time as a dependent variable. We should probably define aphasias as lesion "x" as associated with aphasia profile "y," which changes along dimensions "a" and "b" over time course "t." The dimensions and time courses may be affected by many patient variables unrelated to lesion anatomy (age, sex, handedness, premorbid language capacity, medications with CNS effects, and the like). To avoid this research conundrum we try to restrict analyses to the postacute epoch. We also try to describe aphasia profiles with a time element, but we also believe that many robust relationships hold true or are modified but recognizable over time.

Clinical Correlations of Subcortical Lesions

Striatal lesions (summarized in Fig. 1). Lesions restricted to the striatum do not produce language abnormality. It is not clear that small single lesions even produce speech disturbance. Large lesions may produce dysarthria and hypophonia. The large clinical-anatomic literature on lacunar infarctions supports that assertion. We have seen cases in which striatal damage was extensive, and no aphasia or dysarthria occurred. Further, in Huntington's disease in which bilateral severe striatal atrophy occurs, aphasia is never prominent. With this bilateral process, dysarthria and voicing abnormalities are common.

Capsular lesions (Fig. 1). Lesions restricted to the internal capsule do not produce aphasia, but single, discrete lesions in the posterior portion of the anterior limb of the internal capsule (ALIC) or its junction with the genu (GIC) may produce speech disturbances. When the lesion is on the left, dysarthria (articulatory impairment) occurs. This, too, is supported by the literature on lacunar lesions as well as by our own studies (10,24). A very similar dysarthria can sometimes be seen after lesions restricted to the lower motor cortex, which is the cortical origin of fibers projecting through the posterior ALIC/GIC junction (24). When the lesion is on

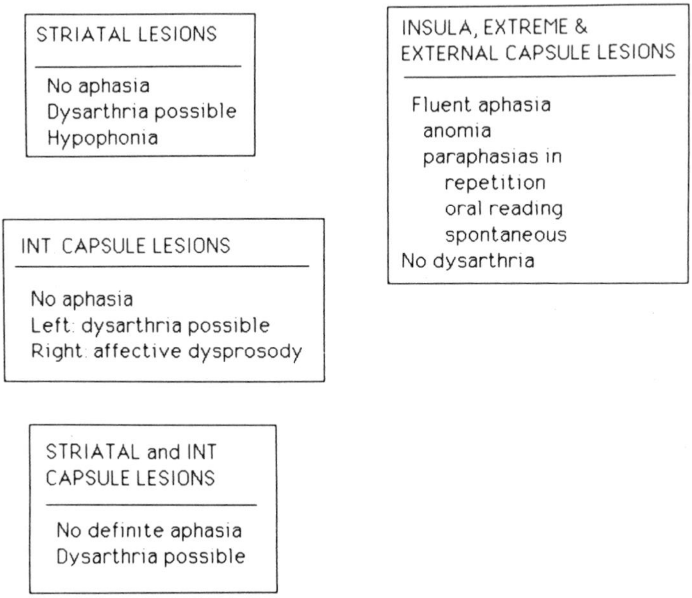

STRIATAL LESIONS
──────────────
No aphasia
Dysarthria possible
Hypophonia

INT. CAPSULE LESIONS
──────────────
No aphasia
Left dysarthria possible
Right affective dysprosody

STRIATAL and INT
CAPSULE LESIONS
──────────────
No definite aphasia
Dysarthria possible

INSULA, EXTREME &
EXTERNAL CAPSULE LESIONS
──────────────
Fluent aphasia
  anomia
  paraphasias in
    repetition
    oral reading
    spontaneous
No dysarthria

FIG. 1.   Summary of the speech and language deficits associated with lesions of the striatum and/or internal or external capsules.

the right, affective dysprosody is produced (23). This abnormality in the melodic, emotional contours of speech also occurs after right frontal cortical lesions. The right and left frontal regions must contribute parallel but differing qualities to speech production, each of which maps onto bulbar motor nuclei by relatively direct convergence of pathways through the ipsilateral ALIC/GIC.

When lesions extend laterally from the putamen, the external capsule, claustrum, extreme capsule, and insular cortex are involved. Damage to posterior insular cortex and to the external/extreme capsule region has been associated with aphasia; the profile is a mild, fluent aphasia (7). There may be phonemic paraphasia, particularly with repetition or oral reading. A similar profile (classically called conduction aphasia) has been described with more extensive lateral suprasylvian lesions (4). It is unclear whether the small posterior insular, extreme capsule lesion damages a portion of the same structures as the larger parietal lesion does or whether damage to the posterior insular cortex alone is sufficient for this syndrome. Both have been suggested on clinical evidence (7,12).

Cases in which lesion extends out of the capsular-striatal limits provide the greatest clinical and theoretical interest. We review evidence from our cases as well as pertinent literature to construct the brain-behavior correlations of these lesions.

Anterolateral white matter damage (Fig. 2). Lesions in this area produce a reduction in spontaneous speech; brief mutism may be present at the outset (11). There are no abnormalities in language content or structure; there is simply reduced

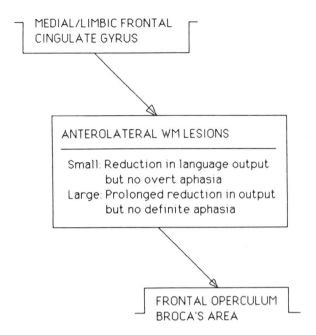

FIG. 2. Summary of the speech and language deficits after damage to the anterolateral paraventricular white matter. The schematic representation indicates that the likely pathophysiology of this lesion is disruption of limbic input to the frontal operculum.

language output. Narratives are sparse; answers are unelaborated and terse; recitation of history may be limited to tabulations. But normal, sentence-length, grammatically rich language is always possible and erratically produced. Recovery is the rule. Even when combined with damage to the caudate or anterior portion of ALIC, this profile is maintained (2). This is the profile of very mild transcortical motor aphasia. It is reminiscent of the syndrome of supplementary motor area injury, although milder. More extensive medial frontal damage produces the same syndrome but to a much more severe extent—much longer mutism and more marked reduction in total language output once speech returns. A similar picture has also been described after middle frontal gyrus lesions (which often extend down into the deep white matter adjacent to the frontal horn of the lateral ventricle) and even after damage to the frontal operculum (11). In these more lateral lesion cases, language abnormalities such as errors in grammatical usage, anomia, and phonemic paraphasias are more prominent. The anterolateral white matter lesion is situated to disrupt connections from medial frontal lobe, including supplementary motor area and cingulate to and from the lateral frontal lobe including Broca's area. We previously (11) hypothesized that damage to these pathways disrupts the limbic activation of speech and language, thus the reduction in the ''drive'' to speak. The degree of overt aphasia depends on the extent of lesion in the lateral elements of the frontal lobe.

Superior white matter damage (Fig. 3). Lesions extending upward into the paraventricular corona radiata directly above the internal capsule and the body of the caudate nucleus have not reliably been associated with any aphasia. Even when coupled with extensive striatal injury, only a reduction in spontaneous language has been observed. Lesion just anterior to the waist of the body of the lateral ventricle has often been associated with dysarthria, presumably damaging the corticobulbar fibers descending to ALIC/GIC from the lower motor cortex. This association has not been invariable in our experience; we do not know why these motor systems are apparently more redundant in some patients. Damage in the most superior paraventricular white matter (PVWM) is almost always associated with right hemiparesis and left limb apraxia (2). Sparing of the immediately paraventricular area just posterior to the waist of the lateral ventricle can allow complete sparing of motor function even with severe aphasia. When there is no right hemiparesis, bilateral limb apraxia is common. The superior PVWM may be an important area of convergence of interhemispheric (callosal sensory-motor) and

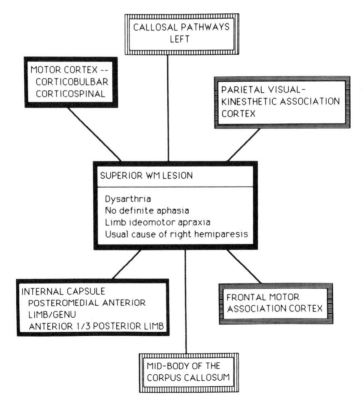

FIG. 3. Summary of the deficits after damage to the superior paraventricular white matter. The schematic represents the three different functional systems that are potentially disrupted by this lesion: motor outflow, motor callosal, and intrahemispheric sensorimotor.

intrahemispheric (parieto-frontal) pathways involved in control of learned motor activities (15).

Anterior white matter extension. Lesions restricted to the white matter anterior to striatum and internal capsule are rare, but are not necessarily associated with any speech or language abnormalities. If the lesion extends broadly and anteriorly deep to operculum, the transcortical motor aphasia syndrome occurs on the same basis as that described above.

Combinations of anterolateral, superior, and anterior extensions. Much more significant disturbances in language occur with lesion combinations. With extensive lesion running through all three white matter zones, deficits in language output are prominent (2). Many cases have dysarthric, slow, effortful, and simplified but usually sentence-length and grammatically correct utterances with anomia and paraphasias. Some cases with lesions in these regions, particularly those cases with anterior lesion extension along the edge of the frontal horn of the lateral ventricle across the corpus callosum into the deep frontal lobe (21), have frankly nonfluent aphasia—short or one-word utterances with impaired grammatical usages. We believe that marked limitations in spoken language output occur when all three white matter areas are damaged. Severely limited language output—short, completely nonpropositional, automatic utterances or stereotypies only—seem to be most clearly associated with damage to the PVWM immediately anterior and adjacent to the head of the caudate nucleus, although only in combination with the more extensive PVWM matter lesions deep to the motor-sensory cortices. These are, of course, important areas of white matter involvement in cases of classic Broca's aphasia (20).

Posterior, superior white matter extension (Fig. 4). Lesions rarely extend from the capsular-putaminal area to the white matter adjacent to the atrium of the lateral ventricle, but lesions deep in the inferior parietal lobule often abut this part of the PVWM. The only deficit specific to spoken language from lesion in the posterio-superior PVWM is one with no known clinical significance. Injury to fibers crossing in the posterior body of the corpus callosum will damage connections between auditory association areas. This disconnection will produce suppression of auditory signals to the left ear during dichotic stimulation, i.e., a loss of auditory information from the right hemisphere to the left auditory association cortex (6). Although of no certain significance when occurring alone, if left hemisphere intrahemispheric auditory pathways are damaged, the callosum can be the sole source of auditory language connections (see below).

Temporal isthmus. Lesions that extend posteriorly from the putamen, external capsule, or internal capsule may travel across the confluent white matter tracts entering and leaving the temporal lobe inferiorally and medially; this area is the temporal isthmus (TI) (Fig. 5). Lesions in this region are associated with impaired language comprehension. This, too, is an area not typically involved in capsular-putaminal infarcts; the vascular anatomy of this region is complex, lying at the boundaries of the lenticulostriate, middle cerebral, and anterior choroidal circulations (13). Occasional capsular-putaminal infarcts extend posteriorly into the temporal isthmus. Putaminal hemorrhages, on the other hand, frequently dissect posteriorly

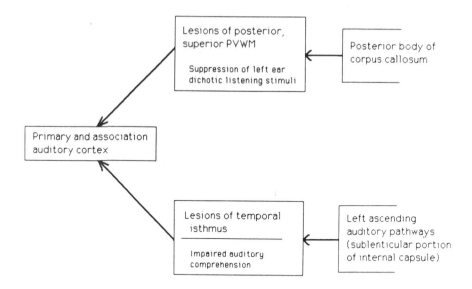

FIG. 4. Summary of the language effects of lesions in the posterior paraventricular white matter. The schematic indicates the two avenues of auditory sensory input to the left temporal lobe, one is ascending from the ipsilateral medial geniculate and the other is callosal from the homologous region of the right temporal lobe. Damage to both pathways has particularly devastating effects upon auditory comprehension.

and produce major comprehension deficits. One of the most unexpected findings of our study of aphasia after intracerebral hemorrhages was that two cases of persistent Wernicke's aphasia were associated with putaminal hemorrhages (1); we had anticipated an association with thalamic hemorrhages. The critical extension across the TI probably accounted for this finding; we were not alert to this structure at the time of that report.

Combination of lesion in TI and posterior-superior PVWM. We have not yet seen a case in which we could unequivocally assert that this combination occurred, although we suppose that more severe comprehension impairment would occur by virtue of the complete isolation of Wernicke's area from auditory input. We have reported two cases of posterior putaminal hemorrhage in which the acute CT suggested this lesion and the clinical course included prolonged severe comprehension impairments, but the late CT did not absolutely confirm that lesion configuration (2).

Combination of all lesions. Global aphasia follows PVWM lesion from the TI around to anterior extension (2). We know of no clinical sign to distinguish this syndrome from the classical cortical-subcortical global aphasia. We also know of no definitive differences in prognosis.

Combination of cortical lesion with additional subcortical lesion. When lesions reach from cortex to ventricle, many structures are potentially involved; the clinical effect of adding another lesion may not be readily computable. It seems likely,

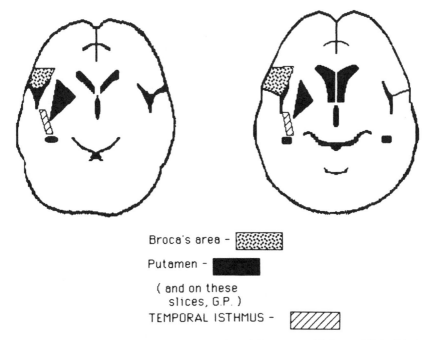

Broca's area –

Putamen –

(and on these
slices, G.P.)

TEMPORAL ISTHMUS –

FIG. 5. Schematic representation of the location of the temporal isthmus (TI) in CT plane. Note that it is the white matter region immediately posterior to the internal capsule and the posterior putamen. It reaches from the posterior limit of the sylvian fissure to the origin of the temporal horn. The anterior TI contains the ascending auditory radiations; the poster TI contains the visual radiations.

however, that many clinical findings that appear anomalous when only cortical lesion is assessed, become transparently accountable when subcortical effects are considered. Broca's original case had damage to the foot of F3, but, as many neurohistorians have pointed out, the bulk of the lesion was deep (20), running posteriorly across almost all of the white matter regions that we considered above (probably excluding TI). His persistent severe aphasia, complete with the famous nonverbal stereotype "tan," was probably most compatible with the subcortical lesion combination associated with severe limitations in spoken language output, as described above. We have reported patients with a different lesion extension but the same clinical lesion, i.e., cortical lesion in Wernicke's area but with subcortical extension anteriorly across all white matter pathways outlined above; the patient had a global aphasia (2) rather than the Wernicke's aphasia that the cortical lesion alone would have predicted.

Summary of Functional Anatomy Suggested by Clinical Studies

Investigation of cases with subcortical vascular lesions has provided little evidence for an important pathophysiologic role of the striatum in language abnormalities.

Large left striatal lesions may cause or contribute to a reduction in total amount of language output and probably cause disturbances in voicing and in rate, initiation, and amplitude of articulatory movements. Beyond these observations, there is little to support a critical position for striatal lesions in any of the subcortical aphasia profiles. This does not mean that the normal striatum does not play a role in normal language.

The ALIC lies between the putamen and the caudate nucleus. The GIC lies at the posterior boundary of the ALIC. Among other important pathways, the ALIC includes the descending fibers from prefrontal and motor association cortex, ascending fibers from the thalamus to the motor association cortex, connections between dorsomedial thalamus and prefrontal cortex, and temporal lobe efferents to the caudate (8). The GIC includes the descending corticobulbar pathways. Damage to the descending motor system in the GIC and immediately adjacent posterior portion of the ALIC results in speech impairment—dysarthria from left hemisphere lesions (24); affective dysprosody from right-sided lesions (23). Positron emission tomography (PET) investigations of the effects upon cortical metabolism of subcortical lesions seem to support the possibility that pathways running through the internal capsule have more direct functional interactions than do striatal pathways (19).

The white matter surrounding the capsular-striatal region is a complex interwoven tapestry. Interhemispheric connections converge toward the corpus callosum in a regular, pincer-like distribution from the forceps major in the occipital lobe to the forceps minor frontally. Long intrahemispheric pathways have a generally fan-like configuration (Fig. 6) as they converge from broad cortical origins into dissectable bundles deep in the hemispheric white matter (22). Finally, the corona radiata converges into the highly topographically differentiated internal capsule (Fig. 7). It is at the margins of the striatum, the lateral ventricles, and internal capsule, i.e., the deep PVWM, that the greatest confluences of converging pathways can be found.

Lesions that stay superior to the capsular-striatal area are not in position to disrupt any visual or auditory input to the hemisphere, nor are they positioned to disrupt the more superficial short perisylvian association pathways. In these cases, comprehension should be intact and, in general, it has been in our cases with superior extension. Among the lesions with only superior lesion extension, the more anterior PVWM damage has been associated with mutism or at least reduced language output. The important projections from supplementary motor area (SMA) and perhaps from the anterior cingulate to the frontal operculum and lower motor cortex run through the anterolateral PVWM (2,5,9).

When the superior lesion includes the middle PVWM region, dysarthria, hemiplegia, and left limb apraxia have been found. The descending motor pathways to the ipsilateral internal capsule and the callosal pathways to the contralateral right sensory-motor association cortices are involved. Lesions situated at the complex white matter intersection immediately posterior to the striatum-capsular area would damage the pathways emerging from the posterior portion of the posterior limb of

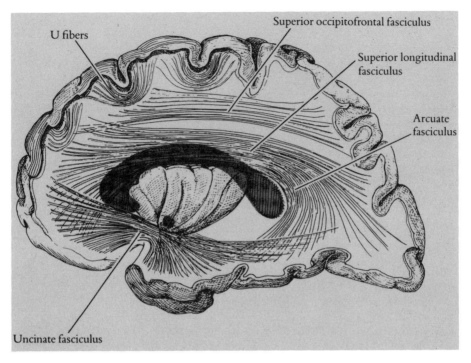

FIG. 6. Schematic representation of the long intrahemispheric association pathways in the left hemisphere. The fan-like origins and terminations can be noted as well as the convergence into dense bundles in the region just lateral to the corpus callosum, that is, just in the superior paraventricular white matter. This figure also demonstrates the more superficial short intrahemispheric pathways (U-fibers). From Nauta and Feirtag (22).

the internal capsule (PLIC); these include the auditory pathways (sublenticular capsule) and the visual pathways (retrolenticular capsule) (22). Damage to this region results in deficits in language comprehension, particularly auditory.

There are several grossly identifiable intrahemispheric white matter bundles (Fig. 6): the superior occipitofrontal fasciculus, the subcallosal fasciculus, the arcuate fasciculus, the uncinate fasciculus, and the inferior occipitofrontal fasciculus (22). These fiber tracts are not situated in a paraventricular manner except for the subcallosal fasciculus (26). They are, instead, more laterally placed, although still deep to the short association pathways. At the present time, it is difficult to subscribe a specific role to any of the long association pathways in aphasia. It is likely that damage to the temporofrontal pathways in the arcuate fasciculus or more inferiorly in the extreme capsule disrupts the integration of function between the anterior and posterior language zones and produces phonemic paraphasias, in spontaneous speech but also, and particularly, in repetition and oral reading. This is not the only lesion that results in phonemic paraphasias. A recent investigation by one of us (M.N.) has suggested that damage to the subcallosal fasciculus is important in the production

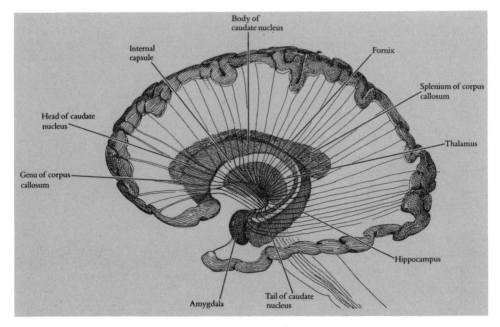

FIG. 7. Schematic of the relationship of the converging fibers of the internal capsule to other important landmarks in subcortical aphasias: the caudate, the thalamus, and the corpus callosum, and by inference, the lateral ventricles. From Nauta and Feirtag (22).

of language initiation deficits (21), perhaps as a result of its role as a conduit of connections between the nearby cingulate and the caudate. Analysis of cases of isolated agraphia has suggested that damage to the superior occipitofrontal fasciculus might be critical in disruption of the transformation of visual letter/word codes into orthographic output (3). Further investigation is needed of the specific effects of lesions in the long association pathways in aphasia.

To end this summary, we again turn to the problem of the interaction of multiple lesions. There is an unwritten rule in the study of aphasia that one should not consider cases with multiple lesions. We suspect that every brain lesion, even the ''single'' lesion, is likely to disrupt multiple functional systems; in that perspective, every case is a multiple lesion case. But here, we are analyzing traditional ''single'' lesions in which the distribution of the lesion is across several functional domains.

Damage to the constellation of anterior, anterolateral, and superior PVWM regions results in severe limitations in language output. This lesion disrupts all descending efferent pathways of motor association cortex, descending corticobulbar pathways, transverse pathways from medial frontal/cingulate (i.e., limbic) to laterofrontal, opercular, and rolandic cortex, the anterior and middle callosal pathways, and the subcallosal fasciculus. There are, presumably, no surviving normal output pathways. When there is extensive posterior, superior PVWM (i.e., deep to parietal lobe) and posterior PVWM (i.e., TI) lesion, much less of the anterior lesion seems to be required for a comparable loss of language output (16).

When the more superficial white matter is involved, there are several important implications about the additional structures that might be damaged. First, it is more problematic to assert that any clinical sign is owing to white matter lesions because the cortex in the deeper gyral folds is also now involved. Second, the white matter pathways affected are overwhelmingly the short association pathways (Fig. 6). Third, the callosal pathways continue to be involved because they obviously course from cortex to contralateral cortex. Fourth, in superficial white matter the involvement of long association structures (including the callosal ones) will not be in the highly converged, dense fiber bundles but in their fanned out and divergent terminations and origins.

Consider now one clinical example of the implications for explicating the aphasias of a lesion that involves cortex and the superficial subcortical white matter. Take the example of the frontal operculum lesion. This is usually the result of an embolic infarction in the territory of the prerolandic branch of the superior division of the middle cerebral artery. Damage will include the posterior inferior and middle frontal gyri, the anterior superior insular cortex, and the white matter immediately deep to those areas. This white matter includes: (a) long association connections of the extreme capsule, of portions of the superior longitudinal fasciculus, of portions of the terminations of the arcuate fasciculus, and of portions of the medial frontal (limbic) projections; (b) short association connections such as to adjacent motor cortex; (c) ascending projection pathways such as from the ventrolateral nucleus of the thalamus; (d) descending projection pathways to the striatum, pons, and contralateral cerebellum; (e) callosal projections to homotopic contralateral neocortex. The clinical syndrome associated with this lesion will be complex, but ultimately, explicable in a theoretical framework of multiple overlapping neural networks.

CONCLUSIONS

There are four important points in this review. First, we summarized some of the evidence that analysis of cases with *subcortical* lesions has led to some robust new rules of clinical-anatomic correlations. Second, we presented the findings that suggest the tentative conclusion that for the special problem of lesions in and around the striatum and capsules, the critical lesions are those to white matter pathways. Third, we tabulated the known white matter bundles conceivably involved by the clinical lesions, and ascribed to them the various individual aphasic signs whenever possible. It is this third step that establishes hypotheses about the pathophysiology of subcortical aphasias. Last, we briefly peered at the nature of the additional complexities involved in the analysis of cases in which the more superficial portions of the white matter are involved.

REFERENCES

1. Alexander, M.P., and LoVerme, S.R. (1980): Aphasia after left intracerebral hemorrhage. *Neurology*, 30:1193–1202.

2. Alexander, M.P., Naeser, M.A., and Palumbo, C.L. (1987): Correlations of subcortical CT lesion sites and aphasia profiles. *Brain (in press)*.
3. Auerbach, S.H., and Alexander, M.P. (1981): Pure agraphia and unilateral optic ataxia associated with a left superior parietal lobule lesion. *J. Neurol. Neurosurg. Psychiatry*, 44:430–432
4. Benson, D.F., Sheremata, W.A., Bouchard, R., Segarra, J.M., Price, D., and Geschwind, N. (1973): Conduction aphasia: A clinicopathological study. *Arch. Neurol.*, 28:339–346
5. Botez, M.I., and Barbeau, A. (1971): Role of subcortical structures and particularly the thalamus in the mechanisms of speech and language. *Int. J. Neurol.*, 8:300–320.
6. Damasio, H., and Damasio, A.R. (1979): "Paradoxic" ear extinction in dichotic listening: Possible anatomic significance. *Neurology*, 29:644–653.
7. Damasio, H., and Damasio, A.R. (1980): The anatomical basis of conduction aphasia. *Brain*, 103:337–350.
8. Damasio, A.R., Damasio, H., Rizzo, M., Varney, N., and Gersh, F. (1982): Aphasia with non-hemorrhagic lesions in the basal ganglia and internal capsule. *Arch. Neurol.*, 39:15–20.
9. Damasio, A.R., and VanHoesen, G.W. (1980): Structure and function of the supplementary motor area. *Neurology*, 30(Suppl. 1):396.
10. Fisher, C.M. (1979): Capsular infarcts: The underlying vascular lesions. *Arch. Neurol.*, 36:65–73.
11. Freedman, M., Alexander, M.P., and Naeser, M.A. (1984): Anatomic basis of transcortical motor aphasia. *Neurology*, 34:409–417.
12. Green, E., and Howes, D.H. (1977): The nature of conduction aphasia: A study of anatomic and clinical features and of underlying mechanisms. *Studies Neuroling.*, 3:123–156.
13. Helgason, C., Caplan, L.R., Goodwin, J. and Hedges, T. (1986): Anterior choroidal artery territory infarction: Report of cases and review. *Neurology*, 43:681–686.
14. Hier, D.B., Hagenlocker, K., and Shindler, A.G. (1985): Language disintegration in dementia: Effects of etiology and severity. *Brain Lang.*, 25:117–133.
15. Kertesz, A., and Ferro, J.M. (1984): Lesion size and location in ideomotor apraxia. *Brain*, 107:921–933.
16. Knopman, D.S., Selnes, O.A., Niccum, N., Rubens, A.B., Yock, D., and Larson, D. (1983): A longitudinal study of speech fluency in aphasia: CT correlates of recovery and persistent nonfluency. *Neurology*, 33:1170–1178.
17. Lomas, J., and Kertesz, A. (1978): Patterns of spontaneous recovery in aphasic groups: A study of adult stroke patients. *Brain Lang.*, 5:388–401.
18. Mesulam, M-M. (1981): A cortical network for directed attention and unilateral neglect. *Ann. Neurol.*, 10:309–325.
19. Metter, E.J., Mazziotta, J.C., Itabaschi, H.H., Markovich, N.J., Phelps, M.E., and Kuhl, D.E. (1985): Comparison of glucose metabolism, x-ray CT, and postmortem data in a patient with multiple cerebral infarcts. *Neurology*, 35:1695–1701.
20. Mohr, J.P., Pessin, M.S., Finkelstein, S., Duncan, G.W., and Davis, K.R. (1978): Broca aphasia: Pathological and clinical aspects. *Neurology*, 28:311–324.
21. Naeser, M.A., Palumbo, C.L., Carlson, L., Helm-Estabrooks, N., and Albert, M.L. (1986): CT scan in nonfluent Broca's aphasia vs. cases with no speech and stereotypies only: Importance of deep subcortical areas. Paper presented at the Academy of Aphasia, Nashville, TN.
22. Nauta, W.J.H., and Freitag, M. (1986): *Fundamental Neuroanatomy*. W.H. Freeman, New York.
23. Ross, E.D. (1981): The aprosodias: Functional-anatomic organization of the affective components of language in the right hemisphere. *Arch. Neurol.*, 38:561–569.
24. Schiff, H.B., Alexander, M.P., Naeser, M.A., and Galaburda, A.M. (1983): Aphemia: Clinical-anatomic correlations. *Arch. Neurol.*, 40:720–727.
25. Selnes, O.A., Knopman, D.S., Niccum, N., Rubens, A.B., and Larson, D. (1983): Computed tomographic scan correlates of auditory comprehension deficits in aphasia: A prospective recovery study. *Ann. Neurol.*, 13:558–566.
26. Yakolev, P.I., and Locke, S. (1961): Limbic nuclei of thalamus and connections of limbic cortex. *Arch. Neurol.*, 4:364–400.

*Language, Communication, and
the Brain*, edited by F. Plum.
Raven Press, New York © 1988.

''It's What You Mean, Not What You Say'': Pragmatic Language Use in Brain-Damaged Patients

Sally T. Weylman, Hiram H. Brownell, and Howard Gardner

*Aphasia Research Center, Department of Neurology, Boston University School of
Medicine, and Boston Veterans Administration Medical Center,
Boston, Massachusetts 02130*

In the late afternoon shadows of the day room on the neurobehavior ward, two gentlemen sat smoking together. Mr. L. was of short stature but commanding presence. With his ever-attentive glance, cordial and prompt smile at visitors, and perfectly coordinated clothes, Mr. L. appeared to be an accommodating host. It was not immediately apparent that he was a severely aphasic patient, one with substantial problems in the comprehension of syntax as well as profoundly impaired output. Sitting down to speak with him on bed rounds that afternoon, the attending physicians immediately learned, through Mr. L.'s diligent use of gestures and pictures, that he was worried that their interview would interrupt his therapy, which was scheduled to start in 15 minutes. After assuring him that he would not miss his appointment, the clinicians quickly assessed Mr. L.'s current language capacities, and then released him for his therapy. They were amazed at the effective range of communication of a man with left hemisphere brain damage whom standard speech and language testing had labeled severely impaired for ''all communication'' (1 out of 5 on the aphasia severity rating scale of the Boston Diagnostic Aphasia Examination) (24).

Across the room, Mr. R., wearing a baggy, dirty pair of blue jeans and untucked flannel workshirt that was buttoned incorrectly, had left his lit cigarette burning on the edge of the ashtray. He appeared totally nonchalant in the face of the doctors' approach to his side of the room. As soon as they reached him, however, he began ribbing one of the junior residents relentlessly. ''You've been eating bullets again, eh?'' he asked in a distinctly flat tone of voice. ''Look, your hair is growing in bangs! That's two-thirds of a pun: P-U!'' Only with firm persuasion could the interview proceed. After a rudimentary mental status check, the physicians examined Mr. R.'s edemic left hand, and asked him how he felt his therapies were progressing. ''How long have you been here?'' a new intern asked him. ''About two and a half minutes,'' Mr. R. answered, and then launched into a tangential discussion that seemed to treat the course of his hospitalization. Moments later, a nurse entered the day room, glanced at Mr. R., and shook her head in frustration. "Mr. R.," she said in exasperation, and pointed at the clock. Still Mr. R. appeared unconcerned. Finally, the nurse went over to him, reminded him he was again late for his physical therapy, and, arm in arm, accompanied him to the elevator. Despite having passed the formal language examination, Mr. R., a right hemisphere-damaged patient, could not fully understand the everyday discourse around him.

Who were these two brain-damaged patients, who presented such sharply contrasting linguistic and behavioral profiles? Mr. L. was a 62-year-old, right-handed man of Middle Eastern descent. He had been admitted to the Neurobehavior Service at the Boston Veterans Administration Medical Center for speech therapy in May 1986 after suffering a left hemisphere embolic stroke the previous September. At the time of onset he was judged to have a "global" aphasia and right hemiplegia, which eventually resolved to a hemiparesis. After the initial hospitalization, Mr. L. lived at home with his family where he was able to walk with a cane, manage the family checking account, play poker and cribbage, and use a children's computer language aid. Mr. L. had graduated from high school, attended roughly 1½ years of college, and subsequently was employed as a computer form designer and salesperson. Throughout the course of his rehabilitation, Mr. L. was always eager to work and to challenge himself. One had the impression, upon observing him on the ward, that even in very trying situations, he continually pushed himself and persevered, an attitude that may well have accelerated the recovery of his communicative powers. He was always correcting himself, ever-vigilant for speech errors, and always considerate in his dealings with staff and other patients. In short, unless he was talking, or unless one saw his hemiparesis, it was virtually impossible to tell that Mr. L. was a brain-damaged patient.

Initially, after his CVA, Mr. L.'s language was characterized by verbal stereotypies, the inability to repeat, and comprehension at the one-step command level. Eight months later, during his admission for speech therapy, his language was similarly characterized by a "nonfluent aphasia with impaired repetition and relative sparing of comprehension." Especially notable was his versatility in pictographic communication. For example, he indicated the breadth of his general current events knowledge by drawing representations of the disasters of the Chernobyl nuclear reactor and the Challenger space shuttle.

In contrast, Mr. R., a 54-year-old, right-handed, college-educated man, who suffered a right hemisphere stroke in the territory of the middle cerebral artery a year ago, had no ostensible linguistic deficits. After several months of rehabilitation following his stroke, he returned to his suburban farm where he attempted to help with the sale of vegetables. Since the onset of his stroke, however, Mr. R. exhibited marked communication problems. In the presence of anyone who would listen, he would rant on for hours in a tangential and perseverative monologue. On three separate testing sessions, he ignored the content of task items and repeated the same rambling story about how, while recovering in the hospital, he had decided to lose weight. Each time, he used the same descriptions and exclamations to unfold the story, without any recognition of having told it before. In the middle of conversations he made casual, mildly inappropriate comments about the examiner's appearance and asked questions that were irrelevant to the testing like "So where did you go to school?" Emotionally he was quite unconcerned and not particularly affected by anything he experienced.

Here, then, we have two instructively contrasting patients. In ordinary terms, Mr. L. is markedly impaired in speaking and understanding language but gets the point of what is said by going beyond the spoken message. In contrast, despite appearing to be conversant and in command of things expressed to him, Mr. R. actually cannot understand or communicate the main point of ideas. But can we go beyond these descriptions in terms of linguistic competence? Can we carry out empirical studies that may clarify the nature and extent of these disorders?

THE PRAGMATICS OF LANGUAGE: FIVE ASPECTS

Everyday language comprises not only the rudiments of speech traditionally probed by linguists—phonology, syntax, and lexical-semantics—but also a broader realm often termed pragmatics (19). The pragmatic portion of language includes the intentions and attitudes conveyed by speech as well as the gestural and prosodic elements that accompany speech. As the above description of Mr. R. indicates, it is possible to retain the traditional elements of language, while becoming insensitive to the uses of language (hereafter, pragmatic language) and to the aspects of tone and gesture that accompany language (hereafter, paralinguistic features). Indeed, as exemplified by the opening vignettes, aphasic patients with unilateral left hemisphere disease (LHDs) characteristically exhibit impairments in the handling of traditional linguistic elements, with relative preservation of pragmatic language and paralinguistic capacities (15,38,41). In contrast, right hemisphere-damaged patients (RHDs) characteristically preserve competence with traditional linguistic elements, in the face of impairments of pragmatic language and paralinguistic competence (4,5,22,29,30,34).

In practice, it is not always easy to draw lines between traditional and pragmatic language, or between linguistic and paralinguistic capacities. For example, is sensitivity to the connotation of a word or phrase better considered a "traditional" or "pragmatic" capacity? Is sensitivity to a pun traditional or pragmatic? Is the use of a tone of voice to ask a question identical to its use in ironic utterances or in the mimicry of an emotion? For present purposes, the precise delineation of these realms is less important than the following claim: There are numerous aspects of communication and language that extend well beyond those units that have thus far occupied most attention in the work of linguists, aphasiologists, and others concerned with communication.

In our own studies of the communicative abilities of brain-injured patients, we have examined a number of pragmatic capacities. Let us consider several in turn.

Following Indirect Requests

To make a request, a person must first take notice of a need and assess what addressing it would entail. S/he must then select the most appropriate way to communicate the request. Polite literal requests are often lengthy and awkwardly constructed (e.g., "I am requesting that you tell me the name of that book"). For greater ease and efficiency, while retaining politeness, speakers tend to use pragmatic language—indirect requests like "Can you tell me the name of that book?"—to request actions. Indirect requests are considered nonliteral utterances; if taken at face value, these questions inquire about an ability or capacity to perform an action and do not specify that the action be carried out.

Although such statements can be interpreted in more than one way, there are clearly preferred readings. The following case illustrates this: When a bewildered driver in a new city asks his wife, "Can you see that house number?", he is making an indirect request for action, i.e., for her to tell him how far along they are on the street. In this case, as in many others of nonliteral language use, the concrete reading of this question would produce the inappropriate response, "Yes, I can," sounding humorous or rude rather than responsive. To reply accurately to requests for action, a listener needs to pay close attention to the cues of the context at hand and actively infer what the speaker actually had in mind.

Understanding Attitudes Expressed Using Figurative Language

Both the comprehension and expression of attitudes are in part mediated by paralinguistic elements such as prosody, gesture, and facial expression, and by nonliteral language use as well. Because attitude is often indicated in paralinguistic or pragmatic ways (scowling, waving a fist, giving extra emphasis to a particular word in a sentence, or using sarcasm), those who would be sensitive to it cannot rely solely on linguistic information. For example, imagine a child who has ignored his mother's pleas to clean his unkempt bedroom. Upon returning from an errand, she remarks to him, "Boy, Johnny, your room looks really clean now." Taking this statement literally would be a significant error, for the mother's remark is meant sarcastically. Sarcasm occurs when a statement is intended to mean its literal opposite. Knowing when an utterance is intended sarcastically, and when it is meant literally, often requires analysis of speaker motivation: Such information may be gleaned from the context surrounding the remark and/or from paralinguistic cues.

Appreciating and Conveying Humor

Humor also requires pragmatic language abilities. Telling a joke necessitates knowing how to sequence parts into a whole and to prepare listeners for the punch-line. Careful, deliberate exposition of narrative (giving enough, but not too much, information) sets up the right cues for the punchline to succeed. To appreciate the humor of someone else's joke, a listener generates expectancies of what will happen while hearing the body of the joke; appreciates that these expectancies are disconfirmed by the punchline; and then recognizes that, in fact, the punchline does fit with the body of the joke in an unanticipated but appropriate way (39). Consider the following joke without its punchline:

> A woman wants to cook a rabbit stew but the hares hanging at the butcher's are quite large. So she says to the butcher, "I'd like to make some rabbit stew, but these things are too big. Could you cut one in two for me?"

After hearing it, one toys with different possibilities, perhaps expecting a food or cooking response (unless the listener is avidly trying to outwit the joketeller or is already familiar with the pun). The butcher's reply—"Sorry, Ma'am, we don't split hares here"—surprises and amuses the listener because of the play on the phrase "splitting hairs." Understanding jokes requires seeing both the coherence and the discontinuity of the punchline and the joke. A listener must understand that at one level the punchline does not make sense but that at a second, more abstract level, it does.

Drawing Inferences

Pragmatic language implicitly assumes that listeners make inferences when necessary. Assuming that others have the ability to infer, a speaker does not have to spell out each aspect of the sequence of ideas in a narrative, but rather can leave the responsibility for inferring the necessary logical and narrative links between ideas to the listener. Consider the following description: "Mr. Smith gave the newspaper boy a tip. He showed him how to fold the newspaper for delivery before throwing it onto the porch." In this instance, a normal reader would first identify the initial meaning of "tip" as payment. Then, using the context, he would see that "tip" here instead means advice.

Interpreting Figurative Language

Pragmatic communication allows, in fact, highlights, the use of nonliteral or figurative forms of speech. Instead of always having to use literal terms to describe the comment on situations, speakers can avail themselves of figurative expressions such as proverbs and metaphors. The use of both proverbs and metaphors entails the ability to dissect a situation into its components and then to compare these elements to those drawn from a seemingly disparate realm of discourse. In both proverbs and metaphors, one uses attributes of another situation to refer to and clarify the one under discussion (e.g., saying "Anyone can hold the helm when the sea is calm," to a corporate executive in the midst of a stockholder uprising). To use metaphor effectively, a speaker must appreciate the literal disparities and nonliteral analogies of the attributes of the two things being compared. The use and comprehension of proverbs entails understanding how the specifics of an event match the more general wisdom captured in a proverb, despite the superficial remoteness of the concrete facts.

With the support of linguistic and paralinguistic cues, pragmatic language extends the range of expression and comprehension possible in discourse. In this chapter, we map out current neuropsychological research in the aforementioned five areas. Then, we attempt to synthesize these findings with our opening clinical impressions in an effort to show how laboratory findings may enhance our understanding of language impairment and language processes.

EMPIRICAL WORK IN PRAGMATIC LANGUAGE CAPACITIES

Neuropsychological research offers a direct route to understanding how the brain mediates cognition. The data yielded by studies of cortically damaged patients elucidate the participation of different brain regions in various cognitive operations. Performance on specific tasks often yields insight for clinical intervention and rehabilitation. To be sure, an impaired performance elicited subsequent to a specific brain lesion may not necessarily represent the perfect inverse of the normal functioning of that brain site. Nonetheless, the study of stroke-lesioned subjects provides one of the clearest ways of unravelling the relationship of anatomy to behavior.

Another important point in neuropsychological research is that performance may not accurately reflect an ability or an underlying competence. For example, an aphasic patient may be perfectly aware of a concept s/he is trying to express but may not be able to produce the appropriate lexical item. A RHD patient may understand a storyline but may get befuddled in reproducing all of its components in correct sequence. Until more precise research techniques are developed, we must assume measures of production and comprehension are conservative estimates of actual ability.

Together, neuropsychology and cognitive science make it possible to distinguish component processes that yield complex behaviors. One way to tease out the different components in an intricate process such as language, and to see if their mode of operation is altered by brain damage, is to devise test items that pit one strategy or mode of analysis against another. One can then see whether, and in what way, the usual (normal) profile is altered by damage to different parts of the brain. To the extent possible, this has been the model design for the work discussed below.

In what follows we describe results obtained from testing RHDs and aphasics in the five pragmatic areas outlined above. Then, more briefly, we present work on several paralinguistic abilities—gesture, intonation, and emotional expression—done with RHDs and aphasics.

In the studies done in our laboratory, subjects were right-handed, unilaterally right or left brain-damaged patients whose infarction localization was confirmed by neurological signs and, in most cases, computerized tomography (CT) scans. All subjects, including patients and controls, were under age 70 and had no previous significant psychiatric or neurologic histories. Control subjects were drawn from the same general population as the patients and roughly matched the patients in age, gender, and educational and socioeconomic status.

Pragmatic Functioning

Following Indirect Requests

Comprehension of an indirect utterance, such as an indirect request, depends on several types of information—including sensitivity to the conventionality of the language form used and to the context in which the remark occurs. For normal listeners, high conventionality utterances (e.g., "Can you . . . ?") in isolation tend to be interpreted as indirect requests, whereas low conventionality questions (e.g., "Are you able to . . . ?") tend to generate interpretations of the remark as a request for information. In past work on indirect request comprehension by Clark (9), normal listeners used conventionality of question form to gauge indirectness when contextual cues were not given. When presented with a question such as "Can you tell me the interest rate on your regular savings account?", subjects interpreted it as meaning "Please tell me the interest rate"; in contrast, the low conventionality question "Are you able to tell me the interest rate?" typically elicited both the literal answer ("Yes" or "No") and then the interest rate. Clark felt that this pattern of responses resulted from a difference in the degree to which the high and low forms were taken seriously (literally).

Evidence from neuropsychology had suggested that the left and right hemispheres assumed separate roles in the comprehension of indirect requests. In particular, sensitivity to the nuances of context seems to aid aphasics, but not RHDs, in the interpretation of the intent of ambiguous utterances like indirect requests. Controls and aphasics have been shown able to use pictorially conveyed context to interpret these remarks; RHDs cannot use this information successfully to bolster their understanding (18).

Seeking to sort out the effects of these two factors on indirect request comprehension, we carried out a study that we reported at the 1986 meeting of the Academy of Aphasia. In this work, we compared the relative attraction of context to that of conventionality of form for aphasics, RHDs, and controls. Both left and right brain-damaged patients were included to pursue further the observed differences between left and right hemisphere contributions to this process (18,28). Previous studies that established a RHD deficit in the use of context had used pictures, thereby possibly confounding contextual insensitivity with visual decrement. Therefore, the present study used purely verbal stimuli.

Subjects were presented with short vignettes, ending in an utterance that could be interpreted either as a request for action or a question about ability. Two contrasting contexts were used, one encouraging an indirect request interpretation, the other a literal question reading. Each item concluded with either a high or low conventionality utterance. In the following example, an indirect context is combined with a low conventionality utterance.

> Tom hears a strange noise coming from the back wheel of his car on Route 95, so he pulls over to the side. Just then a tow truck pulls up. Tom asks the driver, ''Is it possible for you to change a flat tire?''

Relative to normals, and as shown in the studies of Foldi (18) and Hirst et al. (28), RHDs were impaired in their ability to use contextual information to judge the intended indirectness of a remark. Conventionality did not noticeably influence RHDs' decisions. In contrast, for aphasics, whose linguistic deficits prevented their full use of the verbally presented context, high conventionality wording markedly increased the probability of selecting an indirect interpretation over a direct, literally intended response.

The fact that aphasics attempted to use conventionality, whereas RHDs apparently did not, suggests contrasting approaches in the two groups. Aphasics' awareness of their deficits prompts them to make use of all available cues. RHDs' denial of or unconcern about impairment and poor self-monitoring may cause them to overlook information that could be instructive. Whether RHDs *cannot* use or simply *will not* use cues like context remains to be disentangled, but regardless of the answer to this question, our work suggests that aphasics base their comprehension on the use of specific pragmatic language cues such as conventionality of form, and RHDs do not.[1]

The aforementioned study has been described in some detail to convey a feeling for how we test the pragmatic capacities of brain-damaged patients. The studies discussed below were constructed with analogous manipulation of variables. Further information about specifics of particular studies is available in the cited references.

Understanding Attitudes Expressed Using Figurative Language

Although an underlying attitude can be expressed in many ways, it can be conveyed strictly through language. A compelling example can be found in sarcasm. Here a speaker says the opposite of what s/he means, thereby signalling listeners that s/he is mocking the subject or topic (10,23,31). Sarcasm is often signalled by a motivation for the speaker to be hostile. We investigated the extent to which such motivation influences the understanding of sarcasm.

In one situation treated as sarcastic by a normal listener, explicit hostile feelings on the part of a speaker preface an apparently positive comment about a negative performance. In one of our comprehension studies (Jacobs, 1985, *personal communication*; Brownell, *unpublished observations*), subjects heard sarcastic and other types of vignettes, such as:

> Anne and Roger were lawyers in the same law firm. Anne hated Roger because he often teased her for defending clients who couldn't afford to pay her fee. One day Anne saw Roger totally mishandle what should have been a simple case. Anne said to another attorney, ''Roger handled that case well.''

---

[1] After completion of this chapter, more extensive analysis on these and additional data failed to uphold the group (RHD, LHD) by conventionality interaction.

Subjects had to determine whether the final remark was sarcastic: This determination could be accomplished by integrating speaker motivation with the actual performance described in the vignette as either bad (as above) or good.

Relative to controls, RHDs had trouble using information about speaker motivation to guide their decisions. In general, they attributed factually incorrect final comments to error rather than a sarcastic intent. They could not see that the remarks, although apparently stating the opposite of the facts of the vignette, actually referred to the situation at hand.

Appreciating and Conveying Humor

Similar to other narratives, jokes require careful synthesis of parts for full appreciation of meaning, but, like sarcasm, they also demand affective sensitivity. A listener trying to identify the correct punchline must find one that not only meshes with the plotline, but also is surprising and humorous. Most often, the surprise comes about through an unexpected conclusion. In the following example of verbal humor, the correct funny response is both *coherent* and *surprising*, while the other responses lack at least one of these features.

A new housekeeper was accused of helping herself to her master's liquor. She told him, "I'll have you know, sir, I come from honest English parents."

Correct funny: He said, "I'm not concerned with your English parents. What's worrying me is your Scotch extraction."

Humorous nonsequitur: Then the housekeeper saw a mouse and jumped into her master's lap.

Straightforward: He said, "All the same, the next time the liquor disappears, you're fired."

To examine sensitivity to these two aspects of humor, a task of nonverbal humor comprehension was designed (1). Subjects had to choose between competing punchline conclusions, which varied in the degree of surprise and also in the cohesiveness with the narrative. RHDs consistently selected humorous nonsequitur endings over correct funny and other alternatives. Aphasics, in contrast, picked correct funny endings and, when they erred, preferred straightforward endings. This pattern held for both verbal and pictorial jokes (4). Both studies demonstrated a RHD tendency to ignore the coherence demands of narrative humor in favor of exclusive attention to the formal requirement of surprise.

The production of jokes is another area of RHD anomaly. These patients have often been noted to be inappropriately jocular (20,42). In pilot work in our laboratory, we have found that joketelling by RHDs succeeds only when it involves recitation of earlier and overlearned jokes. When asked to relate recently learned jokes, these patients tend to make gross omissions. They fail to supply enough information for listeners to make the appropriate inferences, or to appreciate the connection between the body of the joke and the punchline. One RHD patient related the joke presented above in the following way: "An English housekeeper

. . . uh . . . of Scottish extraction . . . a lot of liquor was missing . . . I presume it was Scotch.''

RHDs' performance on these humor tasks demonstrates the multifaceted nature of their narrative difficulties: Not only do they have trouble creating a cohesive storyline from the pieces given, but they also fail to reproduce narratives in an acceptable manner.

Drawing Inferences

As in jokes and other types of narratives, listeners often have to create links between ideas when these connections have not been explicitly stated. In conversations, for example, the listener's task is to tie together the ideas presented and to revise assumptions when they have been undermined (25). Much of the efficiency of everyday communication rests on the ability to draw inferences from available information and to correct misconceptions.

One factor that influences inferencing in discourse settings is the relative position of the target information in the communication. To investigate the importance of this "position factor," a task was designed in which subjects had to draw the implied conclusion from two associated sentences. In this study (5), RHDs and controls were shown a pair of sentences that, taken together, yielded a correct overall understanding (the correct inference). One of the sentences, however, contained misleading information that, without the disambiguation provided by the second sentence, encouraged an incorrect inference about the action at hand:

> Sally brought a pen and paper with her to meet the movie star.
>   The article would include comments on nuclear power by well-known people.
>
> *Correct inference:*   Sally was going to interview the movie star.
>
> *Incorrect inference:* Sally wanted the movie star's autograph.

RHDs were impaired in their ability to make inferences, particularly when the misleading information was in the first sentence. This so-called position effect may have been the result of RHDs' inability to reject information once it has been accepted as true. The inferencing impairment of RHDs may also emanate from a broader rigidity—an inability to generate alternatives superimposed on an attraction to initial assumptions (30,33).

Interpreting Figurative Language

In the comprehension of single words, normal individuals are sensitive to denotations as well as metaphoric connotations. For example, they can understand that the word "deep" means both "extending down or out from a surface" and "wise." Several types of information may bias the determination of which aspect of word meaning is intended. Contextual information, such as that which can be derived from neighboring words, is one such cue.

In a recent study (6), subjects had to select the two words that were most similar in meaning (or that went together best) from a triad consisting of three adjectives such as "warm"-"loving"-"cold." Compared with aphasic patients and normal control subjects, RHDs were less sensitive to metaphoric equivalences such as "warm" and "loving."

This study did not indicate whether this effect was due to an impaired sensitivity to metaphoric meaning or just a tendency to ignore alternative meanings. Therefore a second study was conducted with the same potentially metaphoric adjectives, as well as nonmetaphoric, polysemous nouns (e.g., suit: garment, trial). As presented by Brownell, Bihrle, Potter, and Gardner in a paper at the 1985 Academy of Aphasia meeting, RHDs performed at the level of aphasic subjects in distinguishing between primary and secondary meanings of the nonmetaphoric word pairs, but showed selective impairment on the metaphoric trials. This result suggests that RHDs' impairment ensues from an insensitivity to metaphoric connotation and not to all alternative meanings—a pattern that would coincide with their hypothesized figurative language deficit.

We secured further support for this hypothesis. In a metaphor comprehension task requiring selection of the correct pictorial description of a metaphoric phrase (44), RHDs tended to choose literal depictions over correct metaphoric interpretations. For the phrase, "he has a heavy heart," for example, these patients were drawn to the picture of a person laboring under the weight of the oversized heart he was carrying. In contrast, aphasics preferred the correct metaphoric drawings. Despite apparent understanding of the metaphors (as demonstrated by a verbal subtest), RHDs persisted in being drawn to the literal pictures in the pictorial subtest. The differing capacities to derive metaphoric meaning in left and right brain-damaged subjects suggest that this process may be in part mediated by the right hemisphere. This general claim regarding the role of the right hemisphere in the comprehension of nonliteral language could be further developed by assessing the influence of specific types of contextual cues on metaphoric comprehension.

Paralinguistic Functioning

By paralinguistic language, we mean those cues that contribute meaning nonlinguistically: in particular, prosody, gesture, and facial expression. As we document briefly below, these abilities seem to be implicated particularly in right hemisphere functioning.

Evidence for significant involvement of the right hemisphere in the production and comprehension of speech prosody derives from several sources. In normal processing of nonverbal emotional aspects of speech prosody, there is a left ear advantage (32). In the neurological literature, RHDs have demonstrated impairment in both the production and comprehension of propositional and emotional prosody (26,27,35–37,40,43). Aphasics seem to have preservation of prosodic production, although intonational styles vary somewhat among aphasic subtypes (12,13). The comprehension of prosodic material by aphasics appears to be mediated by the right hemisphere (19) and is therefore relatively spared when focal left hemisphere damage occurs.

Another paralinguistic ability deficient in RHDs and relatively spared in aphasics is the interpretation of emotional facial expressions (8,14). Moreover, RHDs seem to exhibit parallel impairment in the production of emotional facial expressions (2). Etcoff (16,17) demonstrated that this impairment occurs independent of facial recognition difficulty.

A third paralinguistic feature that complements the communicative value of speech is limb and axial gesture. Aphasics can use gesture to augment their range of expression (7), although their comprehension does not always improve when provided gestural cues (19). Clinical reports suggest that RHDs rarely use gestural information to supplement their comprehension or expression.

CONCLUSIONS

How can we explain the differences between left and right hemisphere contributions to the understanding of language? One school of thought argues that the distinction between the performances of right and left hemisphere patients reflects the attentional deficit in the former group (11). However, this conceptualization is not detailed enough to explain the distinctive error patterns of these groups. Other broad characterizations of the right hemisphere have been invoked previously, labeling it as spatial, musical, and emotional. Each of these has some validity. However, in our view, generalized descriptions of the right hemisphere such as these obscure the range of its abilities and power (3). The present line of research suggests that the right hemisphere may govern a wide realm of sensitivities that has not yet been adequately summarized by any single global deficit.

One sensitivity involves the pragmatic aspects of language. What are some of the ways in which one might try to characterize the demonstrated impairment of the injured right hemisphere in the pragmatics of communication? We here mention four possibilities, which may apply alone or in some combination.

One way of categorizing the impairments of these patients is through an analysis of the size of the language units they can and cannot comprehend. Performance on single-word denotative tasks—such as naming or comprehension—is preserved in most RHDs, impaired in many aphasics. RHDs have difficulty when faced with more than a sentence at a time, whereas aphasics appear to be helped with longer and more redundant texts (22). RHDs have trouble inferring connections and integrating ideas in narratives, whereas left hemisphere patients manage to understand the main idea of narratives, presumably through reliance on the paralinguistic cues described above.

A second conceptualization of left and right hemisphere language capacities orders these performances by the degree to which they rely on suprasentential contextual information. Context-free situations—such as the determination of syntactical correctness or the verification of a word—require minimal additional information. At the opposite end of the spectrum, context-dependent situations are those that exploit information from the surrounding context—such as the relationship of a punchline to its joke. It appears that the right hemisphere mediates context-dependent judgments—ascertaining, for example, when a remark is sarcastic—whereas the left hemisphere is implicated in context-independent language understanding such as single-word comprehension.

A third way of describing the differences between right and left hemisphere patients focuses on distinctions between literal language and its figurative applications. The right hemisphere seems to carry responsibility for discerning the underlying meaning of a proposition and relating it to other propositions that capture the same relationship, as in a metaphor or proverb. RHDs' impairment in handling figurative language may be owing to either an inability to create the link between literal and abstract meanings or a reluctance to accept the nonliteral version in light of the more superficially attractive literal one.

A final way of characterizing these differences also draws support from our own work. Gardner (21) has suggested that much of cognitive activity involves separate analytic modules, which he has termed the "frames of mind." There is a tendency for these frames, such as those subserving language and logical reasoning, to be located in the left hemisphere. An important task in cognition involves separating the kind of analyses carried out by these modules, e.g., the parsing of sentences. At the same time, however, successful communication depends on the additional ability to monitor the different analytic processes, determine when to invoke each, and shift, when needed, from one mode of analysis to another. This ability, which one might call "keeping frames in mind," seems to be typically a capacity of the right hemisphere. We have seen in this chapter many instances in which RHDs carry out specific analyses properly, but fail to appreciate when an alternative mode of analysis is required, when the current one is inappropriate, or when two modes need to be drawn on together.

What are the ramifications of the patterns cited above for treatment and rehabilitation? Despite their frequent placement in neighboring beds on neurology wards, brain-damaged patients are not a homogeneous lot nor can their care be undertaken with indifference to the site of their lesions. Interventions for aphasics—who have distinct ways of understanding commands, relating histories, and interacting—are often inappropriate for right hemisphere patients, and vice versa. Both aphasics and RHDs have functionally specific comprehension disorders that can be circumvented by using alternate vehicles of expression: context, gesture, and figurative language for aphasics; single words and literally construed phrases and sentences for RHDs. Only when these patients' pragmatic competences are taken into account completely can communicative potential be fully realized.

ACKNOWLEDGMENTS

This research was supported by NIH grants NS 11408 and NS 06209, the Research Service of the Veterans Administration, and Harvard Project Zero. We are especially grateful to Nancy Lefkowitz, Director of Speech and Language Pathology, and other personnel of the Spaulding Rehabilitation Hospital for their help and support in the conduct of this research.

REFERENCES

1. Bihrle, A.M., Brownell, H.H., Powelson, J.A., and Gardner, H. (1986): Comprehension of humorous and non-humorous materials in right and left brain-damaged patients. *Brain Cog.*, 5:399–411.
2. Borod, J.C., Koff, E., Perlman, M., and Nicholas, M. Channels of emotional expression in patients with unilateral brain damage. *Arch. Neurol. (in press)*.
3. Bradshaw, J.L., and Nettleton, N.C. (1981): The nature of hemispheric specialization in man. *Behav. Brain Sci.*, 4:51–91.
4. Brownell, H.H., Michel, D., Powelson, J., and Gardner, H. (1983): Surprise but not coherence: Sensitivity to verbal humor in right hemisphere patients. *Brain Lang.*, 18:20–27.
5. Brownell, H.H., Potter, H.H., Bihrle, A.M., and Gardner, H. (1986): Inference deficits in right brain-damaged patients. *Brain Lang.*, 27:310–321.
6. Brownell, H.H., Potter, H.H., Michelow, D., and Gardner, H. (1984): Sensitivity to lexical denotation and connotation in brain-damaged patients: A double dissociation? *Brain Lang.*, 22:253–265.
7. Cicone, M., Wapner, W., Foldi, N.S., Zurif, E., and Gardner, H. (1979): The relation between gesture and language in aphasic communication. *Brain Lang.*, 8:342–349.
8. Cicone, M., Wapner, W., and Gardner, H. (1980): Sensitivity to emotional expressions and situations in organic patients. *Cortex*, 16:145–158.
9. Clark, H. (1979): Responding to indirect speech acts. *Cog. Psychol.*, 11:430–477.
10. Clark, H.H., and Gerrig, R.J. (1984): On the pretense theory of irony. *J. Exp. Psychol. [Gen.]*, 113:121–126.
11. Coslett, H.B., Bowers, D., and Heilman, K.M. (1987): Reduction in cerebral activation after right hemisphere stroke. *Neurology*, 37:957–962.
12. Danly, M., Cooper, W.E., and Shapiro, B. (1983): Fundamental frequency, language processing, and linguistic structure in Wernicke's aphasia. *Brain Lang.*, 19:1–24.
13. Danly, M., and Shapiro, B. (1982): Speech prosody in Broca's aphasia. *Brain Lang.*, 16:171–190.
14. DeKosky, S.T., Heilman, K.M., Bowers, D., and Valenstein, E., (1980): Recognition and discrimination of emotional faces and pictures. *Brain Lang.*, 9:206–214.
15. Delis, D.C., Wapner, W., Gardner, H., and Moses, J.A. (1983): The contribution of the right hemisphere to the organization of paragraphs. *Cortex*, 19:43–50.
16. Etcoff, N.L. (1984): Selective attention to facial identity and facial emotion. *Neuropsychologia*, 22:281–295.
17. Etcoff, N.L. The neuropsychology of emotional expression. *Advances in Clinical Neuropsychology, vol. 3*, edited by G. Goldstein and R.E. Tarter. Plenum, New York *(in press)*.
18. Foldi, N.S. (1987): Appreciation of pragmatic interpretations of indirect commands: Comparison of right and left hemisphere brain-damaged patients. *Brain Lang.*, 31:88–108.
19. Foldi, N., Cicone, M., and Gardner, H. (1983): Pragmatic aspects of communication in brain-damaged patients. In: *Language Functions and Brain Organization*, edited by S. Segalowitz, pp. 51–86. Academic Press, New York.
20. Gardner, H. (1975): *The Shattered Mind*. Knopf, New York.
21. Gardner, H. (1983): *Frames of Mind*. Basic Books, New York.
22. Gardner, H., Brownell, H., Wapner, W., and Michelow, D. (1983): Missing the point: The role of the right hemisphere in the processing of complex linguistic materials. In: *Cognitive Processing in the Right Hemisphere*, edited by E. Perecman, pp. 169–191. Academic Press, New York.
23. Gibbs, R.W. (1986): On the psycholinguistics of sarcasm. *J. Exp. Psychol. [Gen.]*, 115:3–15.
24. Goodglass, H., and Kaplan, E. (1983): *The assessment of aphasia and related disorders, 2nd ed.* Lea & Febiger, Philadelphia.
25. Grice, J. (1975): Logic and conversation. In: *Syntax and Semantics 3: Speech Acts*, edited by P. Cole and J. Morgan, pp. 41–58. Academic Press. New York.
26. Heilman, K.H., Bowers, D., Speedie, L., and Coslett, H.B. (1984): Comprehension of affective and nonaffective prosody. *Neurology*, 34:917–921.

27. Heilman, K.H., Scholes, R., and Watson, R.T. (1975): Auditory affective agnosia: Disturbed comprehension of affective speech. *J. Neurol. Neurosurg. Psychiatry*, 38:69–72.
28. Hirst, W., LeDoux, J., and Stein, S. (1984): Constraints on the processing of indirect speech acts: Evidence from aphasiology. *Brain Lang.*, 28:26–33.
29. Huber, W., and Gleber, J. (1982): Linguistic and nonlinguistic processing of narratives in aphasia. *Brain Lang.*, 16:1–18.
30. Joanette, Y., Goulet, P., Ska, B., and Nespoulos, J-L. (1986): Informative content of narrative discourse in right-brain-damaged right-handers. *Brain Lang.*, 29:81–105.
31. Jorgenson, J., Miller, G., and Sperber, D. (1984): A test of the mention theory of irony. *J. Exp. Psychol. [Gen.]*, 10:1–9.
32. Kimura, D. (1964): Left-right differences in the perception of melodies. *Q. J. Exp. Psychol.*, 16:355–358.
33. Lesser, R. (1986): Comprehension of linguistic cohesion after right brain damage. *J. Clin. Exp. Neuropsych.*, 8:127.
34. Myers, P., and Linebaugh, C. (1981): Comprehension of idiomatic expressions by right hemisphere damaged adults. In: *Clinical Aphasiology—Proceedings of the Conference*, edited by R.H. Brookshire, pp. 254–261. BRK Publishers, Minneapolis.
35. Ross, E.D. (1981): The aprosodias: Functional-anatomical organization of the affective components of language in the right hemisphere. *Arch. Neurol.*, 38:561–569.
36. Ross, E.D., and Mesulam, M.M. (1979): Dominant language functions of the right hemisphere? Prosody and emotional gesturing. *Arch. Neurol.*, 36:144–148.
37. Shapiro, B.E., and Danly, M. (1985): The role of the right hemisphere in the control of speech prosody in propositional and affective contexts. *Brain Lang.*, 25:19–36.
38. Stachowiak, F., Huber, W., Poeck, K., and Kerschensteiner, M. (1977): Text comprehension in aphasia. *Brain Lang.*, 4:177–195.
39. Suls, J.M. (1983): Cognitive processes in humor appreciation. In: *Handbook of Humor Research*, edited by P.E. McGhee and J.H. Goldstein, pp. 39–57. Springer-Verlag, New York.
40. Tucker, D., Watson, R.T., and Heilman, K.M. (1977): Discrimination and evocation of affectively intoned speech in patients with right parietal disease. *Neurology*, 27:947–950.
41. Ulatowska, H.K., Doyel, A.W., Stern, R.F., and Haynes, S.M. (1983): Production of procedural discourse in aphasia. *Brain Lang.*, 18:315–341.
42. Weinstein, E.A., and Kahn, R.C. (1955): *Denial of Illness, Symbolic and Physiological Aspects*. Charles C. Thomas, Springfield, IL.
43. Weintraub, S., Mesulam, M.M., and Kramer, L. (1981): Disturbances in prosody: A right-hemisphere contribution to language. *Arch. Neurol.*, 38:742–744.
44. Winner, E., and Gardner, H. (1977): The comprehension of metaphor in brain-damaged patients. *Brain*, 100:719–727.

Language, Communication, and the Brain edited by F. Plum.
Raven Press, New York © 1988.

Brain Cerebral Metabolic Mapping of Normal and Abnormal Language and Its Acquisition During Development

*†John C. Mazziotta and *‡E. Jeffrey Metter

Department of Neurology, Reed Neurologic Institute, and Division of Nuclear Medicine and Biophysics, Department of Radiological Sciences, University of California, Los Angeles School of Medicine, and †Laboratory of Nuclear Medicine, Los Angeles, California 90024, and ‡Sepulveda Veterans Administration Medical Center, Sepulveda, California 91343

The complex and diverse aspects of human communication and its abnormalities intuitively indicate that it must be a product of multifactorial, integrated, and interdependent functional brain systems. These processes, their anatomical sites of actions, and the disorders that affect them are not well understood. Although more primitive systems of communication may exist and have been investigated in subhuman species, it is not clear how significant such studies will be in understanding human language. Studies of human cerebral anatomy [e.g., postmortem, X-ray computerized tomography (CT), magnetic resonance imaging (MRI)], its alterations by injury and the language disorder syndromes that result, have added to our understanding and knowledge of some aphasic syndromes. However, probably owing to the variable and distributed organization of language in different individuals, these studies have yet to provide a coherent view of human language and its dysfunction.

Initial studies of human cerebral function were performed with xenon-133 measurements of cerebral blood flow in normal individuals performing language related tasks (9,16) and in individuals with language disorders (8,11,32,47). Results of these studies demonstrated an important finding, that is, that functional abnormalities of the brain, demonstrated by measurements of cerebral blood flow, typically showed more widespread abnormalities than those detected by classical anatomical neuroradiological methods (47). These studies, although providing this important insight, were limited in spatial resolution and were highly weighted toward estimates of blood flow in the cerebral cortex.

Positron emission tomography (PET) provides the opportunity to study, in the living human, physiology, biochemistry, and pharmacology in both resting and behavioral states, including the production and reception of language. Thus, functional imaging with PET affords the opportunity to study this most unique human process, language, in health and disease. Such studies need not be static but, in fact, could evaluate a variety of language behaviors in a given normal individual or the recovery of language function in a patient with acute abnormalities of communication. Through these methods one can examine human language acquisition, normal language production and reception, alterations in language acquisition, damage to the adult processes of language processing, and the recovery of function following injury.

PRINCIPLES OF PET

PET is an analytic, noninvasive measurement tool for determining local cerebral function in humans. PET is already able to provide information about local cerebral blood flow (LCBF), oxygen (LCMRO$_2$), and glucose (LCMRGlc) metabolic rates and extraction fractions as well as cerebral blood volume (LCBV) (34,35,37,38). These physiological measurements are made possible by using biologically active compounds labeled with positron-emitting isotopes of carbon, nitrogen, oxygen, fluorine, and others. With these compounds it is possible to label substrates, substrate analogues, and drugs and use them *in vivo* without disturbing their chemical properties or behavior. The basic components that constitute the major methodological elements of PET include analytic PET instruments, positron-labeled compounds, and tracer kinetic mathematical models (Fig. 1).

PET imaging devices make use of the unique physical properties of positron decay that allow for the acquisition of high resolution, quantifiable cross-sectional images of the human brain (Fig. 2) (34,35,37,38). These compounds are administered either by intravenous injection or by inhalation. After a period of time, predicted by the tracer kinetic model, images are obtained that can be mathematically converted to the physiological process of interest. Final image resolution is presently in the range of 5 mm in the plane of section and 8 to 10 mm in slice thickness (Fig. 2). The theoretical limit of resolution is on the order of a few mm. Details about these systems and the resulting accuracy of the quantitative capabilities of PET have been previously described in detail (33,35,37,38).

The short physical half-life of positron-emitting isotopes require that a cyclotron for their production be available at or close to the site of PET imaging. Many labeled compounds are available for measuring biochemical and physiological processes. However, the problem of actually achieving these measurements is far more complex. The measurement of physiological processes requires careful selection of the labeled compound, the process to study, and the use of tracer kinetic models within the limitations imposed by PET for human studies. Most of the studies performed thus far have used oxygen-15 labeled compounds to examine cerebral blood flow, oxygen metabolism and extraction, and fluorine-18 labeled fluorodeoxyglucose (FDG) to examine cerebral glucose utilization. All of the examples provided in this chapter were obtained by using FDG to measure LCMRGlc (34,35,37,38,40). For a detailed description of tracer kinetic methods and positron labeled compounds the reader is referred to recent reviews (34,37).

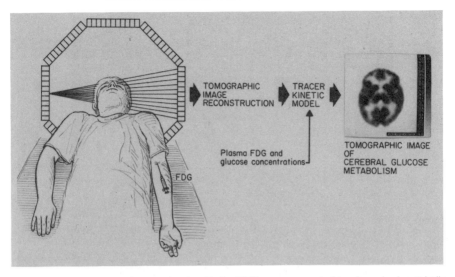

FIG. 1. The sequence of events involved in the PET measurement of local cerebral metabolic rate for glucose with ^{18}F-fluorodeoxyglucose (FDG). About 40 min after intravenous injection of FDG, tomographic data are collected, and cross-sectional images of the fluorine-18 tissue activity distribution are reconstructed. Plasma FDG and glucose concentration are entered into the computer of the tomograph, which also contains the operational equation of the FDG tracer kinetic model. Images are converted to local cerebral metabolic rate for glucose in units of μmole $\times$ min^{-1} $\times$ g tissue^{-1}. Tomographic images are displayed on television screens with a gray scale in proportion to local cerebral metabolic rate for glucose (with black being the highest) and numerical values are shown beside the scale. Lines drawn through the head show that a single detector on the patient's right side can seek out annihilation coincidences occurring in the multiple detectors on the other side of the head. From Phelps et al. (38).

STUDIES OF NORMAL SUBJECTS WITH PET

The measurement of functional brain responses with PET has been clearly demonstrated by the use of sensory, motor, and neurobehavioral stimulation paradigms in normal subjects (17,22). The effects of visual (6,7,14,19,21,33,36,39,43), auditory (7,15,19–21,39,45), somatosensory (2,7), and motor tasks (18,41), have already been reported in normal individuals. The ability to activate functionally cerebral structures in a consistent way using neurobehavioral paradigms and PET allows for the selective stimulation of these areas in patients with minimal abnormalities on "resting" or baseline PET studies (17). Thus, these studies allow, for the first time in humans, local examination of the functional organization of the brain in response to specific stimuli including language. Such investigations provide an opportunity in normal subjects to validate or refute and extend knowledge gained from electrophysiological stimulation of the human brain (i.e., intraoperative), human symptom-lesion studies, and experimental investigations in animals of the functional organization of the brain.

In addition to the evaluation of normal subjects, the comprehensive investigation of sensory, motor, and cognitive tasks in normal populations will provide a set of

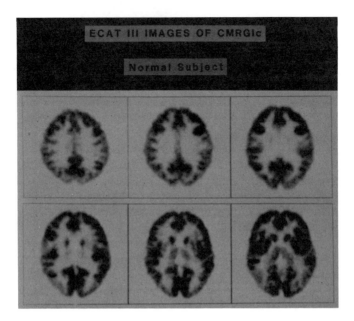

FIG. 2. FDG-PET images obtained with the ECAT III (CTI, Knoxville, TN) tomograph at 5-mm intervals parallel to the canthomeatal plane. This imaging system has a spatial resolution of approximately 5 mm in the transverse direction and 9 mm in the axial direction. Note the improved spatial resolution in comparison with the NeuroECAT (CTI, Knoxville, TN) images seen in Figs. 4–6. In particular, one can see the detailed folding pattern of the cortex, the position of the central sulcus, the clear identification of both the anterior and posterior limbs of the internal capsule as well as the separation of the basal ganglia structures from the overlying insula cortex. With spatial resolution of this quality, detailed functional studies of cortical responses in health and disease can be identified and physiological or pharmacological activations of both cortical and subcortical substructures (e.g., subportions of the striatum and thalamus) could be specifically identified. From Phelps et al. (37).

paradigms that predictively activate specific cortical and subcortical brain regions during language tasks. These paradigms can then be used in patient populations to unmask more subtle alterations in metabolism, flow, or physiological variables that may go undetected in simple resting PET imaging sessions (17). The use of such provocative behavioral stimuli should enhance the specificity and anatomical localization of functional lesions such as those described in patients with various types of language disorders. Lastly, stimulation paradigms can also be used to study the recovery of language function following cerebral injury (17). For example, consider the following situation: First, a task is selected that produces a focal activation of a given brain region, as determined by PET, during a language task. Second, a patient population is identified as containing individuals who can perform the task (perhaps with less efficiency than normal individuals) but who have clear evidence from X-ray CT or resting PET studies of abnormalities within the structures identified as participating in this language task in the normal population. Last, a set of images is obtained when these patients are performing the specific task. The resultant data should provide clues as to how the brain functionally reorganizes or adapts to perform a task even though the system identified for the normal performance of that language function has been compromised by cerebral abnormalities. Such studies should not only provide insights into fundamental processes of cerebral language comprehension and generation after injury but can also potentially provide guidelines for the pathophysiologically oriented rehabilitation of such brain injured individuals. The problems and strategies inherent in designing behavioral paradigms for PET have been reviewed (10,17).

While little information has been obtained with PET for the study of speech production, there have been a number of studies that have examined the local cerebral metabolic and flow responses to verbal and nonverbal auditory stimulation. Initial studies of the auditory system measured LCMRGlc and were performed by Reivich et al. (39) using monaurally presented factual stories. They reported 20% to 25% increases in LCMRGlc in the entire right temporal lobe regardless of the ear stimulated. This was true whether the story was meaningful or nonmeaningful (i.e., foreign language). In six subjects (three left, three right) who listened monaurally to a factual story, Greenberg et al. (7) found a 7.0% ± 2.5% LCMRGlc asymmetry for the temporal cortex. The higher value was consistently contralateral to the ear stimulated.

In contrast to the above studies, Mazziotta et al. (20,21) demonstrated that the stimulus content rather than the side of stimulation determined the site of greatest functional activation (Fig. 3). Right-handed subjects were monaurally presented (equal number in each group had left or right ear stimulation) with either a factual story or one of two types of nonverbal, auditory stimuli. All studies were compared with control LCMRGlc studies obtained in the same subjects with their ears plugged and covered with soundproof headphones. Regardless of the stimulus employed, the distribution of LCMRGlc in the PET images accurately demonstrated the known anatomical asymmetries of the temporal cortex (Fig. 4).

Verbal stimuli produced left-sided (frontal, temporal) metabolic asymmetries, left thalamic activation, and bilateral transverse and posterior temporal cortical activations (Fig. 3) (20,21). Nonverbal stimuli with chord pairs produced right-sided activations and asymmetries as well as bilateral inferior parietal activations. Nonverbal stimuli consisting of pairs of tone sequences produced metabolic responses that correlated with the analysis strategy employed by the subject. Individuals who used stereotyped visual imagery approaches (e.g., "I saw bar graphs of the frequencies in my mind") or who were musically sophisticated had left > right temporal metabolic asymmetries. Conversely, subjects who used less stereotyped strategies and who were musically naive have diffuse right-sided activations and metabolic asymmetries (Fig. 3). Thus, auditory stimulations resulted in changes that varied with the content of the stimulus and the analysis strategy (Fig. 3) (20). It is notable that these were the first studies to demonstrate frontal cortical responses to specific tasks. Like the temporal and parietal responses, the frontal cortical metabolic activations varied with stimulus, causing metabolic asymmetries that followed the left-right responses noted above for the posterior brain regions.

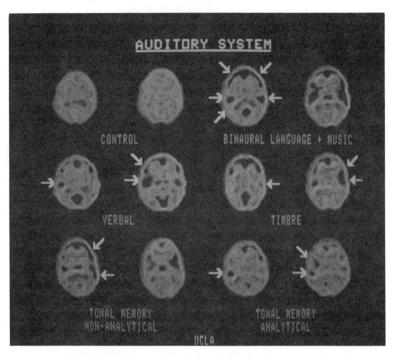

FIG. 3. Examples of LCMRGlc measured with PET and FDG during a variety of states of auditory stimulation. For each state a pair of images is shown, the left image 10 mm above the right. Upper left images represent the control state, with ears closed by rubber stoppers and covered by soundproof headphones (eyes open). Upper right images were obtained during bilateral stimulation with language (Sherlock Holmes story) and music (Brandenburg Concerto). In this state, subjects demonstrated diffuse activations of both posterior temporal and frontal lobes. The verbal stimulation consisted of a monaural presentation of the Sherlock Holmes story alone and resulted in diffuse left-sided activity, with the frontal lobe activation being greater on the left, and bilateral posterior temporal and left temporo-occipital activations. The responses to nonverbal auditory stimuli are also shown. The timbre test required subjects to identify chords that differed only in harmonic composition. All subjects had diffuse right-sided activations and asymmetries, and bilateral temporoparietal activations. Nonverbal stimulation with tone sequences resulted in activations dependent on the subject's analysis strategy. Musical sophistication or use of highly stereotyped visual imagery strategies produced left > right metabolic asymmetries, whereas subjects who were musically naive and used less stereotyped strategies had diffuse right-sided activations similar to the timbre test results. From Mazziotta et al. (20).

It should be noted that PET studies of auditory comprehension of verbal information have shown very complex patterns of metabolic responses. The above described responses indicate the areas of maximal change in the magnitude of LCMRGlc between resting and stimulated states and areas of significant laterality. This is not to say that large numbers of brain regions respond to auditory stimuli of any type. Thus, the most striking impression of any PET study of auditory stimulation is the diversity and complexity of the response (both increases and decreases in metabolic activity) that occur when a subject performs even the most limited auditory task. The time course of these responses is crucial to any stimulation

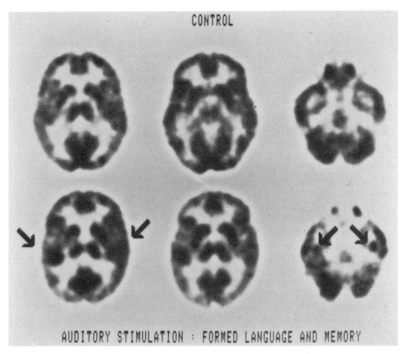

FIG. 4. PET-FDG images of cerebral metabolism of a subject in a control state (ears plugged and covered with soundproof headphones) and of a separate individual during verbal stimulation (Sherlock Holmes story). Note, in the stimulated state, that the increased metabolic activity in the transverse temporal cortex appears to be distributed in an asymmetric fashion between the left and right hemispheres. In the left hemisphere this area was circular and more posterior and encompassed two tomographic levels. The area of activation in the right hemisphere was more discrete and more anterior and had a band-like shape. These asymmetries closely parallel known anatomic asymmetries for Heschl's gyri and the planum temporale. Note also the structure that demonstrated bilateral activation in the inferior (right-most image) tomographic plane. This structure corresponds to the anatomic position of the hippocampus and anterior parahippocampal gyrus. Although not visualized in the control state, this structure was consistently activated and visualized in verbal stimulation studies that have been performed with a memory requirement. Using lower resolution images (as in Fig. 3), it would not be possible to see this structure. It is not yet clear whether activation of the hippocampal area reflects a component of the auditory tasks, specific analysis strategies, some aspect of memory processing and learning employed by the subjects in order to perform well on the poststimulation examination, or some combination of these factors. From Mazziotta et al. (20).

paradigm that one may develop for use with PET either in normal subjects or as a probe to investigate language disorders in patients (45).

Finally, when more than one task is required of the subject, changes in metabolic pattern occur. This was true of subjects studied in our laboratory who were given auditory recognition tasks of verbal information with a specific memory requirement (20) (Fig. 4). PET imaging was obtained from subjects who listened to verbal, monaural auditory stimuli (Sherlock Holmes story) who were required to remember specific aspects of its content. Images from these subjects demonstrated increases in glucose utilization that were similar to subjects asked only to listen to the story without the memory component. However, in addition to the responses noted above for the verbal auditory perception (i.e., large areas of left > right cortical activations in glucose metabolism), bilateral activations of mesial temporal structures were seen only in the stimulated state with the memory requirement and never in control situations (Fig. 4) (20). This was a complex task involving auditory perception, decoding, and encoding of material that the subject was asked to remember, therefore, it was not possible to specifically identify which cerebral structures were responding to which aspects in this complex task. However, in other auditory stimulation paradigms, in which no memory requirement was demanded of the subject, mesial temporal responses (hippocampus, parahippocampus) were not seen. At present, it is unclear whether this mesial temporal response is the result of certain aspects of the auditory task itself, attentional factors, the memory requirement of the task, some combination of these factors, or some other component of the paradigm.

The understanding of how specific language and memory tasks activate brain structures, will be helpful in classifying patients with language disorders and aphasic syndromes. It is interesting to consider how such a strategy might be used with PET. It seems clear that carefully contrived paradigms will have to be developed and slight variations in each paradigm compared with PET to unravel task-related differences in the metabolic or blood flow responses in normal individuals and then apply these to patient populations. Functional activation studies performed with PET, therefore, serve not only to map the normal cerebral responses of human subjects to stimuli, but can also be developed as probes to stress minimally dysfunctioning brain tissue in patients with suspected or known language abnormalities (17).

HUMAN BRAIN METABOLIC DEVELOPMENT AND RELATION TO LANGUAGE ABILITIES

In order to understand fully the cerebral processes that are active in human language information processing, the understanding of language acquisition during development is important. Additionally, this information is a necessary prelude to understanding abnormalities in language acquisition during childhood. In our laboratory at the University of California, Los Angeles, more than 100 children with various neurological disorders were studied with FDG and PET to determine glucose metabolic rates (4,5). Retrospectively, 29 children (age five days to 15.1 years), who had suffered transient neurological events but did not have any significant change in their normal neurological development, were selected as reasonably representative of normal children. These children, therefore, provided an otherwise unobtainable population from which to study the changes in local cerebral metabolic rates for glucose that occur during postnatal brain development (Fig. 5) (4,5).

Glucose metabolism in infants less than five weeks old was highest in sensori-motor cortex, thalamus, brainstem, and cerebellar vermis. By three months, LCMRGlc increased in parietal, temporal, and occipital cortices as well as basal ganglia and the cerebellar cortex. Frontal and dorsolateral occipital cortical regions were the last to display a maturational rise in glucose metabolism with increases in LCMRGlc apparent by approximately six to eight months.

Absolute values of glucose metabolism for various gray matter regions were low at birth and rose to reach adult values by approximately two years of age. Subsequently, metabolic rate continued to rise, until, by two to three years, glucose metabolism in most regions reached values that were equal to or greater than a factor of 2 above normal adult metabolic rates. These high rates were maintained until about 10 to 15 years of age, when they gradually began to decline and reach adult values again by the latter part of the second decade. The highest increases in glucose metabolism over adult values occurred in cerebral cortical structures. Lower increases were seen in subcortical structures and in the cerebellum.

This time course of glucose metabolic changes matches that described for the process of the initial overproduction and subsequent elimination of excessive neurones, synapses, and dendritic spines known to occur in the developing brain. Thus, PET has been and can be used to determine the normal maturational process of cerebral function in the "resting" child.

It may be possible to combine these studies in children with behavioral stimulation paradigms noted in the previous section. Using such a strategy, children with normal neurological development (such as those described above, those being studied with FDG-PET for other reasons, e.g., cardiac disease, or children with systemic malignancies about to undergo total body and cerebral radiation therapy) could be studied at various stages of known language acquisition during maturation and development. Once such studies were completed, and baseline information was available for the structure-function relationships of the developing brain for language tasks, these could be applied to children who had delayed, arrested, or regression of language function during infancy and childhood.

PET has been used for the evaluation of individuals with autism. Rumsey et al. (42) studied 10 men, with a mean age of 26 years, who had well documented histories of infantile autism and compared these PET results for glucose metabolism with 15 age-matched normal male controls. These studies were performed in a resting state with reduced visual and auditory stimulation. Although the patient group, as a whole, showed significantly elevated glucose utilization in widespread regions of the brain, there was considerable overlap between the patients and the controls. No brain regions showed a reduced metabolic rate in the autistic subjects. Significantly more autistic subjects, as compared with controls, showed extreme relative metabolic rates (ratios of regional metabolic rates to whole brain rates and asymmetries) in one or more brain regions.

The finding of elevated glucose metabolism in a disorder that presents during childhood is not unique. Glucose metabolic rates determined with PET in adult subjects with Down's syndrome (44) has been reported. The finding of elevated

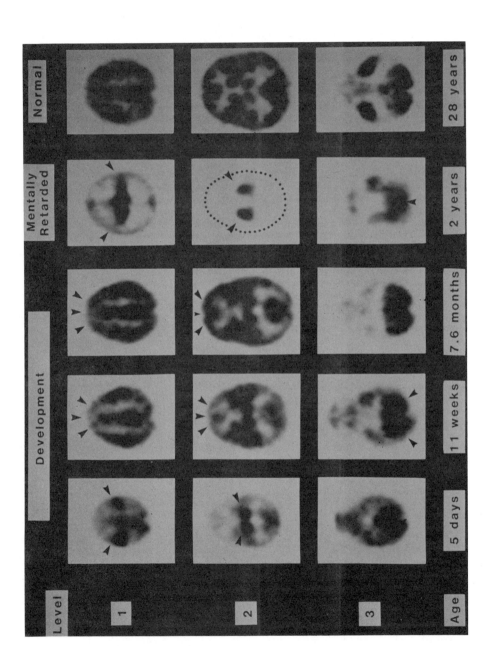

glucose metabolism in Down's and autistic subjects raises an intriguing possibility in light of the maturational data presented above. Is it not possible that a number of developmental disorders, including disorders of language acquisition, are the result of nonselective or absent elimination of neurones and/or synapses during development? Since the PET determination of glucose metabolism is weighted toward a reflection of synaptic activity, the data from the Down's (44) and autism (42) studies would be in keeping with such a hypothesis. Specific paradigms to test this and other hypotheses of altered language acquisition will be of great interest in the future and will undoubtedly be an active area of research with PET.

THE STUDY OF PATIENTS WITH ADULT LANGUAGE DISORDERS

The ability to make functional measurements of physiological or biochemical and hemodynamic processes allows for an earlier and significantly more comprehensive perspective of pathological processes that can be obtained from structural information alone. All neuropathological states affect or are caused by changes in cerebral biochemistry. In general, subtle alterations of these processes precede structural changes that are detectable by more conventional radiological approaches. The measurement of the biochemical process, therefore, should allow for earlier detection of these processes and a better understanding of their fundamental mechanisms. Examples are available that demonstrate the ability of PET to identify functional abnormalities in excess and earlier than those seen structurally (Figs. 6 and 7). In fact, such data indicate that functional images obtained with PET may provide information in excess of that which could be obtained even with the ultimate structural imaging technique, microscopic examination of cerebral anatomy from postmortem specimens (28).

←————————————————————————————————

FIG. 5. Use of PET measurements of LCMRGlc with FDG to map the distribution of functional maturation in humans. Levels 1, 2, and 3 are from superior to inferior. Level 1 is through the cingulate cortex. Level 2 is at midthalamic level and level 3 passes through the suprasellar cistern and cerebellum. During the first month of life (example at five days) glucose utilization is highest in the primary sensory and motor cortices (*arrows*), thalamus (*arrows*), brainstem, and cerebellum, particularly the vermis (*arrow*). Note the relatively low glucose utilization in the neocortex and striatum. As the brain matures, energy requirements of those structures reaching functional neuronal development increase, and at about three months of age glucose utilization has increased in many cortical areas, particularly the neocortical regions, with the exception of frontal cortex (*arrows*). Note that striatal activity has also now increased significantly at a time when the normal physiological chorea of children is also subsiding. By about eight months, the glucose utilization approaches that of the adult. The examples of the cerebral maturation pattern shown with glucose utilization closely parallel, in time, functional (i.e., motor, behavioral, and cognitive) maturation. When the brain sustains a severe insult in the perinatal state, such as a hypoxic-ischemic encephalopathy (fourth column), the cerebral maturation process, at least as indicated by glucose utilization, appears to be halted. Thus, even though the images of child shown in this column are from a two-year-old, the glucose utilization pattern of functional cerebral maturation more closely resembles that of a child a few days of age. This is consistent with the child's state of mental retardation. The apparent lack of glucose utilization throughout the brain is not seen in level 2 because the ratio of thalamus (*arrows*) to the remainder of the cerebral structures is beyond the limits of the photographic gray scale. From Chugani and Phelps (4).

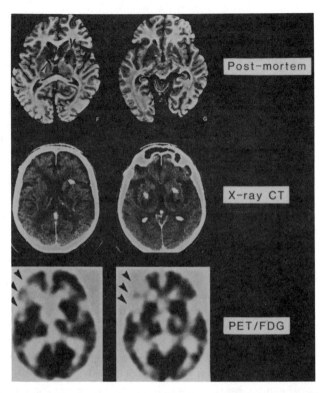

FIG. 6. Structural versus functional anatomy. Images obtained with three different methods from a patient with multiple infarct dementia. Patient had X-ray CT (center row) and PET studies of LCMRGlc with FDG (bottom row) on the same day. Seven days later patient died of non-neurological causes (GI hemorrhage), and gross and microscopic evaluations of the brain (top row) were performed. Both forms of structural imaging (X-ray CT and postmortem) and the metabolic study with PET demonstrated multiple small infarctions of deep structures of the brain (striatum, thalamus, and internal capsule). Neither structural imaging technique demonstrated abnormalities of the cortex. PET, however, demonstrated widespread abnormalities of frontal cortex, particularly on the left. These distant effects probably represent disruption of afferent and efferent fiber systems between the frontal cortical areas and subcortical zones, most likely resulting from small subcortical infarcts seen structurally and metabolically. From Metter et al. (28).

In general, functional lesions identified with PET are greater in extent and magnitude than those seen structurally with techniques such as X-ray CT (Figs. 6 and 7). This more comprehensive view of cerebral pathophysiology, when correlated with specific language signs and symptoms, should provide a better understanding of the structure-function relationships of language in the brain in both health and disease. Therefore, the earliest observations using xenon-133 cerebral blood flow measurements that described functional changes in excess of structural abnormalities in patients (47) have been supported by PET studies of patients with aphasic syndromes.

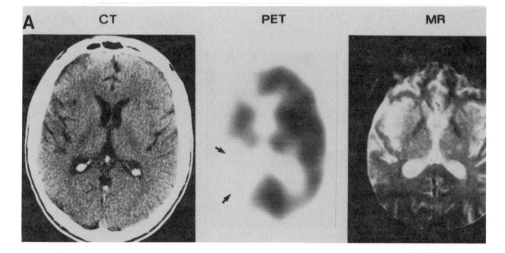

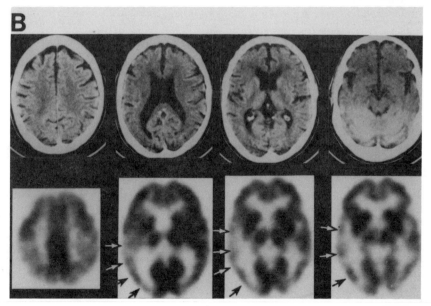

APHASIA

The initial studies of aphasic patients using PET were performed by Metter et al. (23–26,29–31) using FDG to determine cerebral glucose utilization. These and more recent work have provided a number of generalizations about stroke-induced language disorders in adult patients. As was noted above, metabolic abnormalities that result from cerebral infarction and produce language disorders typically have much more widespread regions of functional derangement than structural imaging studies would predict (Figs. 6–10). Thus, whereas a small infarction involving the posterior temporal and inferior parietal cortex might be demonstrated by X-ray CT, PET studies of glucose metabolism might show not only these structural lesions but also the disconnection of deep (thalamus and basal ganglia) and distant cortical (frontal and inferior temporal) brain regions. The composite of these structural and functional effects might be expected to correlate more closely with the resultant language disorder syndrome.

The analysis of patterns of metabolic derangement in language disorders may be instructive and provide insights into the validity and mechanisms underlying various

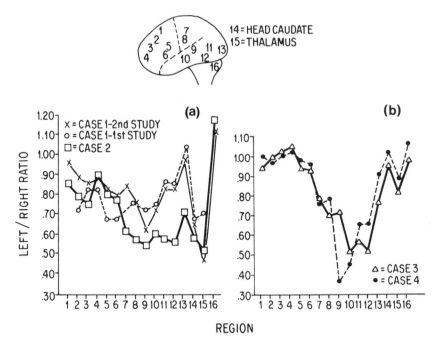

FIG. 8. Regional left to right glucose metabolic ratios from FDG-PET studies of patients with aphasia. The figure at the top indicates that site of the regions indicated on the x-axis of the graphs. In normal subjects, these left-right ratios (for all regions) are in the range of 1.00 ± 0.03. (a) Midputaminal hemorrhage patients whose images are seen in Fig. 9. (b) Patients with hemorrhages of the posterior putamen that have extensions into the temporal region. Images of these patients can be seen in Fig. 10. From Metter et al. (25).

clinical classification schemes of language disorders. For example, Metter and co-workers in our laboratory at the University of California, Los Angeles, have studied patients with Broca's, Wernicke's, and conduction aphasias using FDG and PET (Fig. 11) (23,27). These patients had a variety of structural lesions involving typically the posterior portion of the perisylvian cortex. Metabolically all of these patients had severe reductions in metabolism in the postrolandic cortical regions involving both superior temporal and inferior parietal cortex (<50% of the metabolic value of the presumed normal right hemisphere). Differences, however, between the clinical syndromes correlated with changes in metabolic activity that occurred in inferior frontal and prefrontal dorsolateral cortex. In patients with Broca's aphasia, severe (½–⅓ of the contralateral hemisphere) reductions in glucose metabolism were found in these frontal regions. Patients with Wernicke's aphasia demonstrated abnormalities in glucose metabolism in prefrontal cortex in only 50% of the cases. However, most individuals with Wernicke's aphasia had mild to moderate reductions in glucose metabolism (80% of the contralateral hemisphere) for inferior left frontal zones. Patients with conduction aphasia had the most minimal frontal metabolic abnormalities of the left hemisphere. In such patients the inferior posterior frontal cortex was typically only reduced by 15% or less when compared to the contralateral side. Only two of the 10 patients with conduction aphasia had abnormalities in left prefrontal cortex, and these were mild (5%–10% of the contralateral side) in magnitude. It should be noted that these frontal changes were typically seen in the absence of any structural damage (28). Thus, functional and distant effects of structural lesions may be more highly correlated with clinical syndromes than the structural lesion alone (Fig. 7).

Kushner and colleagues (13) compared PET (glucose metabolism), X-ray CT, and clinical findings in 36 patients with acute cerebral infarctions. Two thirds of these patients were examined within five days of their events, and were followed for an average of three months. Eleven patients were aphasic. They found that the pattern of the metabolic abnormality correlated with the clinical syndrome; that is, regardless of the X-ray CT findings, when the metabolic abnormality was intense, widespread, and multilobar, the clinical syndrome was mixed, heterogeneous, and complex (13). In the majority of cases with multilobar metabolic abnormalities, X-ray CT lesions were confined to only one lobe of a subpart thereof. Of the 11 aphasic patients, 10 had thalamic hypermetabolism despite the fact that thalamic X-ray CT lesions were only seen in three patients. Patients with clinical findings and no structural abnormalities (Fig. 7) had metabolic lesions appropriate to their signs and symptoms (13).

Minimal metabolic alterations were predictive of complete or substantial recovery. Conversely, widespread metabolic changes portended minimal or no improvement. No such relationships were observed between clinical and X-ray CT results (13).

It is clear that the ability to predict a structural lesion in a patient with a clinically demonstrable language disorder is relatively inaccurate. Even more impressive is our inability to predict the presence, absence, or type of language disorder in a patient from merely examining the structural abnormalities of their brain from, for

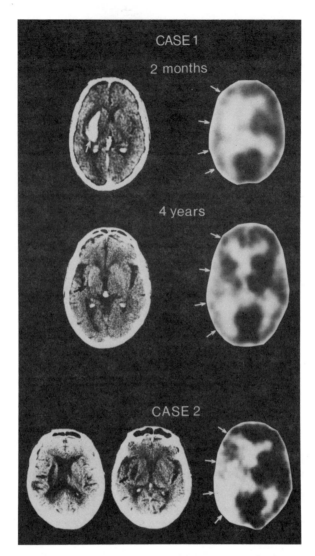

FIG. 9. X-ray CT and FDG-PET studies of two patients with putaminal hemorrhages. Patient 1 was a 51-year-old, right-handed man who developed right hemiparesis and aphasia two months prior to his X-ray CT and PET studies. These studies demonstrate a resolving hemorrhage in the left putamen and left less than right metabolic asymmetries throughout the entire hemisphere. These asymmetries were less in magnitude in frontal than temporal regions. At the time of the study he had a degree of dysarthria with phonemic distortions. Comprehension was normal except for difficulties with complex commands. He was to be categorized as having an anomic aphasia plus dysarthria. Four years later, the patient had only minimal dysphasia and normal memory. X-ray CT at that time showed a slit-like lesion at the site of the original hemorrhage. The PET study showed prominent left less than right metabolic asymmetries. Quantitatively (Fig. 8a), the major metabolic change over four years was a large decline in the thalamic left-right metabolic ratio. Patient 2 was a 67-year-old man with a left putaminal hemorrhage presenting with right hemiplegia and severe aphasia. When studied at six months with PET, his speech was intermittently fluent, including meaningful sentences unrelated to the conversation and at times containing jargon. Articulation was generally accurate, but his voice was weak in intensity. Often, it was difficult to obtain any verbal responses. Verbal and reading comprehension

example, an X-ray CT study. This lack of correlation between clinical presentation, signs and symptoms, and structural anatomy as determined by X-ray CT, MRI, or postmortem examination is indicative of the need for more comprehensive information about structure-function relationships of the brain and their dependent interaction with the formation and residual ability to produce and comprehend language after injury. PET provides this type of information, and when applied in a systematic way may clarify some of the confusing discrepancies between structural lesions and signs and symptoms in patients with language disorders. A number of other language-related deficit syndromes have been reported using PET and FDG to measure glucose metabolism. These have included the study of pure word mutism (12), angular gyrus syndrome (1), crossed dextral aphasic syndrome (3), and pure alexia (46).

CONCLUSION

Functional imaging with PET has already provided new information about the normal response of the human brain to physiological stimuli and to the patterns of pathophysiological derangement that can occur in disease processes associated with language disorders. A number of refinements in techniques and methodology will improve the potential to study these issues in greater detail.

Spatial and temporal resolution of PET methods should improve considerably. Devices are already available that have a spatial resolution capacity for neurologic studies in the range of 4 mm. Such images will provide more accurate quantitative information about physiological processes occurring in smaller cerebral structures.

Techniques that use oxygen-15 labeled compounds to measure cerebral blood flow and oxygen metabolism will provide a means to reduce the measurement time for a stimulation study from 30 to 40 minutes (when using FDG) to 1 to 5 minutes. These stimulus duration reductions will minimize concerns about habituation and acclimatization to the testing environment (17). In addition, the better dosimetry characteristics of short-lived positron-emitting isotopes like oxygen-15 ($t\frac{1}{2}$ = 110 sec) will allow for multiple administrations in the same subject in the same setting. Using such a strategy, a language paradigm could be developed and varied in a way to demonstrate specific components of the complex tasks involved in the perception, decoding, encoding, and production of language-related material. Such paradigms will require sophisticated attention to neuropsychological controls and will need the appropriately sophisticated models for analysis of the resultant data.

---

were also severely impaired. CT and PET studies done at this time demonstrated a persistent large slit-like lesion in the putamen that extended superiorly to cross the internal capsule. This patient had diffuse cortical left less than right metabolic asymmetry most prominent in the temporoparietal regions (Fig. 8a). Thus, these two patients show very similar hemorrhages and metabolic abnormalities although they demonstrated different clinical pictures. The two patients differed metabolically in the posterior temporal and occipital cortices and clinically in the type and severity of their aphasia. From Metter et al. (25).

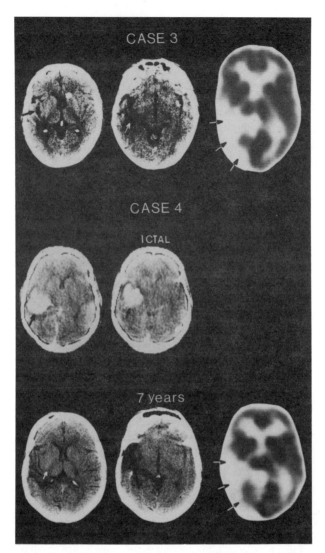

FIG. 10. X-ray CT and FDG-PET studies of patients with posterior putaminal-temporal hemorrhages. Patient 3 was a 62-year-old man studied six months after his intracerebral hemorrhage. At this time he had a conduction aphasia. Memory evaluations showed severe verbal recall problems. X-ray CT and PET studies done at six months posthemorrhage demonstrated encephalomalacia of the posterior putamen, insula, and temporal lobe on the left. The patient had a prominent left less than right metabolic asymmetry of the parietal and temporal lobes. Frontal metabolism was symmetric (Fig. 8b). Patient 4 was a 30-year-old woman with a posterior temporal arteriovenous malformation arising from the anterior choroidal artery. Following her intracerebral hemorrhage, surgical removal of the hematoma resulted in good clinical improvement. When studied seven years later, she had a conduction aphasia and memory abnormalities in verbal, nonverbal, and perceptual domains. X-ray CT demonstrated residual temporal lobe damage extending into and including the posterior putamen. Metabolically, her PET studies showed left less than right metabolic asymmetries throughout the temporoparietal regions. Frontal metabolism was symmetric (Fig. 8b). These two patients showed similar aphasic abnormalities, structural defects, and metabolic patterns. Patients 2 (Fig. 9), 3, and 4 had the most severe persisting aphasias and showed the most prominent posterior temporal metabolic asymmetries. This degree of metabolic asymmetry was not noted in patients with more mild aphasic syndromes. From Metter et al. (25).

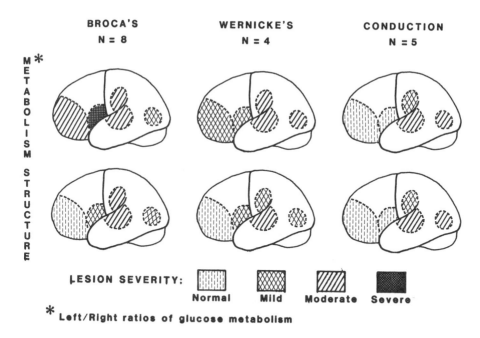

FIG. 11. Structure-function relationships in aphasia. Images depict left hemisphere cortical metabolic (FDG-PET) (top row) and structural (X-ray CT) (bottom row) abnormalities in 17 aphasic patients studied with each approach. Lesion severity was assessed metabolically by the percent reduction in glucose metabolism of the left brain region relative to the contralateral hemisphere. Structural changes were graded by their qualitative appearance on X-ray CT. Note the generally similar patterns of structural damage. The metabolic data are similar in postrolandic regions but correlate with lesion severity (in descending order) relative to Broca's, Wernicke's, and conduction aphasias, respectively.

However, these techniques hold great promise for providing insight into the complex and perhaps heterogeneous functional systems that take part in different language processes.

Once developed, behavioral paradigms that are aimed at language function can be studied, not only in normal adults, but also in children (using the specific ethical considerations noted above). Finally, such paradigms can be transferred to patient populations of individuals with language disorders. As described above, these paradigms would be used as probes to stimulate areas of brain dysfunction and evaluate the functional reserve of damaged tissue and also to examine the recovery of such patients following brain injury. In patients with language disorders secondary to acute events (e.g., cerebral infarction, trauma) behavioral paradigms administered serially over the recovery period may allow for the objective evaluation of the recovery process. Meticulous attention to the control of speech therapy and environmental factors will be crucial in performing a proper study of this sort. Similarly, infant stimulation programs that may or may not benefit language acquisition in children with cerebral disorders could be evaluated using a similar strategy. In patients with degenerative disorders that include abnormalities of language function (e.g., Alzheimer's disease), serial studies should demonstrate functional systems that are operational and act to preserve function in the face of ongoing structural damage.

The study of language function and its abnormalities in adults and children with PET is at a beginning stage. Many problems remain to be investigated and will require methodological improvements and experimental design refinements for their success. However, the available techniques provide previously unattainable information in humans. These issues represent unique and challenging new endeavors for the neurosciences.

ACKNOWLEDGMENTS

The authors extend special thanks to all the various investigators who so generously contributed their time, data, and comments. We are grateful to Lee Griswold for the preparation of the illustrative materials and to Anita Powers and Maggie Marquez for preparing the manuscript. This work was partially supported by DOE contract AMO3-76-SF00012, NIH grants RO1-6M-248388 and PO1-NS-15-654, and NIMH grant RO1-MH-37916. Dr. Mazziotta is the recipient of Teacher Investigator award 1K07-00588-05-NSPA.

REFERENCES

1. Benson, D.F., Cummings, J.L., and Tsai, S.Y. (1982): Angular gyrus syndrome simulating Alzheimer's disease. *Arch. Neurol.*, 39:616–620.
2. Buchsbaum, M.S., Holcomb, H.H., Johnson, J., King, A.C., and Kessler, R. (1983): Cerebral metabolic consequences of electrical cutaneous stimulation in normal individuals. *Hum. Neurobiol.*, 2:35–38.
3. Black, S.E., Gornett, E.S., Nicholson, R.L., Nahmias, C.C., and Kertesz, A. (1984): Nuclear magnetic resonance and PET findings in a crossed dextral aphasic patient. *Ann. Neurol.*, 16:155.
4. Chugani, H.T., and Phelps, M.E. (1986): Maturational changes in cerebral function in infants determined by [18]FDG positron emission tomography. *Science*, 231:840–843.
5. Chugani, H.T., Phelps, M.E., and Mazziotta, J.C. Human brain functional development: A study of local cerebral glucose metabolism with 2-deoxy-2-[18F]-fluoro-D-glucose positron emission tomography. *Ann. Neurol. (in press).*
6. Fox, P.T., and Raichle, M.E. (1984): Stimulus rate dependence of regional cerebral blood flow in human striate cortex demonstrated by positron emission tomography. *J. Neurophysiol.*, 51:1109–1121.
7. Greenberg, J., Reivich, M., Alavi, A., et al. (1981): Metabolic mapping of functional activity in human subjects with the [18F] fluorodeoxyglucose technique. *Science*, 212:678–680.
8. Gustafsan, L., Hagberg, B., and Ingvar, D.H. (1978): Speech disturbances in presenile dementia related to local cerebral blood flow abnormalities in the dominant hemisphere. *Brain Lang.*, 5:103–118.
9. Ingvar, D.H., and Schwartz, M.S. (1974): Blood flow patterns induced in the dominant hemisphere by speech and reading. *Brain*, 97:273–288.
10. Kearfott, K., Rottenberg, D.A., and Volpe, B.T. (1983): Design of steady-state positron emission tomography protocols for neurobehavioral studies: CO[15]0 and [19]Ne. *J. Comput. Assist. Tomogr.*, 7:51–58.
11. Knopman, D.S., Rubens, A.B., Selnes, O.A., Klassen, A.C., and Meyer, M.W. (1984): Mechanisms of recovery from aphasia: Evidence from serial xenon 133 cerebral blood flow studies. *Ann. Neurol.*, 15:530–535.

12. Kushner, M.J., Reivich, M., Alavi, A., Greenberg, J., Stern, M., and Dam, R. (1982): A PET study of the pathophysiology of pure word mutism. *Neurology*, 32:A125.
13. Kushner, M., Reivich, M., Fieschi, C., et al. Metabolic and clinical correlates of acute ischemic infarction. *Neurology*, 34(Suppl. 1):281.
14. Kushner, M.J., Rosenquist, A., Alavi, A., et al. (1982): Macular and peripheral visual field representation in the striate cortex demonstrated by positron emission tomography. *Ann. Neurol.*, 12:89.
15. Kushner, M.J., Schwartz, R., Dann, R., Alavi, A., and Reivich, M. (1984): Cerebral activation by nonmeaningful monaural verbal stimulation: A PET study. *Neurology*, 34(Suppl. 1):117.
16. Larson, B., Skinhoj, E., and Larsen, N.A. (1978): Variations in regional cortical blood flow in the right and left hemispheres during automatic speech. *Brain*, 101:193–209.
17. Mazziotta, J.C., and Phelps, E. (1984): Human sensory stimulation and deprivation. PET results and strategies. *Ann. Neurol.*, 15:S50–S60.
18. Mazziotta, J.C., and Phelps, M.E. (1984): Positron computed tomography studies of cerebral metabolic responses to complex motor tasks. *Neurology*, 34(Suppl. 1):116.
19. Mazziotta, J.C., Phelps, M.E., and Carson, R.E. (1984): Tomographic mapping of human cerebral metabolism: Subcortical responses to auditory and visual stimulation. *Neurology*, 34:825–828.
20. Mazziotta, J.C., Phelps, M.E., Carson, R.E., et al. (1982): Tomographic mapping of human cerebral metabolism: Auditory stimulation. *Neurology*, 32:921–937.
21. Mazziotta, J.C., Phelps, M.E., and Halgren, E. (1983): Local cerebral glucose metabolic responses to audiovisual stimulation and deprivation: Studies in human subjects with positron CT. *Hum. Neurobiol.*, 2:11–23.
22. Mazziotta, J.C., Phelps, M.E., Halgren, E., Carson, R.E., Huang, S.C., and Bayer, J. (1983): Hemispheric lateralization and local cerebral metabolic blood flow responses to physiologic stimuli. *J. Cereb. Blood Flow Metab.*, 3(Suppl. 1):S246–S247.
23. Metter, E.J., and Hanson, W.R. (1985): Brain imaging as related to speech and language. In: *Speech and Language Evaluation in Neurology: Adult Disorders*, edited by J.K. Darby, pp. 123–160. Grune and Stratton, Orlando, FL.
24. Metter, E.J., Jackson, C.A., Kempler, D., et al. (1986): Glucose metabolic asymmetries in chronic Wernicke's, Broca's and conductions aphasias. *Neurology*, 36(Suppl. 1):317.
25. Metter, E.J., Jackson, C.A., Kempler, D., et al. (1986): Left hemisphere intracerebral hemorrhages studied by (F-18)-fluorodeoxyglucose PET. *Neurology*, 36:1155–1162.
26. Metter, E.J., Jackson, C.A., Mazziotta, J.C., et al. (1985): Relationship of temporoparietal lesions and distant glucose metabolic changes in the head of the caudate nucleus in aphasic patients. *J. Cereb. Blood Flow Metab.*, 5(Suppl. 1):S43–S44.
27. Metter, E.J., Kempler, D., Jackson, C.A., Hanson, W.R., Mazziotta, J.C., and Phelps, M.E. Cerebral glucose metabolism: Differences in Wernicke's, Broca's and conduction aphasia. In: *Clinical Aphasiology, 1986*, edited by R.H. Brookshire. BRK Publishers, Minneapolis (*in press*).
28. Metter, E.J., Mazziotta, J.C., Itabashi, H., Mankovich, N.J., Kuhl, D.E., and Phelps, M.E. (1985): Comparison of X-ray CT, glucose metabolism and postmortem data in a patient with multiple cerebral infarctions. *Neurology*, 35:1695–1701.
29. Metter, E.J., Riege, W.H., Hanson, W.R., et al. (1983): Comparison of metabolic rates, language and memory in subcortical aphasia. *Brain Lang.*, 19:33–47.
30. Metter, E.J., Riege, W.H., Hanson, W.R., Phelps, M.E., and Kuhl, D.E. (1982): Role of the caudate nucleus in aphasic language: Evidence from FDG-PET. *Neurology*, 32:A94.
31. Metter, E.J., Waterlain, C.G., Kuhl, D.E., et al. (1981): [18]FDG positron emission computed tomography: A study of aphasia. *Ann. Neurol.*, 10:173–183.
32. Meyer, J.S., Sakai, F., Yamaguchi, F., Yamamoto, M., and Shaw, T. (1980): Regional changes in cerebral blood flow during standard behavioral activation in patients with disorders of speech and mentation compared to normal volunteers. *Brain. Lang.*, 9:61–77.
33. Phelps, M.E., Kuhl, D.E., and Mazziotta, J.C. (1981): Metabolic mapping of the brain's response to visual stimulation: Studies in man. *Science*, 211:1445–1448.
34. Phelps, M.E., and Mazziotta, J.C. (1985): PET: Human brain function and biochemistry. *Science*, 228:799–809.
35. Phelps, M.E., Mazziotta, J.C., and Huang, S.C. (1982): Study of cerebral function with positron computed tomography. *J. Cereb. Blood Flow Metab.*, 2:113–162.
36. Phelps, M.E., Mazziotta, J.C., Kuhl, D.E., et al. (1981): Tomographic mapping of human cerebral metabolism: Visual stimulation and deprivation. *Neurology*, 31:517–529.

37. Phelps, M.E., Mazziotta, J.C., and Schelbert, H.R. (eds.) (1986): *Positron Emission Tomography and Autoradiography: Principles and Applications for the Brain and Heart.* Raven Press, New York.
38. Phelps, M.E., Schelbert, H.R., and Mazziotta, J.C. (1983): Positron computed tomography for studies of myocardial and cerebral function. *Ann. Intern. Med.*, 98:339–359.
39. Reivich, M., Greenberg, J., Alavi, A., et al. (1979): The use of the ^{18}F-fluorodeoxyglucose technique for mapping functional neural pathways in man. *Acta Neurol. Scand.*, 60(Suppl. 72):198–199.
40. Reivich, M., Kuhl, D., Wolf, A., et al. (1979): The [^{18}F] fluorodeoxyglucose method for the measurement of local cerebral glucose utilization in man. *Circ. Res.*, 44:127–137.
41. Roland, P.E., Meyer, E., Shibaski, T., et al. (1982): Regional cerebral blood flow changes in cortex and basal ganglia during voluntary movements in normal volunteers. *J. Neurophysiol.*, 48:467–480.
42. Rumsey, J.M., Duara, R., Grady, C., et al. (1985): Brain metabolism in autism. *Arch. Gen. Psychiatry*, 42:448–455.
43. Schwartz, E.L., Christman, D.R., and Wolf, A.P. (1984): Human primary visual cortex topography imaged via positron tomography. *Brain Res.*, 294:225–230.
44. Schwartz, M., Duara, R., Hoxby, J., et al. (1983): Brain metabolism in Down syndrome. *Science*, 221:181–183.
45. Sidtis, J.J., Kearfott, K.J., Dhawan, V., Jorden, J.O., and Ruttenberg, D.A. (1984): Positron emission tomography measurement of regional cerebral blood flow during auditory stimulation. *Ann. Neurol.*, 16:116.
46. Silver, F.L., Bosley, T.M., Chawluk, T.B., et al. (1985): Resolving metabolic abnormalities in a case of pure alexia. *Neurology*, 35(Suppl. 1):180.
47. Soh, K., Larsen, B., Skinhoj, E., and Lassen, N.A. (1978): Regional cerebral blood flow in aphasia. *Arch. Neurol.*, 35:625–632.

Language, Communication, and
the Brain, edited by F. Plum.
Raven Press, New York © 1988.

Measuring Aphasia Treatment Effects: Large-Group, Small-Group, and Single-Subject Studies

*Audrey L. Holland and †Robert T. Wertz

*Departments of Otolaryngology, Psychiatry, and Communications, University of
Pittsburgh, Pittsburgh, Pennsylvania 15213, and †Veterans Administration Medical
Center, Martinez, California 94553

Individuals who provide speech and language intervention to aphasic adults are continually required to defend their positions regarding the efficacy of those interventions. But generally, the question "Does therapy work?" bores practitioners. For defensive purposes, but also possibly to escape the boredom, clinical researchers who are concerned with aphasia have been meticulous about producing efficacy data, in larger quantities than exist for any other speech or language disorder. Researchers have produced large-group studies addressing the general question, and small-group studies designed to test the efficacy of particular treatment approaches and to determine which methods might best apply to which patients. They have produced a plethora of case reports and single-subject research designs. Further, these clinical researchers have been responsible enough to report failures as well as successes in the matter of treatment. Broadly conceived to include group designs, single-subject designs, and case studies, there are at least 114 studies addressing the efficacy of aphasia rehabilitation (2). Certainly not all, but the clear majority of these studies attest to the efficacy of treatment to *improve* the aphasic condition, but not, of course, to eradicate it. Nevertheless, clinical aphasiologists continue to be asked about efficacy. There are three reasons for the difficulty that others have in evaluating the research that is available on the subject. These reasons are as follows:

1. Failure on the part of clinical investigators, journal reviewers, and consumers of clinical research to appreciate the elements of rigorous experimental design as they apply to large-group studies of aphasia treatment. This results both in flawed research appearing in the literature and uncritical appraisal of published research by its readership.

2. Failure, again on the part of investigators, journal reviewers, and consumers, to understand advances in the techniques of small-group and single-subject research. This results in a tendency by the readership to dismiss a well-controlled small-group

or single-subject study as producing less solid evidence than even a badly conceived large-group study might produce.

3. The third source is a natural consequence of what happens when evidence contradicts a traditional and widely held belief. In this case, it is the medical folk mythology, still inculcated into medical students, that all the language and cognitive return one finds following stroke comes from the undeniably powerful mechanism of spontaneous recovery. Consider these statements for example.

> In light of the foregoing discussion, it will come as no surprise to learn that definitive answers to questions about the degree of recovery possible after an aphasia and the role that therapy may play in augmenting such recovery do not, at the moment, exist (6).
> Speech was a late evolutionary development, distinguishing man from other species, so it is hardly surprising that this complex function has to date defied satisfactory analysis. This is reflected in the multiplicity of classifications of speech disorders of dysphasic type. Hence prognosis is difficult and, in turn, assessment of the value of therapy is virtually impossible (4).

The result is that studies purporting to disprove the efficacy of treatment get bigger and better press than do studies with positive answers.

These three factors probably always interact, with the last being the most potent. Nevertheless, researchers, reviewers, and consumers can be instructed on the first two. The intent of this chapter is to provide a first step in such instruction, using several studies as illustrations. This chapter also considers the fates of efficacy studies when they fly in the face of a contradictory belief system.

LARGE-GROUP STUDIES OF EFFICACY OF TREATMENT

Given the heterogeneity of the aphasic population and the facts of aphasia, a good group study of efficacy of treatment is exceedingly difficult to do. This results in a tendency for researchers to shrug off the difficulties and cut corners on matters of experimental control and design. This, in turn, produces questionable data and logically opens the research to reactions stemming from the belief system. Unfortunately, most of the large-group studies in aphasia have design problems. Let us consider briefly the characteristics of the ideal efficacy study in aphasia.

1. Spontaneous recovery complicates the issue of treated recovery. Therefore, early spontaneous restitution of function must be accounted for in treatment studies. This means that random assignment to treatment and no-treatment groups is a necessity for large-group outcome studies.

2. A number of other biologic, medical, and behavioral variables influence treatment. These include age, etiology, severity, and type of aphasia. Therefore, such factors must be adequately controlled. This means that explicit criteria for selection of study subjects must be used.

3. The most ardent supporter of treatment for aphasia would never state that all therapy for aphasia is equal. One defines a good therapist by the quality of the

treatment he or she provides. To get around the issue of quality, large-group outcome studies must specify, as well as carefully design and control, the treatment regimen.

4. Finally, appropriate statistical methods must be used to analyze the resulting data.

Randomization

Most treatment studies have had to compromise in relation to these four issues. Randomization into treatment and no-treatment groups is a "hell-if-you-do, hell-if-you-don't" problem. Ethical considerations seem to preclude withholding treatment, even by the nonbelievers. The standard solution is to include a self-selected no-treatment group. This is unacceptable because there are many reasons for a person to refuse treatment, and most may bias results. To the best of our knowledge, only the study by Lincoln et al. (5) has assigned patients randomly to a treatment/no-treatment trial. But the recent Veterans Administration (VA) Cooperative Study by Wertz et al. (10) used an ingenious approach to achieve a no-treatment group. The Cooperative study randomly assigned one group of patients to a 12-week treatment trial and delayed treatment in a cohort until 12 weeks had elapsed. This created, by default, a 12-week treatment/no-treatment comparison. Lincoln et al. (5) found no differences between the groups they studied after 24 weeks of treatment. The VA study found statistically significant treatment effects at 12 weeks, with the delayed treatment group catching up by the 24th week. Thus, one study found treatment to be efficacious, the other did not. To examine why these studies produced contradictory results, other experimental design features mentioned earlier must also be examined.

Selection Criteria

Lincoln et al. (5) studied "patients who performed poorly on an aphasia test" following stroke. They excluded those patients whose aphasia was too severe or too mild, or who were too dysarthric. All study subjects were no more than four weeks postonset at entry into the study. This was a good beginning, but unfortunately, Lincoln et al. employed no further selection criteria. The sample mixed first-stroke and multiple-stroke patients, used no criteria to control localization of brain damage, etiology (beyond stroke), sensory acuity, literacy, age, medical complications, and a number of other variables that negatively influence response to treatment. While the Lincoln et al. criteria might produce a representative sample of patients with strokes, they do not produce a representative sample of viable candidates for aphasia therapy following stroke.

The VA Cooperative study also excluded too severe and too mild patients, and controlled time postonset of stroke. In addition, it studied only patients who had had a single thromboembolic stroke confined to the left hemisphere. Further, the study controlled for medical history and status, sensory acuity, literacy, age, and prior treatment. Because of the selection criteria in the VA study, it appears to be a study of treatment for aphasia. Because subjects in the Lincoln study were less stringently selected, it is extremely difficult to call it such. Some of the Lincoln study patients might have had multi-infarct dementia, for example. The high frequency of death and "subsequent illness" reported for both treated and untreated groups, as well as their reported subsequent discovery of a small number of non-stroke etiologies, including tumors, in their sample also testify to the inadequacy of the selection criteria used in a clinical study of "aphasic stroke patients."

Treatment Specificity

The "treated patients" of Lincoln et al. were expected to have two hours per week of treatment for their 24-week treatment period. The form and content of that treatment was neither monitored nor specified. Two hours of treatment per week must be considered minimal, but that is not the central issue. Instead, close examination of their data reveals that less than 13 hours of treatment were given to 38% of the treated patients during the six-month period and only 26% of their total sample received the prescribed amount.

In contrast, closely monitored and carefully specified treatment was given for 8 to 10 hours per week over the 12-week period of interest in the VA study. To make this distinction in treatment even sharper, the majority of the treated group in the Lincoln study would have been dropouts in the VA study.

Statistical Treatment of the Data

Part of the power of random assignment to groups was that it allowed Lincoln et al. to use an analysis of covariance, with severity of aphasia as a covariate. They ignored this power by delaying treatment and using the t statistic instead. This leaves their statistical analysis open to question. This is not necessarily unfortunate in a study that has so many other design flaws; however, the obvious caution is to employ appropriate statistical methods. In contrast, for the VA study, the significance level was set in advance, the N necessary to determine it was specified, and appropriate statistical methods were used.

Group Studies and Belief Systems

It is noteworthy that the VA Cooperative study was rejected by three medical journals before its publication this year. The reasons given for rejection were numerous, including comments that it was "too detailed," "it failed to provide a no-treatment control," and "not of interest to neurologists." *Lancet,* which published the Lincoln study, dealt the VA article a double blow. It not only rejected it but also refused to publish a Letter to the Editor detailing the criticisms of Lincoln outlined above, on the grounds that it had already published enough reactions to the article itself. Incidentally, that Letter to the Editor review finally was published, in the house-organ of the American-Speech-Language and Hearing Association (9), whose readership might have profited from the research criticism, but whose belief systems were already in tune with the article.

SMALL-GROUP STUDIES AND SINGLE-SUBJECT DESIGNS

For some problems that impinge on efficacy, such as the value of a specific approach for managing a specific problem, it is requisite to use small-group or single-subject research designs (3,7). These designs represent a relatively new area of applied technology. In many instances, critics of treatment studies fail to appreciate the extent to which small N designs can circumvent some of the problems inherent in studies of many subjects, for they have provisions for explicit control in areas that continue to plague large group work. For example, the interactive effects of spontaneous recovery and treatment can be averted by using a multiple baseline approach. With this design, the researcher can choose, say, two discrete behaviors that s/he measures until their baselines become stable. At that point, treatment for one behavior is initiated and continued for some time. No treatment is provided for the other behavior, although its baseline continues to be measured. It is obvious that if increases in the trained behavior are disproportionate to changes in second behavior, then training has made the difference. This approach does not require waiting for spontaneous recovery to be complete, and if treatment is initiated during that period, a multiple baseline design provides strong evidence of the value of treatment. This is particularly true when such a study is repeated on a small number of patients.

Single-subject designs can also be used to compare treatments. In a stunningly well-controlled study, Thompson and McReynolds (8) recently compared the effects of a general stimulation approach with a tightly specified prompting approach for retraining the use of wh-interrogatives in agrammatic aphasic patients. Both approaches were used with the same subjects in a counterbalanced design, but involved different training and baseline constructions. For example, training was conducted for ''What?'' constructions, but baselines were also measured for ''Where?'' constructions, and vice versa. The data provided clear-cut evidence of the superiority of the prompting over the stimulation approach. Neither approach generalized to other interrogative forms. This led the authors to speculate about the nature of techniques that must be used to enhance generalization. The point is that this type of fine grain analysis allows clinician-researchers to move from questions such as ''Does therapy work?'' to far more interesting questions such as ''How does therapy work?''.

Details like this are probably not of much interest to those who do not work directly with aphasic patients. Nevertheless, such studies speak to the issue of efficacy of treatment. Pre- and posttraining comparisons concerning specific treatments also are numerous. Their use as efficacy data is affected by the degree to which they satisfy criteria for controlling other explanatory variables, just as is true for large-group studies. It is always fair to ask for more rigorous specification, and seldom are simple pre-post training comparisons sufficient. Some ways to improve pre-post treatment studies are the following:

1. For spontaneous recovery effects, how long poststroke was this treatment procedure instituted? Was a control procedure instituted to address the simple passage of time? For example, as with multiple baselines, in addition to the treated behavior, was behavior on an unrelated task also measured?

2. Were other explanatory variables controlled for? For example, warmth-and-friendliness is frequently cited by critics as an alternative explanation for specific treatment effects. A strong corrective approach is to contrast the effects of only friendliness on another problem with the warm and friendly specific treatment under study.

3. Was treatment specifically described? Such descriptions are necessary to minimize intratherapist effects and increase reliability. Specific description must be an integral part of a new treatment procedure; it also increases the likelihood that resultant data can address the efficacy question.

The bulk of the small, tight studies designed to explore and compare methods of treatment or to develop new ones, are relevant to treatment efficacy. But the efficacy question continues to be asked in its primitive sense, rather than moving on to careful explorations of what works best with whom and at what time. The reason for this has little to do with behavioral science. It has to do with the belief system through which the science is necessarily filtered.

Belief Systems

Scientists have always been required to work in and around the confines of their society's beliefs about the world. The contemporary belief in American medicine is that aphasia therapy is not very useful for aphasic patients. For some aphasic patients such as the elderly victim of a number of strokes that is probably the case. However, for a very substantial segment of the aphasic population, the bulk of the scientific evidence refutes this position, but the evidence is discrepant from the belief. In such a confrontation, evidence typically loses the early rounds.

Mounting evidence coupled with better understanding by the research consumer of the nature of efficacy and treatment research will have a positive effect. A more powerful effect, however, will come from extrascientific experience, such as watching progress in an aphasic family member when his or her language problem is managed directly and well.

But the clinician-researchers have a part to play as well. First it seems necessary for them to abandon the medical impairment model in which aphasia treatment has become mired. By presuming to treat impairments, the profession has become defined as a group of people who fix what is broken, plug up holes in damaged brains, and so forth. This is clearly untenable, and those who practice aphasia rehabilitation know very well that that is not what they do.

The more appropriate framework for clinical aphasiologists involves the concepts of disability and handicap. Beukelman (1) defines disability and handicap in relation to how well and in what ways an impaired individual can participate in his or her normal societal roles. When clinician-researchers begin to discuss intervention effects from these perspectives, confrontation with prevailing beliefs should become easier. For this is what clinical intervention is really all about. Clinical aphasiologists are not naive enough to believe that they fix damaged brains. Rather, they provide alternative compensatory mechanisms or strategies for approximating adequate (if imperfect) means for meeting daily needs. Even though language change is frequently the metric used, the efficacy issue ultimately relates to this domain.

ACKNOWLEDGMENTS

This work was supported by the Veterans Administration Cooperative Studies Program, Medical and Research Service, and by grant NS17495-03 from the National Institutes of Health. We gratefully acknowledge the help of Davida Fromm.

REFERENCES

1. Beukelman, D.R. (1986): Management of dysarthric speakers. Workshop presented at the Annual Meeting, American Speech-Language-Hearing Association, Detroit, MI.
2. Greenhouse, J., Fromm, D. Iyengar, S., Dew, M.A., Holland, A., and Kass, R. (1986): The making of a meta-analysis: A case study of a quantitative review of the aphasia treatment literature. Unpublished Technical Report #379, Department of Statistics, Carnegie Mellon University.
3. Kazdin, A.E. (1982): *Single Case Research Designs: Methods for Clinical and Applied Settings.* Oxford University Press, New York.
4. *Lancet* (1977). Prognosis in aphasia, editorial. 2:24.
5. Lincoln, D.B., Mully, G.P., Jones, A.L., McGuirk, E., Lendrem, W., and Mitchell, J.R.A. (1984): Effectiveness of speech therapy for aphasic stroke patients. *Lancet*, 1:1197–1200.
6. Marshall, J.C., Holmes, J.M., and Newcombe, F. (1975): Fact and theory in recovery from the aphasias. In: *Outcome of Severe Damage to the Central Nervous System.* CIBA Foundation Symposium 34, pp. 245–254. North Holland, New York.
7. McReynolds, L.V., and Kearns, K. (1983): *Single-Subject Experimental Designs in Communicative Disorders.* Pro-Ed., Austin TX.
8. Thompson, C.K., and McReynolds, L.V. (1986): Wh-interrogative production in agrammatic aphasia: An experimental analysis of auditory-visual stimulation and direct-production treatment. *J. Speech. Hear. Res.*, 29:193–205.
9. Wertz, R.T., Deal, J., Holland, A., Kurtzke, G., and Weiss, D. (1986). Comment on an uncontrolled aphasia to treatment trial. ASHA, 28:21–32.
10. Wertz, R.T., Weiss, D., Aten, J., et al. (1986): Comparison of clinic, home, and deferred language treatment for aphasia. *Arch. Neurol.*, 43:653–658.

Language, Communication, and
the Brain, edited by F. Plum.
Raven Press, New York © 1988.

Concluding Remarks: Neuroscience and Cognitive Science in the Study of Language and the Brain

Antonio R. Damasio

*Department of Neurology, The University of Iowa College of Medicine,
Iowa City, Iowa 52242*

The elucidation of the relationships between language and neural function calls for an integration between the sciences of the mind and the brain sciences, understood at multiple levels of structure and operation. The beginnings of such an integration prevailed for a few decades in the second half of the nineteenth century, when psychology and neurology were embodied by the isolated neurologist-scientist. Early in the twentieth century, however, the bond broke down, for a variety of historical reasons having to do with the evolution of the two disciplines. Later, in the period following World War II, the proliferation of new techniques and approaches on both sides of the mind-brain equation gradually introduced even greater distances among areas of endeavor that just barely maintained contact until then. It is reasonable to ask where we stand now, and my own answer is that we are in a transition period that may well lead to a new phase of convergence and integration. This view, I must admit, is likely to be controversial. For instance, not everybody will agree that an integration between cognitive science and neuroscience is timely or even desirable. Others will claim that scientists working on language and brain align themselves more rigidly than ever along different and competing models. Within the limited scope of my remarks, I only discuss the latter claim briefly, in the hope of establishing, with some epistemological reflection, that we are closer than generally agreed to bringing together seemingly disparate domains of knowledge.

Theoretical discussion of research on language and the brain often makes appeal to one of three prominent and competing models: (a) the "lesion" model, generally associated with the names of Wernicke and Geschwind to the point that, unfortunately, they have become virtually synonymous; (b) the "electrophysiological" model, which dates back to the early work of Penfield on the electrical stimulation of cortical language areas and has been given special prominence by Ojemann; and (c) the "linguistic" model, an umbrella that invokes the work of the most influential theoretical linguist of the postwar period, Noam Chomsky, but refers to the activity of a number of cognitive psychologists and psycholinguists.

In my brief remarks I would like to establish the following. First, the so-called electrophysiological and linguistic ''models'' do not have the inherent constitution or status of models. They are approaches, clusters of methodologies applied to a purpose, and as such they generate data that can be used to design a variety of theoretical accounts with greater or lesser explanatory power and heuristic value. As for the Wernicke-Geschwind model, it is a model indeed but the approach that permitted its conceptualization, the lesion method, must be firmly separated from it. In other words, the alleged three models are a somewhat superficial and misleading shorthand for a multitude of approaches and specific methods, and secondarily derived theoretical accounts. Second, these approaches and methods are definitely not in competition. To the contrary, they can and should be combined at a variety of levels of scientific inquiry. I attempt to support these opinions in the following discussion.

DISTINGUISHING THE WERNICKE-GESCHWIND MODEL FROM THE LESION METHOD APPROACH

The work of the brilliant nineteenth-century neurologists as well as the work of many contemporary neuroscientists concerned with aphasia is based on the possibility of a reliable relationship between a set of describable changes in language and speech on the one hand, and the presence of a region of focal cerebral damage with a specifiable anatomical position on the other. The validity of this type of relationship is no longer in question, and it constitutes the central tenet of the lesion method. More than 100 years of consistently replicated observations as well as corroborating evidence obtained by methods based on entirely different assumptions indicate that the relation between certain types of cognitive disorder and the destruction of certain brain structures is unassailably robust, especially in the domain of language. Now, that does not mean that the lesion method, in language research as well as in other domains of cognition (and in humans as well as experimental animals), is itself unassailable, nor does it legitimize any theoretical constructs regarding neural structure or cognitive function based on findings obtained by the lesion method, i.e., it gives no guarantee that models constructed on the basis of lesion method data are necessarily correct (or incorrect). The lesion method is one thing, with its inherent limitations, pitfalls, and virtues; theoretical constructs that make use of it, such as the Wernicke-Geschwind model, be they good, bad, or indifferent, are another. As with any methodology the lesion method can lead to invalid data and misleading interpretations if improperly used. First, the method is only as good as the finest level of cognitive characterization and anatomical resolution it uses. In other words, the yield of the method is limited by: (a) the sophistication of the neuropsychological assessment and/or experimentation with which anatomical lesions are correlated; (b) the sophistication of the theoretical constructs and hypotheses being tested by the lesion probes; (c) the degree of sophistication with which the nervous tissue is conceptualized, i.e., how are the missing processing units viewed anatomically and physiologically, what type of network are they missing from?, at what level do those neurally defined networks establish contact with the cognitively defined structures?; and (d) the anatomical resolution of the procedures used. It is clear that, until quite recently, because of historical technical limitations, several of these methodological features have been weak. Perhaps the prime example is that cognitive structures have not been teased apart componentially but rather taken as conflated units. The gross conflation, commonly referred to as "auditory comprehension" in the study of aphasia, is as good an example as any of how numerous cognitively separable structures and processes have been conceptualized as unitary and measured as one. However, it is just as clear that a new generation of investigators, often working in multidisciplinary teams, is striving for a novel approach that overcomes these shortcomings. In the work of Bellugi (2,7; *this volume*), Alexander and Naeser (*this volume*), or Baynes and Gazzaniga (*this volume*) there are examples of this new type of effort.

Furthermore, the history of the lesion method contains genuine errors of procedure. Examples that can be cited are (a) the use of inappropriate neuropathological specimens, e.g., cerebral tumors, that led to incorrect correlations; (b) the use of appropriate specimens such as stroke but at inappropriate epochs in the evolution of the disease process; (c) the incorrect anatomical placement of lesions, either because their position was improperly interpreted or the true extent of the lesion at microscopic level could not be properly estimated from gross postmortem study or neuroimaging; and (d) the abusive averaging of individual measurements in group studies, cognitive as well as anatomical, that creates artifactual views of some aspects of the data and conceals others.

Finally, and perhaps no less important, is the intrinsic limitation of a method in which investigators are asked to conceive "normal function" on the basis of the subtraction of a given set of inoperative processing units from a network, rather than on the basis of the regular working of those units themselves. The intellectual pirouette necessary to conceptualize normal structure and function from damaged structure and deviant function is risky indeed. The danger can only be reduced by the quality of the theoretical framework and the tight formulation of hypotheses under scrutiny.

As should be clear, there is no inherent need for the lesion method to be gross or to lead to gross results, and no inherent need either for lesion method users to agree or disagree with the conceptualizations we inherited from Wernicke (20) or Geschwind (12). *In vivo* neuroimaging techniques, as well as postmortem techniques permitting microscopic analysis of biologically labeled neural tissue, now allow the definition of lesions with precision at a fine anatomical level. On the other hand, new cognitive experimentation techniques have increased the "resolution" of the cognitive phenomena being correlated with lesions. As is reiterated later in this chapter, the lesion method is *not* in competition with the so-called "linguistic" or "cognitive" approaches. On the contrary, it often needs the assistance of the latter if it is to be practiced properly. In other words, if certain researchers correlate large lumps of missing brain with equally large and highly conflated psychological processes, that error cannot be attributed to an intrinsic fault of the lesion method but rather to the incompetence of the researchers in question. The lesion method can be used to test, in firmly controlled ways, well-defined hypotheses about the structure of neural networks at a level of organization appropriate to the dimension of the lesion probes, no more and no less.

In language research as well as in other cognitive domains, the lesion method has not only provided fundamental tokens of knowledge with which to think our way through the mind and brain question, but it has continued to deliver numerous observations that, in turn, generate hypotheses testable with other approaches. In fact, the lesion method is especially helpful for work with the new generation of more direct and physiological methods of brain imaging that use emission tomography [positron emission tomography (PET) and single photon emission tomography (SPET)]. For instance, it is possible to test claims derived from lesion method data regarding the putative function of a certain brain region. An example of this is the finding of regions in the human superior visual association cortex that activate in response to the perception of random-dot stereograms (P. Fox and J. Allen, 1986, *personal communication*, 9) in the same areas where the lesion method had predicted that stereoptically active cortex should lie (17). It is also possible to take subjects with well-defined lesions and abnormal cognitive processes, and study the functional state of specific *nondamaged* areas of their brains with the help of the new dynamic techniques (8). Clearly, the lesion method still has a contribution to make to the otherwise brilliant future of research with emission tomography.

The Wernicke view of language and brain (20), quite in keeping with a prevalent conceptualization during the 1870s [but hardly the only game in town as Sigmund Freud's 1891 treatise on aphasia clearly proves (10)], attributed concatenations of language-related processes to the operation of large, single, and fairly isolated sectors of dominant cerebral cortex (e.g., Wernicke's area, Broca's area, and so forth) joined by sizable but discrete connecting pathways. The model was added to by the work of many other European neurologists, most notably Lichtheim, Dejerine, Liepmann, and Goldstein, and later revised and amplified by Geschwind during the 1960s (12). Geschwind's version added novel features to the model, such as connections between language cortices and medial temporolimbic structures with an assigned role in learning, and a role for bilateral sensory-motor receptors and effectors conjoined by interhemispheric connections. The combined "Wernicke-Geschwind view" that held sway for the past two decades was a rich and testable account of both normal language and aphasia. It inspired investigators to assess its validity and in so doing enlarged our knowledge. That the account was unsatisfactory is not surprising. What is somewhat startling is the way its historical errors have been highlighted rather than exculpated, unlike the way in which, say, Gordon Holmes' erroneous views on the organization of the central visual system very justly and frequently are (6,13). Equally startling is that the errors have been blamed on the use of the lesion method itself rather than on the conceptualization secondary to it, as if data collected by this approach would irrevocably have led investigators to conceive nothing but discrete processing centers, major interconnecting pathways, and simple psychological processes. In truth nothing prevents the lesion method from helping to test or modify a hypothetical model in which *overlapping networks of distributed information operate the activation of and the selective attention to neural representations.* Nothing in the lesion method binds innocent investigators to "diagram-maker" centers, "single-purpose" pathways, or "grandmother" neurons.

THE ELECTROPHYSIOLOGICAL APPROACH

Few methods for understanding brain function can be more appealing than those that permit the observation of results of electrical stimulation of a small cortical region or the direct recording of an event-related potential over the cortical surface. Wilder Penfield was not the first to use the method, but he steered it to the language areas and gave it fame (16). In recent decades, George Ojemann has further refined the methodology and explored painstakingly the language cortices of epileptic patients prior to their therapeutic corticectomies. In so doing he has provided the literature with an alternative set of data about language and the brain (15).

Because of its particular procedural demands, this research has few practitioners. There are, furthermore, numerous unresolved questions mostly related to the fact that all subjects are epileptic patients whose brain structure and function are likely to be, in some respects, different from normal. How confidently the results obtained in these patients can be extrapolated to the situation of normals is a disquieting and still unanswered question. Be that as it may, the view on the neural organization of language that has been based on electrophysiological data is highly deserving of attention. However, the notion that either the findings or the model are in radical opposition to the classical views based on the lesion method is, in my view, incorrect. Certainly there is no way to equate the findings of both methods. How can the consequences of temporarily stimulating a small area of cortex be compared with those of destroying permanently a sizable region of cortex and underlying white matter? The notion that electrical stimulation produces a transient minilesion is not really acceptable, i.e., we certainly do not know how extensive the physiological inactivation is, nor do we know its boundaries. The problem of the "remote" effects of the stimulation, in spite of all the technical attention it currently gets, is not smaller than with destructive lesions. Likewise, the notion that electrical stimulation mimics some type of normal neural operation is not tenable, for nothing even faintly indicates that cortical stimulation resembles normal firing patterns within a given region of cortical columns. The extant account derived from these findings is certainly different from the Wernicke-Geschwind views, but it really has nothing to say, positive or negative, about the lesion method. On the contrary, some of its hypotheses are directly testable by the lesion method. When Ojemann proposed that there is a perisylvian ring of cortex concerned with phonemic processing, encircled by yet another ring concerned with short-term memory related to speech, there is absolutely no reason why those captivating notions should not be addressed by the study of appropriately placed lesions in the territory so defined. Furthermore, there is no *a priori* reason why those same hypotheses could not have been generated on the basis of data collected by other means, including the lesion method itself, provided the theoretical framework would have been conducive to such an interpretation. By the same token, Ojemann's interpretation of his findings might not have been the same had his theoretical framework been different, and his conclusions are not the only ones that may be responsive to his data. The point that I want to stress is that methods are often not the issue that should be argued but rather the theoretical framework or the adequacy and creativity of the interpretation of the findings. In short, models and hypotheses derived on the basis of lesion method data can be counterchecked with the electrophysiological method and vice versa.

THE COGNITIVE APPROACH

We have witnessed during the past three decades a notable development of a variety of theories and methodologies of a highly diverse nature that are loosely bound together by their focus on the phenomena of the mind. Linguistics and psycholinguistics, numerous brands of cognitive psychology, artificial intelligence, and the newer computational modeling approaches to psychological processes are all part of this broad and still evolving field known, for lack of a better name, as cognitive science (1,4,5,14,18,19; V.A. Fromkin, *this volume*; S.E. Blumstein, *this volume*; and E. Bates and V.A. Marchman, *this volume*). The invisible bond among such disparate sciences and scientists was the prospect of finally liberating neuropsychology from the suffocation of behaviorism, centering all efforts on the analysis of representations and rules for their operation. Howard Gardner (11) has proposed that the scope and historical meaning of this development constitutes a true revolution, and that may well be the case. Even broadly defined, it is apparent that the cognitive sciences offer the possibility of pursuing and eventually achieving a true biology of the mind.

If the lesion method and the electrophysiological method are not in conflict with each other, it is even less clear why the methods developed in the multidisciplinary field of cognitive science should be in competition with either. One can imagine a struggle for subjects to be studied with these different approaches or a competition for the limelight where the most seductive breakthroughs would be displayed but not, at least not reasonably, a competition among methodologies. As noted above, most studies of neural structure or function directly related to language (using lesion method, electrophysiology, or emission tomography) require, if they are to be at all interesting and valid, a high degree of sophistication in psychological experimentation. On the other hand, with some fair symmetry, the most interesting revelations on cognitive processes as they relate to the human brain should be linked in some fashion to neuroanatomy and neurophysiology. Once again, integration, not competition, is the key word. However, the remarkable lack of conflict goes even further. It is entirely legitimate to address numerous issues of cognitive research without making any appeal whatsoever to the neural underpinnings of the cognitive processes under consideration. In other words, it is possible to build and test theoretical models of, say, recognition or syntactical processing, without being directly concerned with the neural structures that embody and implement those processes. By the same token, it is also possible to analyze the structural definition and operation of neural networks and inquire, at a computational and psychologically naive level, about the possible functions that such neural networks might carry out, independently of what is or is not known about the *real* performance of such networks.

This epistemological issue becomes transparent when one realizes that as investigators ponder the relation between language and the brain, they have the option of considering numerous different levels of structure and function. Some structures and levels of operation are approachable and describable with the armamentarium of neuroscience, ranging from molecular neurobiology to classical neuroanatomy and physiology (which now include the modern neuroimaging techniques). Some structures and levels of operation are only approachable and describable with the methods developed with the equally revolutionary cognitive sciences. Nonetheless, cognitive descriptions are not truer than neural descriptions, nor vice versa. *Neither* can have "preferred" status. Fortunately, *both* neural and cognitive descriptions can be translated in the language of mathematics and ideally scrutinized with computational methodologies.

If it is true that the integration of neuroscience and cognitive science is not with us yet, it is no less true that the procedural means for it to occur are immediately available and that it has even begun to occur, to some limited extent. The success of the integration clearly depends on a rejection of traditional single-discipline perspectives and on the recognition that the broad range of currently existing approaches aim at different angles of complex, multilevel processes. Depending on the eye of the beholder, these processes may appear to be "purely" cognitive or "purely" neural, but they are, quite simply, merely biological.

ACKNOWLEDGMENTS

This work was supported by NINCDS grant P01 NS19632.

REFERENCES

1. Arbib, M.A., and Caplan, D. (1979): Neurolinguistics must be computational. *Behavioral and Brain Sciences*, 2:449–483.
2. Bellugi, U., Poizner, H., and Klima, E.A. (1983): Brain organization for language: Clues from sign aphasia. *Human Neurobiology*, 2:155–170.

3. Black, P., Black, S., and Droge, J. (1986): Three models of human language. *Neurosurgery*, 19:308–315.
4. Bradley, D.C., Garrett, M.E., and Zurif, E.B. (1980): Syntactic deficits in Broca's aphasia. In: *Biological Studies of Mental Processes*, edited by D. Caplan. MIT Press, Cambridge, MA.
5. Chomsky, N. (1980): Rules and representations. *The Behavioral and Brain Sciences*, 3:1–61.
6. Damasio, A. (1985): Disorders of complex visual processing. In: *Principles of Behavioral Neurology. Contemporary Neurology Series*, edited by M.M. Mesulam, pp. 259–288. F.A. Davis, Philadelphia.
7. Damasio, A., Bellugi, U., Damasio, H., Poizner, H., and Van Gilder, J. (1986): Sign language aphasia during left-hemisphere Amytal injection. *Nature*, 322:363–365.
8. Damasio, H., Rezai, K., Eslinger, P., Kirchner, P., and Van Gilder, J. (1986): SPET patterns of activation in intact and focally damaged components of a language related network. *Neurology*, 36:316.
9. Fox, P., Raichle, M., and Allman, J. (1987): Abstracts to ARVO and Society for Neuroscience 1987.
10. Freud, S. (1891): *On Aphasia*. Translated by E. Stengel (1953). International University Press, New York.
11. Gardner, H. (1985): *The Mind's New Science, A History of the Cognitive Revolution*. Basic Books, New York.
12. Geschwind, N. (1965): Disconnexion syndromes in animals and man. *Brain*, 88:237–294.
13. Holmes, G. (1918): Disturbances of visual orientation. *Br. J. Ophthalmol.*, 2:449–468.
14. Kean, M.L. (1977): The linguistic interpretation of aphasic syndromes: Agrammatism in Broca's aphasia, an example. *Cognition*, 5:9–46.
15. Ojemann, G.A. (1983): Brain organization for language from the perspective of electrical stimulation mapping. *The Behavioral and Brain Sciences*, 189:230.
16. Penfield, W., and Roberts, L. (1959): *Speech and Brain Mechanisms*. Princeton University Press, Princeton.
17. Rizzo, M., and Damasio, H. (1985): Impairment of stereopsis with focal brain lesions. *Ann. Neurol.*, 18:112.
18. Saffran, E.M., Schwartz, M.F., and Marin, O.S.M. (1980): The word order problem in agrammatism. II. Production. *Brain Lang.*, 10:249–262.
19. Schwartz, M.F., Saffran, E.M., and Marin, O.S.M. (1980): The word order problem in agrammatism. I. Comprehension, *Brain Lang.*, 10:249–262.
20. Wernicke, C. (1874): *Der Aphasische Symptomencomplex*. Cohn and Weigert, Breslau.

Subject Index

A

Agnosia, verbal auditory, 64–65
Agrammatism
  agrammatic patterns in, 201
  in aphasia, 121–122,124
    Broca's, 201–203,208–211
  productive, 201
Alexia, pure, 261
American Sign Language, 39–56
  acquisition, 42–45
  event-related brain potentials and, 90–91
  linguistic mechanisms, 39–40
  phonology, 40
  pronomial signs, 40,42–43
  syntax, 40–41,43–45
  use by brain lesioned signers, 45–54
    apraxia/aphasia separation, 51–52
    left-lesioned signers, 45–46,47,48,49–50,52,53,54
    right-lesioned signers, 45–46,48–49,50–51,52–53,54
    spatial cognition, 48–50
    spatial mapping, 50–51
    spatial syntax, 50–51
  verb agreement, 43
  verb signs, 40–41
  vertically arrayed morphology, 40
Angular gyrus syndrome, 261
Anomia, 219. See also Naming
  as aphasia syndrome, 61
  electrical stimuli-evoked, 103,104
Aphasia
  acquired, brain lesion-related, 171, 172
  agrammatical, 121–122,124
  anomic, 61,70–71
  auditory comprehension in, 277
  borderzone, 60
  brain lesion-related, 58–59
  brain localization in, 58–59
  Broca's, 58,60,61
    agrammatism in, 201–203,208–211

    cerebral glucose metabolism, 257,258–259,263
    comprehension deficits, 201–203
    cortical-subcortical lesions, 223
    lexical-semantic deficits, 203–204,206,207,208
    phonetic deficits, 199–201
    phonologic-syntactic deficit syndrome versus, 68–69
    processing deficits, 204,205,206,208,209–210,211
    speech production, 199–201
    structural deficits, 204,206,207,208–211
    syntactic deficits, 201–203,208,209,210,211
  cerebral metabolic abnormalities, 256–261,263
  cognitive systems, 4–6
  conduction, 61,218
    cerebral glucose metabolism, 258,259,262,263
    lexical-syntactic deficit syndrome versus, 70–71
    paraphasia, 68
  cortical-subcortical lesion differences in, 215–228
    capsular lesions, 217–218,220,224–225,226
    lesion clinical correlations, 217–227
    multiple lesions, 226–227
    striatal lesions, 217,218,223–224
    temporal isthmus, 221–222,223
    white matter lesions, 218–221,222,224–227
  crossed dextral syndrome, 261
  dysfluent, 58,61
  dysphasia syndrome parallels, 63–71
  epileptic, 65
  expressive. See Aphasia, Broca's
  fluent, 58,61
    in brain-lesioned children, 185

Verbal processes (*contd.*)
  naming effects, 103–106,108–
    109,110–114
  subcortical, 110–112
  thalamic mechanisms, 110–114
  verbal memory effects, 106–110
Verbal proficiency, sex factors, 60
Verbal stimulation, metabolic response,
  249,250–252
Verb omission, in language acquisition,
  23–25
Verb signs, in American Sign Language,
  40–41
Visuospatial language. *See* American
  Sign Language
Vocalization, frontal lobe lesion-related,
  159

W
Wechsler Intelligence Scale for Children
  score, of unilateral brain-lesioned
  children, 177,178,181,191,193

Wechsler Preschool and Primary Scale of
  Intelligence score, of unilateral
  brain-lesioned children,
  177,178,181,191,193
Wernicke's area, 6. *See also* Aphasia,
  Wernicke's
  language zones, 105
Wernicke-Geschwind model, of brain/
  language research, 275,276–279
White matter lesions, in aphasia, 218–
  221,222,224–227
  anterior extension, 221
  anterolateral, 218–220
  posterior-superior extension, 221,
    222
  superior, 220–221
  superior paraventricular, 220–
    221,222,224–225,226
Word deafness, 64–65
Word expectancy, in language
  comprehension, 87–100
Word order, in language comprehension,
  25–27